Antiseizure Medication Interactions

Philip N. Patsalos

Antiseizure Medication Interactions

A Clinical Guide

Fourth Edition

Springer

Philip N. Patsalos
Department of Clinical and Experimental Epilepsy
UCL Queen Square Institute of Neurology
London, UK

ISBN 978-3-030-82789-2 ISBN 978-3-030-82790-8 (eBook)
https://doi.org/10.1007/978-3-030-82790-8

This Springer imprint is published by the registered company Springer Nature Switzerland AG
The registered company address is: Gewerbestrasse 11, 6330 Cham, Switzerland

Preface

The third edition of this book, published in February 2016, included 29 antiseizure medications (ASMs). Since then, four new ASMs have been licensed for clinical use (cannabidiol, cenobamate, everolimus, and fenfluramine), and one ASM (retigabine) is no longer licensed for clinical use. Consequently, there has been a surge of publications reporting on interactions, particularly interactions involving the newer ASMs. In this fourth edition, a total of 32 ASMs are reviewed, in alphabetical order, including ASMs that are not necessarily licensed worldwide but that are prescribed to patients in different countries (e.g., acetazolamide, methsuximide, piracetam, and sulthiame).

ASM interactions present a major challenge in the management of epilepsy, and even though our understanding of these interactions has increased substantially, the sheer size of available data has discouraged many physicians from taking an effective approach to minimize adverse consequences, which may result from these interactions. The purpose of this book is to provide, in a systematic fashion, a description of the drug interactions that occur between ASMs and between ASMs and non-ASMs, which may present problems for patients and that often require a drug dose adjustment. With this information, it is anticipated that medical practitioners, who treat patients with epilepsy or patients with morbidities who also require ASM use, will be better placed to allow a more rational drug choice when polytherapy regimens are indicated. In addition, the content of this book will allow for a more informed rationale as to how drugs will interact and, therefore, the dosage adjustment that would be consequently necessary to maintain an appropriate therapeutic response (maximal efficacy, minimal adverse effects).

The book is divided into four sections:

- The "Introduction" is a general introduction which explains the basic mechanisms of drug interactions, how to anticipate and predict interactions, and how to prevent and manage adverse interactions.
- Part I describes the interactions that occur between ASMs.

- Part II describes the interactions that occur between ASMs and non-ASMs whereby the interaction affects ASMs. The non-ASMs are listed in drug classes in alphabetical order.
- Part III describes the interactions that occur between ASMs and non-ASMs whereby the interaction affects non-ASMs. The non-ASMs are listed in drug classes in alphabetical order.

Because pharmacokinetic interactions represent the majority (>98%) of described interactions involving ASMs, it is inevitable that the focus of this book is on pharmacokinetic interactions. Nevertheless, pharmacodynamic interactions are equally important and are therefore also described. As a drug class, the number of known interactions involving ASMs is substantial, and while it has been the author's aim to be as complete as possible, the listings may not be exhaustive and the possibility exists that clinically significant interaction will occur with other drugs.

The data used in compiling this book were identified by searches of Medline and PubMed with the terms "antiepileptic drug interactions" or "antiseizure medication interactions" combined with individual drug names and drug groups, references from relevant articles, and searches of the author's files. No gender or age limits were imposed but searches, last conducted in March 2021, were limited to human subjects. Publications' preference in descending order was as follows: formal interaction studies in patients; formal interaction studies in healthy volunteers; case studies/reports; population pharmacokinetic modeling databases; and therapeutic drug monitoring databases. Papers published in English were preferred, but non-English articles were used if they were the sole reference source. Abstracts were included only when a complete published article was not available.

All statements in this book as to the nature of an interaction (pharmacokinetic, pharmacodynamic, or no interaction) are referenced so that the reader can readily identify the appropriate publication. For most such statements, one reference is included (representing the key reference), but where the interaction is controversial, two or three references are cited.

The pharmacokinetic interactions presented in this book are described in terms of a change in plasma (blood) levels because physicians and allied health professionals treating patients with epilepsy are very familiar with drug plasma levels and how changes in these levels are reflective of a drug's pharmacokinetic characteristics and efficacy/adverse effect profile. However, in some studies, blood levels are not reported, and instead clearance, half-life, area under the concentration versus time curve (AUC), and/or maximum blood level (C_{max}) values are quoted. Thus, for these studies, the interactions are described in terms of changes in clearance, half-life, AUC, and/or C_{max} values. Whenever available, pharmacokinetic changes in mean values are quoted; otherwise a value representing the most significant change reported, for example, in small case series, is quoted. Finally, some studies do not quote any pharmacokinetic variables and instead describe the interaction in terms of a change in the clinical status; for example, patient(s) experienced an enhanced or a reduced therapeutic response or enhanced toxicity. For these interactions, the interactions are described generically, for example, "enhances the metabolism" or "inhibits the metabolism" of the affected drug. Wherever the data are available, interactions are also described in relation to their effects on hepatic enzyme activity, for example, cytochrome P450, uridine glucuronyl transferases, and epoxide hydrolase. This will allow the reader to ascertain the propensity of similar interactions occurring with other drugs that may have similar enzyme activities to substrates, inhibitors, and/or inducers. Where pharmacokinetic interactions have been studied but no interaction observed, they are reported as "does not affect the pharmacokinetics of drug…."

When using the information detailed in this book, the reader should remember that although a drug interaction is considered clinically relevant when it results in the need for dosage adjustment or other medical intervention in the majority of patients, a marked deviation in an unusually susceptible individual is also important. Also, one needs to consider the end result because a marked elevation in a low ASM/drug level may improve seizure control/therapeutic response while a small elevation of a nearly toxic level may actually precipitate toxicity. Finally, while an interaction involving a 10% change in a drug blood level may have little, if any, clinical relevance in the majority of patients, it may be of profound clinical relevance in a significant minority of patients.

London, UK
March 2021

Philip N. Patsalos

Contents

Part I
Drug Interactions Between ASMs

Interactions between antiseizure medications (ASMs): expected changes in plasma concentrations (levels) when an ASM is added to a preexisting ASM regimen.

ASM added	Preexisting ASM										
	BRV	**CNB**	**CBZ**	**CLB**	**CZP**	**ESL-a**	**ESM**	**FBM**	**GBP**	**LCM**	**LTG**	**LEV**
BRV	–		CBZ↓	↔	↔	NA	NA	NA	NA	↔	↔	↔
			CBZ-E⇑									
CNB	?	–	↔	CLB⇑	↔	ESL↑	↔	?	NA	↔	↔	↔
				DMCLB⇑								
CBZ	BRV↓	?	AI	CLB⇓	CZP⇓	ESL↓	ESM⇓	FBM⇓	↔	↔	LTG⇓	LEV↓
				DMCLB⇑								
CLB	NA	CNB⇑	CBZ↑	–	NA	↔	?	NA	NA	NA	↔	↔
			CBZ-E↑									
CZP	NA	NA	↔	NA	–	NA	NA	↔	NA	NA	↔	↔
ESL-a	NA	?	↔	↔	NA	–	NA	NA	↔	NA	LTG↓	↔
ESM	NA	NA	↔	NA	NA	NA	–	NA	NA	NA	↔	↔
FBM	NA	?	CBZ↓	CLB⇑	CZP↑	?	?	–	NA	NA	LTG↑	↔
			CBZ-E↑	DMCLB⇑								
GBP	NA	NA	↔	NA	NA	↔	NA	FBM↑	–	NA	↔	↔
LCM	NA	NA	↔	NA	↔	NA	NA	NA	↔	–	↔	↔
LTG	↔	?	↔	↔	CZP↓	↔	↔	↔	NA	↔	–	LEV↓
LEV	↔	NA	↔	↔	↔	↔	↔	NA	↔	↔	↔	–
OXC	↔	?	CBZ↓	?	?	NCCP	?	?	NA	NA	LTG↓	LEV↓
PMP	NA	?	CBZ↓	CLB↓	↔	?	NA	NA	NA	NA	LTG↓	↔
PB	BRV↓	?	CBZ⇓	CLB⇓	CZP⇓	?	ESM⇓	↔	↔	LCM↓	LTG⇓	LEV↓
				DMCLB⇑								
PHT	BRV↓	?	CBZ⇓	CLB⇓	CZP⇓	ESL↓	ESM⇓	FBM⇓	↔	LCM↓	LTG⇓	LEV↓
				DMCLB⇑								
PGB	NA	NA	↔	NA	NA	NA	NA	NA	↔	NA	↔	↔
PRM	?	?	CBZ⇓	?	CZP⇓	?	ESM⇓	?	NA	?	LTG⇓	↔

RFN	NA	?	CBZ↓	↔	NA	NA	NA	NA	NA	NA	LTG↓	NA
STP	?	H-CBD↑	CBZ⇑	CLB⇑	?	?	ESM↑	?	NA	NA	?	NA
				DMCLB ⇑								
TGB	NA	NA	↔	NA	NA	NA	NA	NA	NA	NA	↔	↔
TPM	↔	?	↔	?	?	ESL↓	NA	?	NA	↔	↔	↔
VPA	↔	H-CBD↑	CBZ-E⇑	↔	?	↔	ESM↑↓	FBM↑	↔	↔	LTG⇑	↔
VGB	NA	NA	CBZ↑↓	NA	NA	NA	NA	↔	NA	NA	↔	↔
ZNS	**NA**	?	CBZ-E↑	?	?	NA	?	?	NA	NA	↔	NA

BRV brivaracetam, *CNB* cannabidiol, *CBZ* carbamazepine, *CBZ-E* carbamazepine-10,11-epoxide (active metabolite of *CBZ*), *CLB* clobazam, *CZP* clonazepam, *DMCLB* N-desmethylclobazam (active metabolite of CLB), *ESL-a* eslicarbazepine acetate, *ESL* eslicarbazepine (active metabolite of ESL-a), *ESM* ethosuximide, *FBM* felbamate, *GBP* gabapentin, *H-OXC* 10-hydroxy-carbazepine (active metabolite of OXC), *H-CBD* 7-hydroxy-cannabidiol (active metabolite of CBD), *LCM* lacosamide, *LEV* levetiracetam, *LTG* lamotrigine, *OXC* oxcarbazepine, *PMP perampanel, PB* phenobarbital, *PHT* phenytoin, *PGB* pregabalin, *PRM* primidone, *RFN* rufinamide, *STP* stiripentol, *TGB* tiagabine, *TPM* topiramate, *VPA* valproic acid, *VGB* vigabatrin, *ZNS* zonisamide.

OXC	PMP	PB	PHT	PGB	PRM	RFN	STP	TGB	TPM	VPA	VGB	ZNS	
↔	NA	↔	PHT↑	↔	NA	NA	NA	NA	↔	↔	NA	↔	**BRV**
↔	↔	↔	↔	↔	?	RFN↑	↔	NA	TPM↑	↔	↔	ZNS↑	**CNB**
H-OXC↓	PMP⇓	↔	PHT↑↓	↔	PRM↓ PB↑	RFN↓	STP⇓	TGB⇓	TPM⇓	VPA⇓	↔	ZNS⇓	**CBZ**
↔	↔	↔	PHT↑	NA	PRM↑	↔	STP↑	?	?	VPA↑	NA	NA	**CLB**
NA	↔	↔	PHT↑↓	NA	↔	NA	NA	?	NA	↔	NA	↔	**CZP**
NCCP	?	↔	PHT↑	NA	NA	NA	NA	NA	TPM↓	VPA↓	NA	NA	**ESL**
NA	NA	↔	↔	NA	PRM↑	NA	NA	NA	NA	VPA↓	NA	NA	**ESM**
↔	?	PB⇑	PHT⇑	NA	?	?	?	?	?	VPA⇑	VGB↓	?	**FBM**
NA	NA	↔	↔	PGB↓	NA	↔	NA	NA	↔	↔	NA	NA	**GBP**
H-OXC↓	?	NA	↔	NA	NA	NA	NA	NA	↔	↔	NA	↔	**LCM**
↔	↔	↔	↔	↔	↔	↔	NA	NA	↔	VPA↓	NA	↔	**LTG**
NA	↔	↔	↔	↔	↔	NA	NA	NA	↔	↔	↔	NA	**LEV**
–	PMP⇓	PB↑	PHT↑	NA	?	RFN↓	?	?	TPM↓	↔	NA	NA	**OXC**
OXC↑	–	↔	↔	NA	NA	NA	NA	NA	↔	VPA↓	NA	↔	**PMP**
H-OXC↓	?	AI	PHT↑↓	↔	NCCP	RFN↓	STP⇓	TGB⇓	TPM⇓	VPA⇓	↔	ZNS⇓	**PB**
H-OXC↓	PMP⇓	PB↑	AI	PGB↓	PRM↓ PB↑	RFN↓	STP⇓	TGB⇓	TPM⇓	VPA⇓	↔	ZNS⇓	**PHT**
NA	NA	↔	↔	–	NA	NA	NA	TGB↓	↔	↔	NA	NA	**PGB**
?	?	NCCP	↔	NA	–	RFN↓	STP⇓	TGB⇓	TPM⇓	VPA⇓	↔	ZNS⇓	**PRM**
NA	NA	PB↑	PHT↑	NA	NA	–	NA	NA	↔	↔	NA	NA	**RFN**
\	?	PB⇑	PHT⇑	NA	PRM⇑	?	–	?	?	VPA⇑	NA	?	**STP**
NA	?	NA	↔	↔	NA	NA	NA	–	NA	VPA↓	NA	NA	**TGB**
↔	PMP⇓	↔	PHT↑	↔	↔	↔	NA	?	–	VPA↓	NA	NA	**TPM**

↔	↔	PB⇑	PHT↓*	↔	PB⇑	RFN↑	↔	↔	TPM↓	–	↔	↔	**VPA**
NA	NA	↔	PHT↓	NA	↔	RFN↓	NA	NA	NA	↔	–	NA	**VGB**
?	↔	↔	↔	NA	↔	?	?	NA	NA	↔	NA	–	**ZNS**

AI autoinduction, *NA* none anticipated, *NCCP* not commonly co-prescribed, ↔ no change, ↓ a usually minor (or inconsistent) decrease in plasma level, ⇓ a usually clinically significant decrease in plasma level, ↑ a usually minor (or inconsistent) increase in plasma level, ⇑ a usually clinically significant increase in plasma level.

[a]Free (pharmacologically active) level may increase;? = unknown, an interaction could occur.

Introduction

Epilepsy, which affects approximately 1% of the world's population, is a chronic disorder that usually persists for many years and often for a lifetime [1]. Antiseizure medications (ASMs) are the mainstay of epilepsy treatment, and complete seizure control can be achieved in the majority (65%) of newly diagnosed patients by prescribing a single ASM, and this is the ideal situation [2]. For the remaining 35% of patients, the prescribing of polytherapy regimens (the use primarily of two ASMs but often three or four ASMs), so as to achieve optimal seizure control, is a common practice. However, for the majority of these patients, little additional benefit is achieved from the use of polytherapy ASMs as intolerable adverse effects commonly occur as a consequence of pharmacokinetic and/or pharmacodynamic interactions. Furthermore, for those patients who respond to monotherapy, they too may experience the consequences of ASM interactions as ASMs are added and withdrawn during the optimization of their monotherapy drug regimen [3–5]. A further confounding factor is that since epilepsy is a chronic condition many patients will inevitably develop comorbid diseases or other debilitating conditions and disorders, which will require the coadministration of non-ASMs. In this setting, the potential for drug interactions is considerable [6]. A further source of potential clinically significant interactions that is being increasingly recognized relates to the increasing use of over-the-counter medications and supplements, many of which have unknown constituents and inconsistent quality [7]. Finally, ASMs are increasingly used to treat other non-epilepsy conditions such as mood disorders, migraine, and pain, thereby further increasing the possibility of combined use with other drugs [8].

The pharmacokinetic properties of ASMs make them particularly susceptible to pharmacokinetic interactions. Furthermore, many ASMs have a narrow therapeutic index in that the plasma (serum) level (concentration) associated with a desirable antiseizure effect is close to the plasma level that is associated with undesirable adverse effects. Thus, even a relatively small change in their plasma level, consequent to inhibition or induction, may readily result in signs of intoxication or loss of seizure control, respectively. In addition, some ASMs exert a major influence on the

P. N. Patsalos, *Antiseizure Medication Interactions*,
https://doi.org/10.1007/978-3-030-82790-8_1

activity of hepatic drug-metabolizing enzymes, stimulating (e.g., carbamazepine, phenytoin, phenobarbital, and primidone) or inhibiting (e.g., valproic acid, stiripentol, and sulthiame) their activity, thereby leading to a wide variety of pharmacokinetic interactions with other drugs that are also metabolized and eliminated by the same enzymes. Conversely, because most ASMs undergo extensive hepatic metabolism (e.g., cannabidiol, carbamazepine, cenobamate, eslicarbazepine acetate, everolimus, fenfluramine, lamotrigine, perampanel, phenytoin, phenobarbital, primidone, tiagabine, topiramate, oxcarbazepine, valproic acid, and zonisamide), they too are vulnerable to the effect of other drugs with inhibiting or inducing properties [9].

Mechanisms of Drug Interaction

Drug interactions can be divided into two groups: pharmacodynamic and pharmacokinetic:

- Pharmacodynamic interactions
- Pharmacodynamic interactions occur at the cellular level where drugs act and can occur between drugs that have either similar or opposing pharmacological mechanisms of action. Because these interactions are not associated with any change in plasma drug level, they are less well recognized and documented. Nevertheless, they are of major clinical significance and are invariably concluded by default whereby a change in the clinical status of a patient consequent to a drug combination cannot be ascribed to a pharmacokinetic interaction.
- Pharmacokinetic interactions
- Pharmacokinetic interactions are characterized by a change in plasma level of either the drug or its metabolite(s) or both. They are particularly prevalent, and their magnitude and time course can be readily determined and involve a change in their absorption, usually gastrointestinal; distribution, usually binding to plasma albumin; metabolism, usually by isoenzymes of cytochrome P450 [CYP] and uridine glucuronyl transferases [UGTs]); or elimination, usually renal excretion. Consequently, there is an alteration in the level of the affected drug at the site of drug action.

Pharmacodynamic Interactions

Although pharmacodynamic interactions have been traditionally neglected in epilepsy therapy, increasing evidence indicates that their recognition is essential so as to maximize ASM efficacy and minimize ASM toxicity. Most pharmacodynamic interactions simply involve additive neurotoxicity and may be explained by superimposition of adverse events caused by ASMs sharing the same modes of action. For example, combinations of two sodium-channel blockers, such as carbamazepine and oxcarbazepine, or carbamazepine and lamotrigine, are less well tolerated than combinations of drugs acting through different mechanisms. Combinations of drugs that enhance GABAergic inhibition, such as valproic acid and phenobarbital, may result in profound sedation that cannot be explained solely by a pharmacokinetic interaction. Lamotrigine and valproic acid in combination may produce disabling tremor [10]. Examples of potential favorable drug combinations include valproic acid and ethosuximide in the management of refractory absence seizures [11]; valproic acid and lamotrigine in the management of partial and generalized seizures [12]; and carbamazepine and valproic acid in the management of partial seizures [13].

Pharmacodynamic interactions between AEDs and non-AEDs can also result in increased toxicity. For example, the concurrent use of lithium and carbamazepine has been associated with a syndrome characterized by somnolence, confusion, disorientation, and ataxia and other cerebella symptoms consequent to a pharmacodynamic interaction [14, 15]. Also, the delirium observed in some patients when quetiapine is coadministered with valproic acid is considered to be the consequence of a pharmacodynamic interaction [16]. Finally, combining carbamazepine with clozapine is generally contraindicated due to concerns about potential additive hematological adverse effects [17].

Pharmacokinetic Interactions

Interactions Affecting Drug Absorption

Interactions affecting the absorption of ASMs are uncommon, although occasionally they do occur and can be important. For example, antacids reduce the absorption of phenytoin, gabapentin, valproic acid, and sulthiame. Furthermore, phenytoin absorption is impaired when the drug is given together with certain nasogastric feeds (e.g., Isocal) so that plasma phenytoin levels are reduced by 72% [18]. In both examples, it is thought that the formation of insoluble complexes may be responsible for the reduced absorption. Other such interactions include a reduction of absorption of primidone by acetazolamide [19] and a reduction in absorption of carbamazepine by colestipol and cisplatin [20, 21].

Plasma Protein-Binding Displacement Interactions

Plasma protein-binding displacement interactions are considered particularly important with the highly protein-bound (>90%) ASMs (e.g., phenytoin, perampanel, cannabidiol, stiripentol, tiagabine, and valproic acid) [22]. Because these drugs have a low intrinsic hepatic clearance, their displacement causes an initial transient increase in total drug plasma level prior to re-equilibration and a subsequent decrease. However, the pharmacologically relevant free non-protein-bound plasma level is unaffected, and thus, the clinical effects of the affected ASM are unchanged. Consequently, a dosage adjustment is usually unnecessary following displacement of highly protein-bound ASMs from their plasma protein binding sites. A well-characterized plasma protein-binding displacement interaction is that of phenytoin by valproic acid [23]. However, it is important to recognize that the clinical effects of phenytoin will now correspond to lower total plasma levels, and patient management may benefit from monitoring free non-protein-bound phenytoin levels [24].

Interactions at the Renal Level

Interactions at the level of renal elimination can be expected to occur with drugs that are predominantly renally eliminated, and although rare, such clinically relevant interactions have been described including a decrease in renal clearance and an increase in plasma carbamazepine-10,11-epoxide levels by zonisamide [25] and the decrease in felbamate elimination by gabapentin [26].

Metabolic Interactions

Interactions involving changes in hepatic metabolism represent, by far, most of the pharmacokinetic interactions described with ASMs and involve both induction and inhibition of drug metabolism. Because most ASMs undergo hepatic metabolism, they are susceptible to inhibitory and/or induction interactions. These processes are catalyzed by various enzyme systems, which can occur in series, and are referred to as Phase I (functionalization) and Phase II (conjugation) enzyme systems. Phase I reactions include hydroxylation (the addition of a polar functional group) or N-demethylation (deletion of a nonpolar alkyl group) by oxidation, reduction, or hydrolysis. Phase II reactions serve to further increase the water solubility of the drug/metabolite and involve conjugation with glucuronic acid, sulfate, acetate, glutathione, or glycine. Although metabolic drug interactions may involve changes in any one of the numerous enzymes involved in drug metabolism, by far the most important are those associated with the CYP and UGT systems. The CYP system is particularly important because it is not only responsible for the oxidative metabolism of many drugs and exogenous compounds but also of many endogenous compounds such as prostaglandins, fatty acids, and steroids. Metabolic processes serve to convert a drug into one or more metabolites, which are more water soluble than the parent drug and thus facilitate urinary excretion.

CYP Enzymes

The CYP enzyme system consists of a superfamily of isoenzymes that are located in the smooth endoplasmic reticulum, primarily in the liver but also in many other tissues (e.g., intestine, kidney, brain, and placenta). They are classified into families (the first Arabic number; there is a > 40% amino acid sequence identity within family members), subfamilies (the capital letter that follows; there is a > 59% amino acid sequence identity within subfamily members), and individual isoenzymes (the second Arabic number). Although in humans approximately 60 different CYP isoenzymes have been identified, five isoenzymes (CYP3A4, CYP2D6, CYP2C9, CYP1A2, and CYP2C19) are known to be responsible for the metabolism of 95% of all drugs, and three (CYP2C9, CYP2C19, and CYP3A4) are of particular importance in relation to ASM interactions [27]. Because the activity of these isoenzymes is genetically determined, genetic polymorphism resulting in enzyme variants with higher, lower, or no activity, or even resulting in the absence of an isoenzyme, can have a profound effect on the pharmacological expression of an interaction (vide infra). In relation to ASMs, those polymorphisms that have clinical consequences relate primarily to CYP2C9 and CYP2C19.

Epoxide Hydrolases

Epoxide hydrolases are a family of enzymes whose function is to convert arene oxides to trans-dihydrodiols and simple epoxides to vicinal diols by hydration and consequently are involved in detoxification processes, although sometimes they are involved in bioactivation reactions [28]. Only the microsomal form of epoxide hydrolase is involved in xenobiotic metabolism and plays an important role in the metabolism of carbamazepine, phenobarbital, and phenytoin. Epoxide intermediates have been implicated in teratogenic events and hypersensitivity reactions, and in relation to carbamazepine, carbamazepine-10,11-epoxide is considered to be equipotent to carbamazepine and contributes both to its antiseizure and adverse effects. Furthermore, epoxide hydrolase inhibition has been implicated in various important interactions involving carbamazepine metabolism (e.g., valproic acid, brivaracetam, and quetiapine inhibit its activity and increase plasma carbamazepine-10,11-epoxide levels, while phenobarbital enhances its activity and decreases plasma carbamazepine-10,11-epoxide levels [29–31]).

Uridine Glucuronyl Transferases

In humans, three families of UGTs have been identified, of which UGT1 and UGT2 appear to be the most important in drug metabolism [32]. The UGT1A3 and UGT2B7 isoforms are involved in the O-glucuronidation of valproic acid, while a variety of isoforms (UGT1A6, UGT2B7, UGT2B17, UGT2B4) are involved in the metabolism of eslicarbazepine. UGT1A4 has been found to be the major isoform responsible for the metabolism (N-glucuronidation) of lamotrigine. Although any substrate of UGT has the potential to competitively inhibit the glucuronidation of other substrates by the same isoform, there are few data in this regard. Furthermore, unlike the CYP system, no specific UGT inhibitors have been identified. Nevertheless, valproic acid inhibits several UGTs, while carbamazepine, phenobarbital, and phenytoin are inducers (e.g., interactions with lamotrigine).

Enzyme Inhibition

Enzyme inhibition is the consequence of a competition by drugs to bind to the same enzymic site resulting in a reduction of enzyme activity and a decrease in the rate of metabolism of the affected drug. Inevitably, plasma levels are elevated, and this is commonly associated with clinical toxicity. Inhibition is usually competitive in nature and therefore dose dependent and tends to begin as soon as sufficient levels of the drug inhibitor are achieved, and this usually occurs within 24 h of inhibitor addition. The time to maximal inhibition will depend on the elimination half-life of the affected drug and the inhibiting agent. When the inhibitor is withdrawn, the time course of de-inhibition is dependent on the elimination half-life of the inhibitor. Among the ASMs valproic acid, stiripentol, sulthiame, topiramate, and felbamate have been associated with inhibitory interactions. Furthermore, while topiramate and felbamate are primarily selective inhibitors of CYP2C19, valproic acid is considered to be a broad-spectrum inhibitor of hepatic metabolizing enzymes as it inhibits CYP2C9, UGTs, and microsomal epoxide hydrolase. Stiripentol inhibits CYP2C19 and CYP3A4, while the isoenzymes inhibited by sulthiame are probably CYP2C9 and CYP2C19.

In some circumstances, inhibitory interactions are complicated and problematic. For example, interactions involving the active metabolite(s) of the coadministered drugs may not always be obvious if concurrent plasma level changes of the parent drug do not occur. Because it is not common practice to monitor plasma metabolite levels, if one is unaware of the interaction, plasma level monitoring of the parent drug could be misleading. Such problematic interactions are associated with carbamazepine-10,11-epoxide, the pharmacologically active metabolite of carbamazepine. For example, during carbamazepine combination therapy with either valproate or quetiapine, patients can experience adverse effects as a result of an elevation of carbamazepine-10,11-epoxide levels resulting from an inhibition of epoxide hydrolase, without concurrent changes in plasma carbamazepine levels [29, 31].

An ASM may be the affected drug or the cause of an interaction. In fact, with some drug combinations, both the hepatic metabolism of the ASM and that of the other drug are altered. For example, during co-medication with ketoconazole and carbamazepine, carbamazepine plasma levels are increased due to inhibition of carbamazepine metabolism [33]. Conversely, the effectiveness of standard dosages of ketoconazole is reduced because carbamazepine enhances the metabolism of ketoconazole [34]. Other bidirectional interactions include those between topiramate and phenytoin, and between valproic acid and lamotrigine.

Several drugs including macrolide antibiotics (e.g., erythromycin and troleandomycin) and hydrazines (e.g., isoniazid) undergo metabolic activation by CYP enzymes so that the formed metabolites bind to the prosthetic hem of CYPs to form stable metabolic intermediates rendering the CYP inactive. As CYP activity can only be restored by synthesis of a new enzyme, the effect of such inhibitors may persist well after the elimination of the precursor (parent) drug. This mechanism is involved in the interaction between erythromycin and troleandomycin with carbamazepine (via inhibition of CYP3A4) and between isoniazid and phenytoin (via inhibition of CYP2C9) [35].

Finally, inhibitory interactions can be irreversible in nature in that drugs containing certain functional groups can be oxidized by CYPs to reactive intermediates that subsequently cause irreversible inactivation of the CYP by alteration of hem or protein or a combination of both. An example of these "suicide inhibitors" is the furanocoumarins that are contained in grapefruit juice and irreversibly inhibit CYP3A4. Thus, grapefruit juice inhibits the metabolism of carbamazepine so that mean plasma carbamazepine C_{max} and AUC values are increased by 40% [36] (Table 1).

Enzyme Induction

Enzyme induction is the consequence of an increase in enzyme protein resulting from an increase in gene transcription that is mediated by intracellular receptors. However, enzyme induction may also occur by an inducer-mediated decrease in the rate of enzyme degradation, through stabilization of proteins, as occurs with ethanol induction. Thus, although there are several different mechanisms of enzyme induction, the phenobarbital "type" has been best characterized. Indeed, even though phenobarbital is the prototype enzyme-inducing drug, many other drugs (e.g., carbamazepine, phenytoin, primidone, and rifampicin) also enhance drug-metabolizing enzymes with induction patterns that overlap that of phenobarbital. The enzymes associated with phenobarbital "type" induction include CYP1A2, CYP2B6, CYP2C8, CYP3C9, and CYP3A4, epoxide hydrolase, and some UGTs.

Enzyme induction results in an increase in enzyme activity, which in turn results in an increase in the rate of metabolism of the affected drug and therefore leads to a decrease in plasma level and possibly a reduction in the therapeutic response. If the affected drug has a pharmacologically active metabolite, induction can result in increased metabolite levels and possibly an increase in drug toxicity. The amount of enzyme induction is generally proportional to the dose of the inducing drug. As enzyme induction requires synthesis of new enzymes, the time course of induction (and indeed the reversal of induction upon removal of the inducer) is dependent on

Table 1 Antiseizure medications effects on hepatic enzymes

Drug	Effect	Enzymes/transporters affected
Acetazolamide	None	–
Brivaracetam	Inhibitor	EH
Cannabidiol	Inhibitor	CYP1A2, CYP2B6, CYP2C8, CYP2C9, CYP2C19,
Carbamazepine	Inducer	UGT1A9, UGT2B7
Cenobamate	Inducer	CYP2C, CYP3A, CYP1A2, EH, UGT, PGP, CYP2B6, CYP2C8, CYP3A4
Clobazam	Inhibitor None	CYP2B6, CYP2C19, CYP3A –
Clonazepam	None	–
Eslicarbazepine acetate	Inducer (weak)	CYP3A4
	Inducer (moderate)	UGT1A1
	Inhibitor (moderate)	CYP2C9, CYP2C19
Ethosuximide	None	–
Everolimus	Inhibitor	CYP3A4, PGP
Felbamate	Inducer	CYP3A4
	Inhibitor	CYP2C19, β-oxidation
Fenfluramine	Inhibitor	CYP2D6
Gabapentin	Inducer None	CYP2B6, CYP3A4 –
Lacosamide	None	–
Lamotrigine	None/weak inducer	UGT
Levetiracetam	Inhibitor None	UGT, CYP2C19
Methsuximide	None	–
Oxcarbazepine	Inducer (weak)	CYP3A4, UGT
Perampanel	None	–
Phenobarbital	Inducer	CYP2C, CYP3A, EH, UGT
Phenytoin	Inducer	CYP2C, CYP3A, EH, UGT, PGP
Piracetam	None	–
Pregabalin	None	–
Primidone	Inducer	CYP2C, CYP3A, EH, UGT, PGP
Rufinamide	None	–
Stiripentol	Inhibitor	CYP2D6, CYP2C19, CYP3A2
Sulthiame	Inhibitor	CYP2C9, CYP2C19
Tiagabine	None	–
Topiramate	Inducer (weak)	CYP3A4, β-oxidation
	Inhibitor (weak)	CYP2C19
Valproic acid	Inhibitor	CYP2C9, EH, UGT
Vigabatrin	None	–
Zonisamide	Inhibitor	CYP2C9, CYP2C19, CYP2A6, CYP2E1

The above data are based on both in vitro and in vivo data
CYP cytochrome P450, *EH* epoxide hydrolase (microsomal), *UGT* uridine glucuronyl transferases, *PGP* P-glycoprotein transporter

the rate of enzyme synthesis and/or degradation and the time to reach plasma steady-state levels of the inducing drug. The latter is usually the rate-limiting step and only occurs at a time which is approximately five elimination half-lives of the inducing drug. Thus, the time course of induction is usually gradual and dose dependent.

Enzyme induction represents a common problem in the management of epilepsy. Carbamazepine, phenobarbital, phenytoin, and primidone are potent inducers of CYPs, although phenytoin and carbamazepine appear to be less potent inducers at doses used clinically. The elderly appear to be less sensitive than younger adults to inducers, and thus there is reduced induction of drug metabolism in the elderly, although the evidence for this is contradictory. The reason for the age-dependent response to inducers is not fully understood. Although enzyme induction generally reduces the pharmacological effect of a drug because of increased drug metabolism, sometimes the formed metabolite has the same pharmacological activity as the parent drug. Thus, the clinical consequence of enzyme induction will be determined by the relative reactivity of the parent drug and the formed pharmacologically active metabolite.

Of the ASMs presently used in clinical practice, carbamazepine, oxcarbazepine, phenobarbital, phenytoin, primidone, and topiramate (at doses of ≥200 mg/day) are the only drugs that are associated with clinically important hepatic enzyme-inducing properties.

Anticipating and Predicting Metabolic Interactions

In the clinical setting, an important objective of the ASM treatment is to anticipate and minimize the risks of interactions with other agents. An unexpected loss of seizure control or development of toxicity during ASM therapy often accompanies the addition or removal of a concurrently administered drug.

In the past, drug interactions were identified essentially by serendipity. Typically, patients would complain of adverse effects or an increase in seizure frequency subsequent to the introduction of an additional drug to their drug regimen and upon investigation a drug interaction would be confirmed or refuted. In the late 1980s, formal drug interaction studies became an integral component of ASM clinical trial development programs, but most drug interaction studies were conducted relatively late in Phase II and Phase III clinical development programs and were based on a strategy that was in turn based on the therapeutic indices of drugs and the likelihood of their concurrent use. More recently, with the availability of human hepatic tissue and recombinant CYP enzymes, in vitro systems have been used as screening tools to predict the potential for in vivo drug interaction at a much earlier stage of drug development. The use of in vitro systems for investigating the ability of a drug to inhibit the metabolism of other drugs provides some of the most useful information in predicting potential drug–drug interactions. Nevertheless, the in vitro and clinical evaluation of all drugs with the potential to interact with an ASM is not possible prior to licensing, and thus interactions continue to come to light subsequent to licensing and during the drugs' availability for general clinical use. Particular sources of such interaction data include case reports, therapeutic drug monitoring databases, and population pharmacokinetic modeling databases [36].

In recent years, our understanding of how individual drugs are metabolized has greatly facilitated the prediction of metabolic interactions. While ASMs are metabolized in the liver via numerous pathways such as β-oxidation (e.g., valproic acid) and conjugation involving UGTs (e.g., eslicarbazepine, cenobamate, lamotrigine, oxcarbazepine, and valproic acid), by far the most important system for ASM metabolism is the CYP system (e.g., cannabidiol, clobazam, clonazepam, carbamazepine, everolimus, ethosuximide, felbamate, fenfluramine, perampanel, phenytoin, phenobarbital, stiripentol, topiramate, tiagabine, and zonisamide). For an accurate prediction of a drug's potential to interact, it is essential to identify the enzyme(s) responsible for the metabolism of the drug. Furthermore, in order to be able to anticipate the possible clinical relevance of an interaction, it is important to determine the relative contribution of the metabolic pathway(s) being inhibited or induced to the overall elimination of the drug. In some cases, a single metabolic reaction may involve multiple isoforms or different enzyme systems, while in other cases all the metabolic reactions of a drug are catalyzed by a single enzyme. The metabolism (S-oxidation) of 10-(*N*, *N*-dimethylaminoalkyl) phenothiazines is an example of the first scenario in which numerous CYP isoforms, including CYP2A6, CYP2C8, and CYP2D6, are involved in its metabolism. On the other hand, the metabolism of indinavir, an HIV protease inhibitor, via four oxidative metabolic reactions (N-oxidation, N-dealkylation, indan hydroxylation, and phenyl hydroxylation), is catalyzed by a single isoform of CYP, namely, CYP3A4.

While in vitro data can be used to anticipate in vivo inhibitory interactions, such data are of very limited value in assessing the enzyme-inducing properties of a drug. For ASMs that do not undergo hepatic metabolism (e.g., gabapentin, levetiracetam, pregabalin, and vigabatrin), or those that are metabolized by non-CYP isoenzymes (e.g., lacosamide, rufinamide) and neither inhibit nor induce CYP isoenzymes, these characteristics provide a powerful predictor that these ASMs are unlikely to be associated with pharmacokinetic interactions. Indeed, clinically these ASMs are observed to be minimally interacting or noninteracting.

The clinical consequences of enzyme inhibition depend on the plasma level of the inhibitor, its inhibition constant for the enzyme, and the relative contribution of the pathway to the elimination of the affected drug. If the inhibited pathway accounts for only a small fraction (e.g., <30–40%) of the drug's total clearance, the impact of the interaction on the drug's plasma level and clinical effect will be small. Age, genetics, and environmental factors may also influence the extent of inhibition. The effects of inhibition interactions are usually apparent within 24 h of addition of the inhibitor, with time to the maximal increase in plasma levels determined by the time required for both the inhibitor and affected drug, which will now have a more prolonged half-life, to achieve steady state. After discontinuation of the inhibitor, the time course for the decrease in plasma levels depends on the same factors.

In contrast to inhibitory interactions, interactions involving induction can be substantial even if induction involves a minor pathway of drug elimination. In this setting, the minor pathway may become the major pathway responsible for drug clearance causing a clinically relevant decrease in plasma levels (e.g., topiramate).

Interactions with phenytoin, whereby the hepatic enzyme primarily responsible for the metabolism of phenytoin is the isoenzyme CYP2C9 (>80%) while CYP2C19 contributes <20% to the metabolism of phenytoin, need more thoughtful consideration. Thus, if amiodarone, fluconazole, miconazole, ketoconazole, propoxyphene, or valproic acid (which inhibit CYP2C9) are coadministered with phenytoin, they will have a substantial potential to inhibit phenytoin metabolism and elevate plasma phenytoin levels. In contrast, if topiramate, cimetidine, felbamate, omeprazole, fluoxetine, or ticlopidine (which inhibit CYP2C19) are coadministered with phenytoin, they will only have a small potential to inhibit phenytoin metabolism and elevate plasma phenytoin levels. However, while CYP2C19 is a minor pathway for phenytoin metabolism, its relative contribution increases at higher plasma phenytoin levels due to saturation of the primary phenytoin pathway, CYP2C9. Thus, interactions with CYP2C19 inhibitors, while of minor importance at low phenytoin plasma levels, assume greater significance as plasma phenytoin levels increase. Consequently, patients with phenytoin plasma levels above the saturable level for CYP2C9, which occur at or below the reference range (therapeutic range), are more prone to significant elevations in phenytoin plasma levels with the addition of CYP2C19 inhibitors.

Many interactions are associated with large intersubject variability. In the case of interactions involving phenytoin, this can be explained by various factors. Firstly, there is significant intersubject variability in the contribution of CYP2C9 and CYP2C19 to its metabolism. Secondly, it is known that drugs that inhibit CYP2C19 (without inhibiting CYP2C9), including carbamazepine, omeprazole, ticlopidine, felbamate, and topiramate, produce inconsistent elevations in phenytoin plasma levels. Thirdly, there is pharmacogenetic variability in CYP expression and a significant proportion of Caucasians and Asians exhibit the "poor metabolizer phenotype" of CYP2C19. In such subjects, inhibition of CYP2C19 is not manifested. Lastly, in the case of the interaction with carbamazepine, carbamazepine may increase the clearance of phenytoin through induction of CYP2C9 and/or CYP2C19.

A further confounding factor relates to the fact that drug interactions may relate to specific competitive inhibition of polymorphic enzymes. For example, omeprazole and diazepam are predominantly metabolized by CYP2C19. The CYP2C19 isoform is known to be polymorphic and approximately 2–6% of Caucasians and 18–22% of Asians have been found to be poor metabolizers. Thus, patients who are extensive metabolizers of omeprazole, and consequently have a higher baseline metabolism of omeprazole, are more susceptible to enzyme inhibition interactions than are patients who are poor metabolizers of omeprazole. Similarly, extensive metabolizers are more susceptible to enzyme induction than poor metabolizers.

Databases listing substrates, inhibitors, and inducers of different CYP isoenzymes provide an invaluable resource in helping the physician to predict and eventually to avoid potential interactions (Table 2). For example, knowledge that carbamazepine is an inducer of CYP3A4 allows one to predict that it will reduce the plasma level of CYP3A4 substrates such as ethosuximide, tiagabine, steroid oral

Table 2 Metabolic characteristics of antiseizure medications (ASMs) and their propensity to affect hepatic metabolism and cause a pharmacokinetic interaction with other ASMs

ASM	Hepatic metabolism (%)	Enzymes involved in metabolism	Elimination by renal excretion (%)	Propensity to interact
Carbamazepine	Substantial (98)	CYP1A2, CYP2C8, CYP3A4	Minimal (2)	Substantial
Phenytoin	Substantial (95)	CYP2C9, CYP2C19	Minimal (2)	Substantial
Phenobarbital	Substantial (80)	CYP2E1, CYP2C19	Minimal (20)	Substantial
Primidone	Minimal (35)	CYP2E1, CYP2C9, CYP2C19	Moderate (65)	Substantial
Stiripentol	Substantial (73)	CYP1A2, CYP2C19, CYP3A4	Minimal (27)	Substantial
Sulthiame	Moderate (68)	Not identified but involve CYP isoenzymes	Minimal (32)	Substantial
Valproic acid	Substantial (97)	CYP2A6, CYP2C9, CYP2C19, CYP2B6, UGT1A3, UGT2B7	Minimal (3)	Substantial
Everolimus	Substantial (95)	CYP3A4	Minimal (5)	Substantial
Cannabidiol	Substantial (88)	CYP3A4, CYP2C19, UGT1A7, UGT1A9,UGT2B7	Minimal (12)	Moderate
Cenobamate	Substantial (93)	UGT2B7,UGT2B4, CYP2E1, CYP2A6, CYP2B6, CYP2C19, CYP3A4/5	Minimal (7)	Moderate
Fenfluramine	Substantial (75)	CYP1A2, CYP2B6, CYP2D6, CYP2C9, CYP2C19, CYP3A4	Moderate (25)	Moderate
Lamotrigine	Substantial (90)	UGT1A4, UGT1A1, UGT2B7	Minimal (10)	Moderate
Brivaracetam	Substantial (91)	Amidase, CYP2C19	Minimal (9)	Minimal
Clobazam	Substantial (100)	CYP3A4	None (0)	Minimal
Clonazepam	Substantial (99)	CYP3A4	Minimal (1)	Minimal
Eslicarbazepine acetate	Substantial (>99)	Not identified but UGTs are involved	Minimal (1)	Minimal
Ethosuximide	Substantial (80)	CYP2B, CYP2E1, CYP3A4	Minimal (20)	Minimal
Felbamate	Moderate (50)	CYP3A4, CYP2E1	Moderate (50)	Minimal
Methsuximide	Substantial (99)	CYP2C19	Minimal (1)	Minimal
Oxcarbazepine	Substantial (>99)	Not identified but UGTs are involved	Minimal (<1)	Minimal
Perampanel	Substantial (98%)	CYP3A4, CYP3A5	Minimal (2)	Minimal
Rufinamide	Substantial (96)	Unknown (but not CYP-dependent)	Minimal (4)	Minimal

Table 2 (continued)

ASM	Hepatic metabolism (%)	Enzymes involved in metabolism	Elimination by renal excretion (%)	Propensity to interact
Tiagabine	Substantial (98)	CYP3A4	Minimal (<2)	Minimal
Topiramate	Moderate (50)	Not identified but involve CYP isoenzymes	Moderate (50)	Minimal
Zonisamide	Moderate (65)	CYP3A4	Minimal (35)	Minimal
Acetazolamide	Not metabolized	None	Substantial (100)	Noninteracting
Gabapentin	Not metabolized	None	Substantial (100)	Noninteracting
Lacosamide	Moderate (60)	Demethylation	Minimal (40)	Noninteracting
Levetiracetam	Minimal (30) – non-hepatic, occurs in whole blood	Type-B esterase	Moderate (66)	Noninteracting
Piracetam	Not metabolized	None	Substantial (100)	Noninteracting
Pregabalin	Not metabolized	None	Substantial (98)	Noninteracting
Vigabatrin	Not metabolized	None	Substantial (100)	Noninteracting

contraceptives, and cyclosporine. Likewise, the ability of ketoconazole to inhibit CYP3A4 explains the clinically important rise in plasma carbamazepine levels after ingestion of this antifungal agent.

Factors That Impact on the Relevance of a Metabolic Interaction

Although the number of theoretically possible interactions based on knowledge of the CYP and other enzyme systems (Table 3) is increasing, it must be appreciated that not all will be of clinical importance. The factors to be considered when evaluating the practical relevance of a potential interaction are as follows:

1. The nature of the interaction at the enzyme site—is it a substrate, an inhibitor, or an inducer?
2. The spectrum of isoenzymes that are induced or inhibited by the interacting agent.
3. The potency of the inhibition/induction—a potent effect will result in a more ubiquitous interaction affecting many/most patients.

4. The level (concentration) of the inhibitor/inducer at the isoenzyme site—drugs that achieve low levels in blood may never reach the level threshold necessary to elicit an interaction.
5. The extent of metabolism of the substrate through the particular isoenzyme—if the affected enzyme is only responsible for a small fraction of the drug's clearance, its inhibition is not going to result in a substantial interaction. Conversely, enzyme induction may increase the activity of the affected enzyme manyfold, and therefore, it may increase substantially the total clearance of the drug.
6. The saturability of the isoenzyme—isoenzymes that are saturable at drug levels encountered clinically are more susceptible to significant inhibitory interactions.
7. The route of administration—for drugs showing extensive first-pass metabolism, any change in plasma drug level caused by enzyme induction or inhibition will be much greater after oral than after parenteral administration.
8. The presence of pharmacologically active metabolites—such metabolites complicate the outcome of a potential interaction and may themselves act as enzyme inducers or inhibitors.

Table 3 ASM and non-ASM drug substrates, inhibitors, and inducers of the major CYP and UGT isoenzymes involved in drug metabolism

Isoenzymes	Substrates	Inhibitors	Inducers
CYP1A2	**ASMs**: carbamazepine, fenfluramine, stiripentol **Non-ASMs**: aminophylline, amitriptyline, caffeine, chlorpromazine, clomipramine, clozapine, dacarbazine, fluvoxamine, haloperidol, imipramine, lidocaine, melatonin, mirtazapine, olanzapine, paracetamol, phenacetin, propranolol, ropivacaine, ***R***-warfarin, sulindac, tacrine, tamoxifen, theophylline, tizanidine, verapamil, zolpidem, zopiclone	***ASMs*** Cannabidiol ***Non-ASMs*** Ciprofloxacin Clarithromycin Enoxacin Fluvoxamine Furafylline Methoxsalen Oral contraceptives Rofecoxib	***ASMs*** Carbamazepine Phenobarbital Phenytoin Primidone ***Non-ASMs*** Rifampicin Ritonavir St. John's wort[b]
CYP2C9	**ASMs**: fenfluramine, phenobarbital, phenytoin, primidone, valproic acid **Non-ASMs**: amitriptyline, celecoxib, diclofenac, dicoumarol, fluoxetine, fluvastatin, ibuprofen, losartan, miconazole, naproxen, olanzapine, phenylbutazone, piroxicam, quetiapine, theophylline, tolbutamide, torasemide, voriconazole, *S*-warfarin, zidovudine, zolpidem	***ASMs*** Cannabidiol Valproic acid Zonisamide[a] ***Non-ASMs*** Amiodarone Chloramphenicol Delavirdine Efavirenz Fluconazole Fluoxetine Fluvoxamine Miconazole Sulfaphenazole Voriconazole	***ASMs*** Carbamazepine Phenobarbital Phenytoin Primidone ***Non-ASMs*** Hyperforin Rifampicin Ritonavir St. John's wort

Table 3 (continued)

Isoenzymes	Substrates	Inhibitors	Inducers
CYP2C19	**ASMs**: brivaracetam, cannabidiol, cenobamate, diazepam, fenfluramine, phenobarbital, phenytoin, primidone, stiripentol, valproic acid **Non-ASMs**: amitriptyline, citalopram, clomipramine, esomeprazole, imipramine, lansoprazole, moclobemide, omeprazole, pantoprazole, proguanil, propranolol, *R*-warfarin, voriconazole	***ASMs*** Cannabidiol Eslicarbazepine Felbamate Oxcarbazepine Stiripentol Topiramate[a] Zonisamide[a] ***Non-ASMs*** Cimetidine Delavirdine Efavirenz Esomeprazole Fluconazole Fluvoxamine Lansoprazole Miconazole Omeprazole Ticlopidine Voriconazole	***ASMs*** Carbamazepine Phenobarbital Phenytoin Primidone ***Non-ASMs*** Rifampicin Ritonavir
CYP2D6	***ASMs:*** fenfluramine ***Non-ASMs***: alprenolol, amitriptyline, bufuralol, chlorpromazine, citalopram, clomipramine, clozapine, codeine, debrisoquine, desipramine, dextromethorphan, encainide, flecainide, fluoxetine, fluphenazine, fluvoxamine, haloperidol, imipramine, maprotiline, metoprolol, mianserin, mirtazapine, nefazodone, nortriptyline, olanzapine, paroxetine, perphenazine, phenformin, pindolol, propafenone, propranolol, quetiapine, risperidone, ritonavir, sertindole, tamoxifen, thioridazine, timolol, tramadol, venlafaxine, zuclopenthixol	***ASMs*** Everolimus Fenfluramine Stiripentol ***Non-ASMs*** Cimetidine Fluoxetine Haloperidol Lansoprazole Paroxetine Perphenazine Propafenone Quinidine Terbinafine Thioridazine Verapamil	*No inducer known*
CYP2E1	***ASMs***: cenobamate, ethosuximide, felbamate, phenobarbital, primidone ***Non-ASMs***: chlorzoxazone, dapsone, ethanol, halothane, isoniazid	***ASMs*** Zonisamide[a] ***Non-ASMs*** Disulfiram	***Non-ASMs*** Ethanol Isoniazid

(continued)

Table 3 (continued)

Isoenzymes	Substrates	Inhibitors	Inducers
CYP3A4	***ASMs***: cannabidiol, carbamazepine, cenobamate, clobazam, clonazepam, diazepam, ethosuximide, everolimus, felbamate, fenfluramine, perampanel, stiripentol, tiagabine, valproic acid, zonisamide ***Non-ASMs***: alfentanil, amiodarone, amitriptyline, astemizole, atorvastatin, cisapride, citalopram, clarithromycin, clomipramine, clozapine, cyclophosphamide, cyclosporine A, dexamethasone, diltiazem, docetaxel, doxorubicin, erythromycin, etoposide, felodipine, fentanyl, fluoxetine, fluvoxamine, glucocorticoids, haloperidol, ifosfamide, imipramine, indinavir, irinotecan, isoniazid, itraconazole, ketoconazole, lacidipine, lercanidipine, lidocaine, lopinavir, lovastatin, methadone, mirtazapine, nefazodone, nevirapine, nifedipine, nimodipine, olanzapine, oral contraceptives, paclitaxel, procarbazine, proguanil, quetiapine, quinidine, rifampicin, risperidone, ritonavir, saquinavir, sertindole, sertraline, sildenafil, simvastatin, steroids, tacrolimus, tamoxifen, teniposide, terfenadine, theophylline, thiotepa, topotecan, trazodone, troleandomycin, venlafaxine, verapamil, vinblastine, vincristine, vindesine, voriconazole, ziprasidone, zolpidem	***ASMs*** Everolimus Stiripentol ***Non-ASMs*** Amprenavir Cimetidine Clarithromycin Cyclophosphamide Cyclosporine A Delavirdine Dexamethasone Dextropropoxyphene Diltiazem Docetaxel Doxorubicin Efavirenz Erythromycin Etoposide Fluconazole Fluoxetine Fluvoxamine Grapefruit juice Ifosfamide Indinavir Isoniazid Itraconazole Ketoconazole Lidocaine Lopinavir Methadone Miconazole Nefazodone Nelfinavir Nifedipine Paclitaxel Posaconazole Propoxyphene Ritonavir Teniposide Troleandomycin Venlafaxine Verapamil Vinblastine Vindesine Zidovudine	***ASMs*** Carbamazepine Eslicarbazepine Felbamate[a] Fenfluramine, Oxcarbazepine[a] Phenobarbital Phenytoin Primidone Topiramate[a] ***Non-ASMs*** Cyclophosphamide Dexamethasone Docetaxel Efavirenz Glucocorticoids[a] Nefazodone Nevirapine Paclitaxel Rifabutin Rifampicin St. John's wort Tamoxifen Teniposide

Table 3 (continued)

Isoenzymes	Substrates	Inhibitors	Inducers
UGT1A4	**ASMs**: lamotrigine, eslicarbazepine **Non-ASMs**: amitriptyline, clozapine, imipramine, olanzapine	**Non-ASMs** Sertraline **ASMs** Valproic acid	**ASMs** Carbamazepine Phenobarbital Phenytoin Primidone **Non-ASMs** Oral contraceptives
UGT1A6	**ASMs**: valproic acid **Non-ASMs**: acetaminophen	**Non-ASMs** Probenecid	**ASMs** Carbamazepine Phenobarbital Phenytoin Primidone **Non-ASMs** Oral contraceptives
UGT1A7 **UGT1A9**	**ASMs**: cannabidiol **ASMs**: cannabidiol, eslicarbazepine, valproic acid **Non-ASMs**: acetaminophen, propofol, tolcapone	**ASMs** Cannabidiol **Non-ASMs** Probenecid	**ASMs** Carbamazepine Phenobarbital Phenytoin Primidone **Non-ASMs** Oral contraceptives
UGT2B7	**ASMs**: cannabidiol, cenobamate, eslicarbazepine, valproic acid **Non-ASMs**: codeine, ibuprofen, morphine, naloxone, naproxen, zidovudine	**ASMs** Cannabidiol **Non-ASMs** Atovaquone Fluconazole Probenecid	**ASMs** Carbamazepine Phenobarbital Phenytoin Primidone **Non-ASMs** Oral contraceptives
UGT2B17	**ASMs**: eslicarbazepine		**ASMs** Carbamazepine Phenobarbital Phenytoin Primidone
UGT2B4	**ASMs**: cenobamate, eslicarbazepine		**ASMs** Carbamazepine Phenobarbital Phenytoin Primidone

The list is not exhaustive and is intended for guidance only. Prediction of drug interactions based on this table (see text) is involved in determining whether a clinically significant drug interaction will or will not occur

CYP cytochrome P450, *UGT* uridine glucuronyl transferases

[a]These drugs are weak inducers or inhibitors

[b]Only an inducer in females

9. The therapeutic window of the substrate—interactions affecting drugs with a narrow therapeutic window are more likely to be of clinical significance.
10. The plasma level of the affected drug at baseline—any change in plasma drug level will have greater consequences if the baseline level is near the threshold of toxicity (or near the threshold required to produce a desirable therapeutic effect).
11. The genetic predisposition of the individual patient—for example, subjects who show deficiency of a genetically polymorphic isoenzyme (e.g., CYP2D6 or CYP2C19) will not exhibit interactions mediated by induction or inhibition of that isoenzyme.
12. The susceptibility and the sensitivity of the individual in relation to adverse effects—the elderly are more susceptible to interactions because as a patient group they are more likely to receive multiple medications. Also the elderly are more sensitive to the adverse effects of drugs.
13. The probability of the potential interacting drugs being co-prescribed—if a particular combination is unlikely to be co-prescribed, then any potential interaction will be of no clinical relevance.

Prevention and Management of Adverse ASM Interactions

From a therapeutic viewpoint, drug interactions are best avoided by use of drugs that are not potent CYP inhibitors or inducers and are not readily inhibited by other drugs. In reality, drug interactions caused by mutual inhibition are almost inevitable, because CYP-mediated metabolism represents a major route of elimination of many drugs and because the same CYP enzymes can metabolize numerous drugs. The clinical significance of a metabolic drug interaction will depend on the magnitude of the change in the concentration of the active species (parent drug and/or metabolites) at the site of pharmacological action and the therapeutic index of the drug. The smaller the difference between toxicity and efficacy, the greater the likelihood that a drug interaction will have serious clinical consequences.

Prevention of ASM interactions is best achieved by avoiding unnecessary polytherapy or by selecting alternative agents that have less potential to interact. The management of interactions begins with anticipating their occurrence and being familiar with the mechanisms involved (Fig. 1). Indeed, awareness of the mechanism of a drug interaction can be used to clinical advantage. For example, when one drug decreases the rate of elimination of another and increases the half-life of the affected drug, this can have an impact on the frequency of dosing, which in turn may improve compliance, or it may mean that a reduction of the dose of the affected drug is necessary. Also, in patients with a sub-therapeutic plasma drug level, elevation of the level may actually result in better seizure control. By following a few simple rules, potential adverse consequences of ASM interactions can be minimized or even avoided:

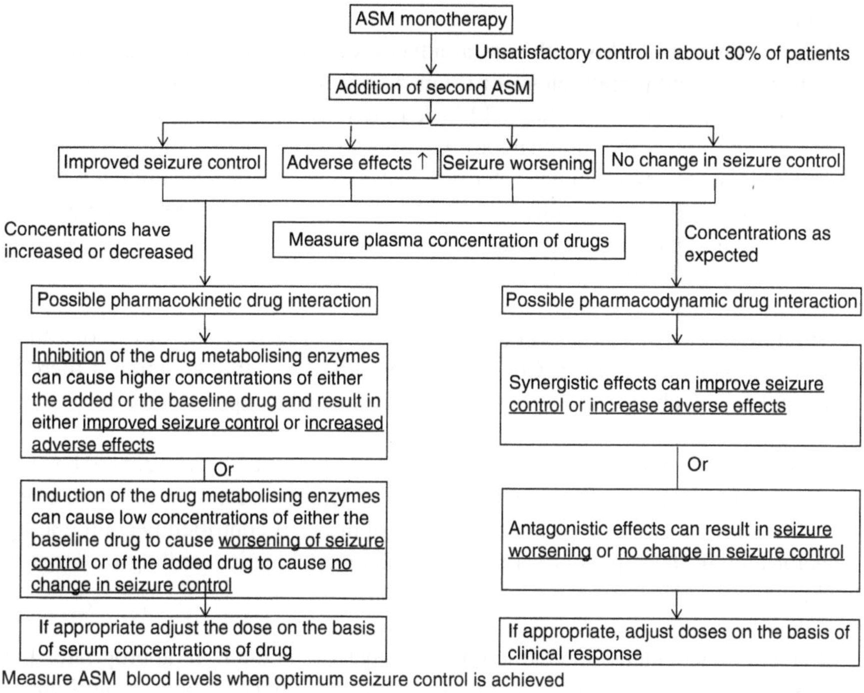

Fig. 1 Effect of ASM interactions on therapeutic outcome (Adapted from Patsalos et al. [3] with permission John Wiley and Sons)

- Rule 1
  Utilize multiple drug therapy only when it is clearly indicated. Most patients with epilepsy can be best managed with a carefully individualized dosage of a single ASM.
- Rule 2
  If a patient suffers from comorbidities requiring multiple medications, it is preferable to treat the seizure disorder with an ASM having a low interaction potential. Brivaracetam, eslicarbazepine acetate, ethosuximide, lamotrigine, topiramate, lacosamide, levetiracetam, perampanel, tiagabine, gabapentin, and pregabalin have little or no ability to cause enzyme induction or inhibition. Among ASMs, the lowest interaction potential is associated with the renally eliminated agents acetazolamide, gabapentin, levetiracetam, piracetam, pregabalin, and vigabatrin.
- Rule 3
  Be aware of the most important interactions and their underlying mechanisms and any corrective action required (e.g., altered dosing requirements). Most interactions are metabolically based and can be predicted from knowledge of the isoenzymes responsible for the metabolism of the most commonly used drugs and the effects of these drugs on the same isoenzymes.

- Rule 4
  Avoid combining ASMs with similar adverse effect profiles—for example, benzodiazepines and barbiturates—or drugs associated with additive neurotoxicity, for example, two sodium-channel blockers (carbamazepine and oxcarbazepine, or carbamazepine and lamotrigine). Combining drugs acting through different mechanisms are much better tolerated. Always choose drug combinations for which there is clinical evidence of favorable pharmacodynamic interactions (e.g., ethosuximide and valproate in refractory absence seizures or valproate and lamotrigine in the management of a wide variety of refractory seizures).
- Rule 5
  Observe clinical response carefully whenever a drug is added or discontinued from the patient's regimen. Consider the possibility of an interaction if there is an unexpected change in response. Adjust dosage when appropriate.
- Rule 6
  Be aware that some patient groups (e.g., the elderly, patients with renal or hepatic insufficiency, and during pregnancy) may be more susceptible to interactions and/or more sensitive to the adverse effects of drugs. A contributing confounding factor among these patients is that their pharmacokinetic handling of drugs is altered.
- Rule 7
  If a pharmacokinetic interaction is anticipated, monitor, if appropriate, the plasma level of the affected drug. Be aware that under certain circumstances (e.g., in the presence of drug displacement from plasma proteins), routine total drug level measurements may be misleading and patient management may benefit from monitoring of free non-protein-bound drug levels (e.g., the interaction between valproic acid and phenytoin). In some cases, dosage adjustments may have to be implemented at the time the interacting drug is added or removed. Also, with some drugs, monitoring of surrogate therapeutic markers is preferable over blood level monitoring [e.g., with warfarin and dicoumarol, it is advisable to monitor the INR (international normalized ratio) whenever a significant change in therapy of a concomitant enzyme-inducing ASM is made].
- Rule 8
  When adding a drug to treat intercurrent or concomitant conditions, choose the one which within a given class is least likely to be involved in worrisome problematic interactions. For example, famotidine would be preferable to cimetidine as an H_2 antagonist, and atenolol would be preferable to metoprolol as a β-adrenoceptor blocker.
- Rule 9
  Ask patients to report any symptoms or signs suggestive of overdosage or insufficient therapeutic cover.

- Rule 10
  Inform patients of potential hazards associated with over-the-counter medicines, vitamin supplements, and herbal products. Many such products are known to interfere with the metabolism of ASMs. Discuss in advance with patients and appropriate alternatives should be suggested, e.g., cold or allergy preparations containing a sympathomimetic amine rather than antihistamines, nonalcoholic formulations of medications, and use of parenteral or oral nonsteroidal anti-inflammatory drugs rather than narcotic analgesics for mild-to-moderate pain control.

The Role of Therapeutic Drug Monitoring in the Management of ASM Interactions

Since ASM interactions are primarily pharmacokinetic in nature and therefore characterized by a change in drug plasma levels, the role for therapeutic drug monitoring in managing these interactions is very important [24, 37–39]. For most ASMs, there are well-accepted reference ranges; however, this is not the case for non-ASMs. Indeed, for many non-AEDs there is still debate as to what would be the best parameter for measurement (trough [C_{min}] or peak [C_{max}] blood level or the area under the concentration versus time curve [AUC]). The best approach, in most clinical settings, is to undertake a drug level measurement before adding a second drug and then to undertake further drug level measurements and to use the latter values, as necessary, to adjust dosage to achieve the previously effective plasma level and response. It should be remembered, however, that for plasma protein-binding displacement interactions, patient management may be best guided by the use of free (non-protein-bound) plasma drug levels [25] (Fig. 2).

With some drug interactions, surrogate markers other than plasma drug levels are better suited as a guide to clinical management. For example, it is advisable to monitor the INR (international normalized ratio) with warfarin and dicoumarol whenever a significant change in therapy of a concomitant enzyme-inducing ASM is made. Also, the determination of the viral load of HIV patients prescribed ASMs and antiviral medication may provide an invaluable indicator of an underlying interaction.

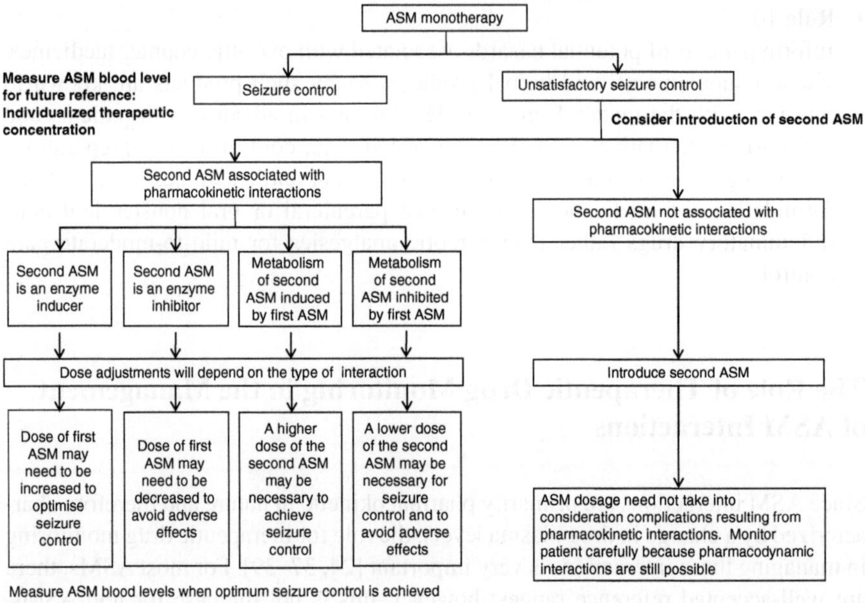

Fig. 2 Strategies for managing interactions: dosage adjustments based on the mechanism of drug interaction (Adapted from Patsalos et al. [3] with permission John Wiley and Sons)

References

1. Kwan P, Sander JW. The natural history of epilepsy: an epidemiological view. J Neurol Neurosurg Psychiatry. 2004;75:1376–81.
2. Kwan P, Brodie MJ. Early identification of refractory epilepsy. N Engl J Med. 2000;342:314–9.
3. Patsalos PN, Froscher W, Pisani F, van Rijn CM. The importance of drug interactions in epilepsy therapy. Epilepsia. 2002;43:365–85.
4. Patsalos PN, Perucca E. Clinically important drug interactions in epilepsy: general features and interactions between antiepileptic drugs. Lancet Neurol. 2003;2:347–56.
5. Patsalos PN. Drug interactions with the newer antiepileptic drugs (AEDs) - Part 2: Pharmacokinetic and pharmacodynamic interactions between AEDs and drugs used to treat non-epilepsy disorders. Clin Pharmacokin. 2013;52:1045–1061.
6. Patsalos PN, Perucca E. Clinically important drug interactions in epilepsy: interactions between antiepileptic drugs and other drugs. Lancet Neurol. 2003;2:473–81.
7. Johannessen Landmark C, Patsalos PN. Interactions between antiepileptic drugs and herbal medicines. Bol Latinoam Caribe Plant Med Aromaticas. 2008;7:116–26.
8. Johannessen LC. Antiepileptic drugs in non-epilepsy disorders: relations between mechanisms of action and clinical efficacy. CNS Drugs. 2008;22:27–47.
9. Patsalos PN, St Louis EK. The epilepsy prescriber's guide to antiepileptic drugs. Cambridge: Cambridge University Press; 3nd Ed, 2018.
10. Reutens DC, Duncan JS, Patsalos PN. Disabling tremor after lamotrigine with sodium valproate. Lancet. 1993;342:185–6.
11. Rowan AJ, Meijer JW, de Beer-Pawlikowski N, van der Geest P, Meinardi H. Valproate-ethosuximide combination therapy for refractory seizures. Arch Neurol. 1983;40:797–802.

12. Pisani F, Oteri G, Russo MF, Di Perri R, Perucca E, Richens A. The efficacy of valproate-lamotrigine comedication in refractory complex partial seizures: evidence for a pharmacodynamic interaction. Epilepsia. 1999;40:1141–6.
13. Brodie MJ, Mumford JP. Double-blind substitution of vigabatrin and valproate in carbamazepine-resistant partial epilepsy. 012 Study group. Epilepsy Res. 1999;34:199–205.
14. Shukla S, Godwin CD, Long LEB, Miller MG. Lithium-carbamazepine neurotoxicity and risk factors. Am J Psychiatry. 1984;141:1604–5.
15. McGinness J, Kishimoto A, Hollister EA. Avoiding neurotoxicity with lithium-carbamazepine combinations. Psychopharmacol Bull. 1990;26:181–4.
16. Huang CC, Wei IH. Unexpected interaction between quetiapine and valproate in patients with bipolar disorder. Gen Hosp Psychiatry. 2010;32:446.e1–2.
17. Junghan U, Albers M, Woggon B. Increased risk of haematological side-effects in psychiatric patients treated with clozapine and carbamazepine? Pharmacopsychiatry. 1993;26:262.
18. Bauer LA. Interference of oral phenytoin absorption by continuous nasogastric feedings. Neurology. 1982;32:570–2.
19. Syversen GB, Morgan JP, Weintraub M, Myers GJ. Acetazolamide-induced interference with primidone absorption. Case reports and metabolic studies. Arch Neurol. 1977;34:80–4.
20. Neef C, de Voogd-van der Straaten I. An interaction between cytostatic and anticonvulsant drugs. Clin Pharmacol Ther. 1988;43:372–5.
21. Neuvonen PJ, Kivisto K, Hirvisalo EL. Effects of resins and activated charcoal on the absorption of digoxin, carbamazepine and frusemide. Br J Clin Pharmacol. 1988;25:229–33.
22. Patsalos PN, Zugman M, Lake C, James A, Ratnaraj N, Sander JW. Serum protein binding of 25 antiepileptic drugs in a routine clinical setting: A comparison of free non-protein-bound concentrations. Epilepsia. 2017;58:1234–43.
23. Perucca E, Hebdige S, Frigo GM, Gatti G, Lecchini S, Crema A. Interaction between phenytoin and valproic acid: plasma protein binding and metabolic effects. Clin Pharmacol Ther. 1980;28:779–89.
24. Patsalos PN, Berry DJ, Bourgeois BFD, Cloyd JC, Glauser TA, Johannessen SI, Leppik IE, Tomson T, Perucca E. Antiepileptic drugs—best practice guidelines for therapeutic drug monitoring: a position paper by the Subcommission on Therapeutic Drug Monitoring. ILAE Commission on Therapeutic Strategies. Epilepsia. 2008;49:1239–76.
25. Ragueneau-Majlessi I, Levy RH, Bergen D, Garnet W, Rosenfeld W, Mather G, Shah J, Grundy JS. Carbamazepine pharmacokinetics are not affected by zonisamide: in vitro mechanistic study and in vivo clinical study in epileptic patients. Epilepsy Res. 2004;62:1–11.
26. Hussein G, Troupin AS, Montouris G. Gabapentin interaction with felbamate. Neurology. 1996;47:1106.
27. Li AP, Kaminski DL, Rasmussen A. Substrates of human hepatic cytochrome P4503A4. Toxicology. 1995;104:1–8.
28. Guengerich FP. Epoxide hydrolase: properties and metabolic roles. Rev. Biochem Toxicol. 1982;4:5–30.
29. Pisani F, Caputo M, Fazio A, Oteri G, Russo M, Spina E, Perucca E, Bertilsson L. Interaction of carbamazepine-10,11-epoxide, an active metabolite of carbamazepine, with valproate: a pharmacokinetic ionteraction. Epilepsia. 1990;31:339–42.
30. Rambeck B, May T, Juergens U. Serum concentrations of carbamazepine and its epoxide and diol metabolites in epileptic patients: the influence of dose and comedication. Ther Drug Monit. 1987;9:298–303.
31. Fitzgerald BJ, Okos AJ. Elevation of carbamazepine-10,11-epoxide by quetiapine. Pharmacotherapy. 2002;22:1500–3.
32. Mackenzie PI, Owens IS, Burchell B, Bock KW, Bairoch A, Belanger A, Fournel-Gigleux S, Green M, Hum DW, Iyanagi T, Lancet D, Louisot P, Magdalou J, Roy Chowdhury J, Ritter JK, Schachter H, Tephly TR, Tipton KF, Nebert DW. The UDP glucosyltransferase gene subfamily: recommended nomenclature based on evolutionary divergence. Pharmacogenetics. 1997;7:255–69.

33. Spina E, Arena S, Scordo MG, Fazio A, Pisan F, Perucca E. Elevation of plasma carbamazepine concentrations by ketoconazole in patients with epilepsy. Ther Drug Monit. 1997;19:535–8.
34. Tucker RM, Denning DW, Hanson LH, Rinaldi MG, Graybill JR, Sharkey PK, Pappagianis D, Stevens DA. Interaction of azoles with rifampin, phenytoin, and carbamazepine: in vitro and clinical observations. Clin Infect Dis. 1992;14:165–74.
35. Miller RR, Porter J, Greenblatt DJ. Clinical importance of the interaction of phenytoin and isoniazid. Chest. 1979;75:356–8.
36. Garg SK, Kumar N, Bhargava VK, Prabhakar SK. Effect of grapefruit juice on carbamazepine bioavailability in patients with epilepsy. Clin Pharmacol Ther. 1998;64:286–8.
37. Johannessen SI, Bettino D, Berry DJ, Bialer M, Kramer G, Tomson T, Patsalos PN. Therapeutic drug monitoring of the newer antiepileptic drugs. Ther Drug Monit. 2003;25:347–63.
38. Johannessen Landmark C, Patsalos PN. Methodologies used to identify and characterise interactions among antiepileptic drugs. Exp Rev. Clin Pharmacol. 2012;5:281–92.
39. Patsalos PN, Spencer EP, Berry DJ. Therapeutic drug monitoring of antiepileptic drugs: A 2018 update. Ther Drug Monit. 2018;40:526–48.

Acetazolamide

Acetazolamide (Fig. 1) corresponds chemically to *N*-(5-(aminosulfonyl)-1,3,4-thiadiazol-2-yl)-acetamide with an empirical formula of $C_4H_6N_4O_3S_2$ and a molecular weight of 222.25.

Pharmacokinetic Characteristics

Absorption and Distribution

After oral ingestion, acetazolamide is rapidly absorbed (T_{max} = 2–4 h) with a bioavailability of >90%. Its volume of distribution is 0.3 L/kg, and plasma protein binding is 90–95%.

Biotransformation

Acetazolamide is not metabolized.

Renal Excretion

Approximately 100% of an administered dose is excreted as unchanged acetazolamide in urine.

Elimination

Plasma elimination half-life values in adults are 10–15 h.

Fig. 1 Acetazolamide

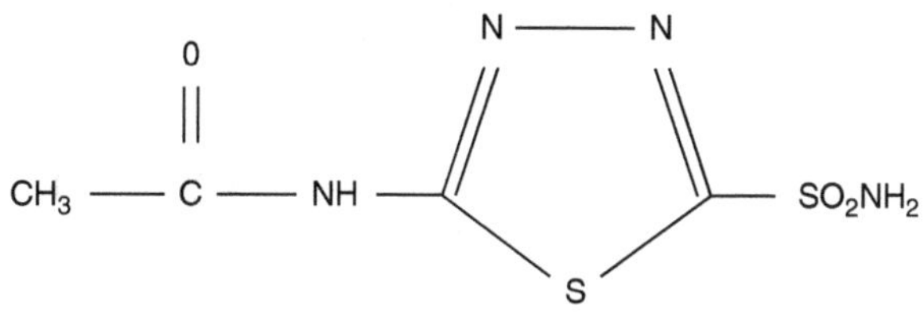

P. N. Patsalos, *Antiseizure Medication Interactions*,
https://doi.org/10.1007/978-3-030-82790-8_2

Effects on Isoenzymes

No in vitro data on the induction or inhibition potential of acetazolamide on human CYP or UGT isoenzymes have been published.

Therapeutic Drug Monitoring

Optimum seizure control in patients on acetazolamide monotherapy is most likely to occur at plasma acetazolamide levels of 10–14 mg/L (45–63 μmol/L). The conversion factor from mg/L to μmol/L is 4.50 (i.e., 1 mg/L = 4.50 μmol/L).

Propensity to Be Associated with Pharmacokinetic Interactions

- Acetazolamide affects the pharmacokinetics of other drugs—does not interact.
- Other drugs affect the pharmacokinetics of acetazolamide—does not interact.

Interactions with ASMs

Brivaracetam	The interaction has not been investigated. Theoretically, a pharmacokinetic interaction would not be anticipated
Cannabidiol	The interaction has not been investigated. Theoretically, a pharmacokinetic interaction would not be anticipated
Carbamazepine	The interaction has not been investigated. Theoretically, a pharmacokinetic interaction would not be anticipated
Cenobamate	The interaction has not been investigated. Theoretically, a pharmacokinetic interaction would not be anticipated
Clobazam	The interaction has not been investigated. Theoretically, a pharmacokinetic interaction would not be anticipated
Clonazepam	The interaction has not been investigated. Theoretically, a pharmacokinetic interaction would not be anticipated
Eslicarbazepine acetate	The interaction has not been investigated. Theoretically, a pharmacokinetic interaction would not be anticipated
Ethosuximide	The interaction has not been investigated. Theoretically, a pharmacokinetic interaction would not be anticipated
Everolimus	The interaction has not been investigated. Theoretically, a pharmacokinetic interaction would not be anticipated
Felbamate	The interaction has not been investigated. Theoretically, a pharmacokinetic interaction would not be anticipated
Fenfluramine	The interaction has not been investigated. Theoretically, a pharmacokinetic interaction would not be anticipated
Gabapentin	The interaction has not been investigated. Theoretically, a pharmacokinetic interaction would not be anticipated
Lacosamide	The interaction has not been investigated. Theoretically, a pharmacokinetic interaction would not be anticipated
Lamotrigine	The interaction has not been investigated. Theoretically, a pharmacokinetic interaction would not be anticipated
Levetiracetam	The interaction has not been investigated. Theoretically, a pharmacokinetic interaction would not be anticipated
Methsuximide	The interaction has not been investigated. Theoretically, a pharmacokinetic interaction would not be anticipated
Oxcarbazepine	The interaction has not been investigated. Theoretically, a pharmacokinetic interaction would not be anticipated

Perampanel	The interaction has not been investigated. Theoretically, a pharmacokinetic interaction would not be anticipated
Phenobarbital	The interaction has not been investigated. Theoretically, a pharmacokinetic interaction would not be anticipated
Phenytoin	The interaction has not been investigated. Theoretically, a pharmacokinetic interaction would not be anticipated
Piracetam	The interaction has not been investigated. Theoretically, a pharmacokinetic interaction would not be anticipated
Pregabalin	The interaction has not been investigated. Theoretically, a pharmacokinetic interaction would not be anticipated
Primidone	The interaction has not been investigated. Theoretically, a pharmacokinetic interaction would not be anticipated
Rufinamide	The interaction has not been investigated. Theoretically, a pharmacokinetic interaction would not be anticipated
Stiripentol	The interaction has not been investigated. Theoretically, a pharmacokinetic interaction would not be anticipated
Sulthiame	The interaction has not been investigated. Theoretically, a pharmacokinetic interaction would not be anticipated.
	Sulthiame and acetazolamide are both weak inhibitors of carbonic anhydrase and as a direct result may independently increase the risk of renal calculi. Consequently, there is a theoretical potential that when they are administered together, an adverse pharmacodynamic interaction will occur [1]
Tiagabine	The interaction has not been investigated. Theoretically, a pharmacokinetic interaction would not be anticipated
Topiramate	The interaction has not been investigated. Theoretically, a pharmacokinetic interaction would not be anticipated
	Topiramate and acetazolamide are both weak inhibitors of carbonic anhydrase and as a direct result may independently increase the risk of renal calculi. Consequently, there is a theoretical potential that when they are administered together, an adverse pharmacodynamic interaction will occur [1]
Valproic acid	The interaction has not been investigated. Theoretically, a pharmacokinetic interaction would not be anticipated
Vigabatrin	The interaction has not been investigated. Theoretically, a pharmacokinetic interaction would not be anticipated
Zonisamide	The interaction has not been investigated. Theoretically, a pharmacokinetic interaction would not be anticipated
	Zonisamide and acetazolamide are both weak inhibitors of carbonic anhydrase and as a direct result may independently increase the risk of renal calculi. Consequently, there is a theoretical potential that when they are administered together, an adverse pharmacodynamic interaction will occur [1]

Reference

1. Patsalos PN, St Louis EK. The epilepsy prescriber's guide to antiepileptic drugs. 3rd ed. Cambridge: Cambridge University Press; 2018.

Perampanel	The interaction has not been investigated. Theoretically, a pharmacokinetic interaction would not be anticipated
Phenobarbital	The interaction has not been investigated. Theoretically, a pharmacokinetic interaction would not be anticipated
Phenytoin	The interaction has not been investigated. Theoretically, a pharmacokinetic interaction would not be anticipated
Piracetam	The interaction has not been investigated. Theoretically, a pharmacokinetic interaction would not be anticipated
Pregabalin	The interaction has not been investigated. Theoretically, a pharmacokinetic interaction would not be anticipated
Primidone	The interaction has not been investigated. Theoretically, a pharmacokinetic interaction would not be anticipated
Rufinamide	The interaction has not been investigated. Theoretically, a pharmacokinetic interaction would not be anticipated
Stiripentol	The interaction has not been investigated. Theoretically, a pharmacokinetic interaction would not be anticipated
Sulthiame	The interaction has not been investigated. Theoretically, a pharmacokinetic interaction would not be anticipated Sulthiame and acetazolamide are both weak inhibitors of carbonic anhydrase and as a direct result may independently increase the risk of renal calculi. Consequently, there is a theoretical potential that when they are administered together, an adverse pharmacodynamic interaction will occur [1]
Tiagabine	The interaction has not been investigated. Theoretically, a pharmacokinetic interaction would not be anticipated
Topiramate	The interaction has not been investigated. Theoretically, a pharmacokinetic interaction would not be anticipated Topiramate and acetazolamide are both weak inhibitors of carbonic anhydrase and as a direct result may independently increase the risk of renal calculi. Consequently, there is a theoretical potential that when they are administered together, an adverse pharmacodynamic interaction will occur [1]
Valproic acid	The interaction has not been investigated. Theoretically, a pharmacokinetic interaction would not be anticipated
Vigabatrin	The interaction has not been investigated. Theoretically, a pharmacokinetic interaction would not be anticipated
Zonisamide	The interaction has not been investigated. Theoretically, a pharmacokinetic interaction would not be anticipated Zonisamide and acetazolamide are both weak inhibitors of carbonic anhydrase and as a direct result may independently increase the risk of renal calculi. Consequently, there is a theoretical potential that when they are administered together, an adverse pharmacodynamic interaction will occur [1]

Reference

1. Patsalos PN, St Louis EK. The epilepsy prescriber's guide to antiepileptic drugs. 3rd ed. Cambridge: Cambridge University Press; 2018.

Brivaracetam

Brivaracetam (Fig. 1) corresponds chemically to (2S)-2-[(4R)-2-oxo-4-propylpyrrolidinyl] butanamide with an empirical formula of $C_{11}H_{20}N_2O_2$ and a molecular weight of 212.15.

Pharmacokinetic Characteristics

Absorption and Distribution

After oral ingestion, brivaracetam is rapidly absorbed (T_{max} = 0.5–1.0 h) with a bioavailability of ~100%. Its volume of distribution is 0.5 L/kg, and plasma protein binding is 17%.

Biotransformation

Brivaracetam is extensively metabolized in the liver (91%), primarily by hydrolysis of the acetamide group, via an amidase, resulting in the formation of an acid metabolite (34.2% of dose). A secondary pathway, oxidation primarily mediated by CYP2C19, forms a hydroxy metabolite (15.9% of dose) and a combination of these two pathways leads to the formation of a hydroxyacid metabolite (15.2% of dose). None of the metabolites are pharmacologically active.

Renal Excretion

Approximately 9% of an administered dose is excreted as unchanged brivaracetam in urine.

Elimination

Following both single and multiple doses, plasma elimination half-life values in adults are 7–8 h.

P. N. Patsalos, *Antiseizure Medication Interactions*,
https://doi.org/10.1007/978-3-030-82790-8_3

Fig. 1 Brivaracetam

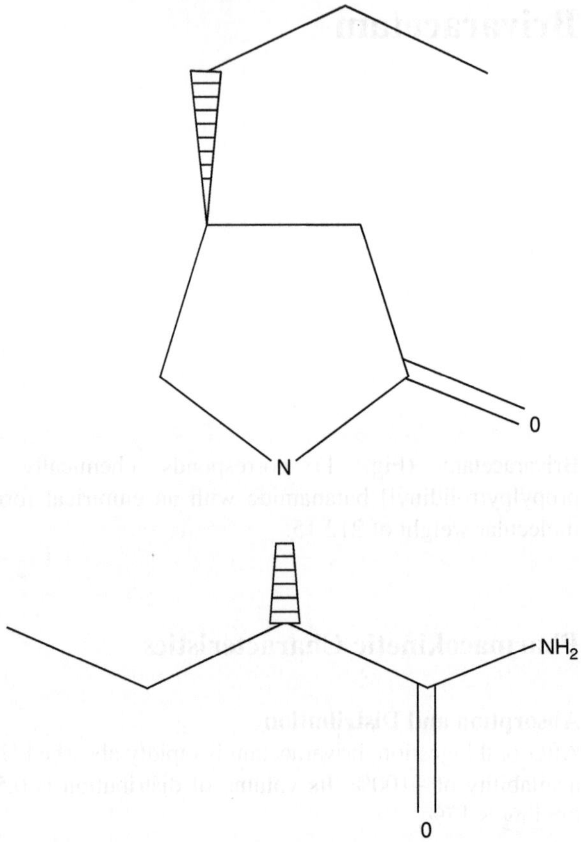

Time to new steady-state blood levels consequent to an inhibition of metabolism interaction:

- Brivaracetam = 2 days later

Effects on Isoenzymes
In vitro brivaracetam is not an inhibitor of CYP1A2, CYP2A6, CYP2B6, CYP2C8, CYP2C9, CYP2D6, CYP3A4 or the transporters PgP, BCRP, BSEP, MRP2, MATE-K, MATE-1, OATP1B1, OATP1B3, OAT1, and OCT1 at clinically relevant concentrations. Brivaracetam, in vitro, does not induce CYP1A2.

Therapeutic Drug Monitoring
There are no data relating plasma brivaracetam levels with that of seizure suppression or adverse effects.

Propensity to Be Associated with Pharmacokinetic Interactions
- Brivaracetam affects the pharmacokinetics of other drugs—minimal.
- Other drugs affect the pharmacokinetics of brivaracetam—minimal.

Interactions with ASMs

Acetazolamide	The interaction has not been investigated. Theoretically, a pharmacokinetic interaction would not be anticipated
Cannabidiol	Inhibits the metabolism of brivaracetam
Consequence	Plasma brivaracetam concentrations can increase, probably via inhibition of CYP2C19, by 95–280% [1]
Carbamazepine	Enhances the metabolism of brivaracetam
Consequence	Mean plasma brivaracetam levels can decreased by 49% [2]
Cenobamate	The interaction has not been investigated. Theoretically, a pharmacokinetic interaction could occur
Clobazam	The interaction has not been investigated. Theoretically, a pharmacokinetic interaction would not be anticipated
Clonazepam	The interaction has not been investigated. Theoretically, a pharmacokinetic interaction would not be anticipated
Eslicarbazepine acetate	The interaction has not been investigated. Theoretically, a pharmacokinetic interaction would not be anticipated
Everolimus	The interaction has not been investigated. Theoretically, a pharmacokinetic interaction would not be anticipated
Ethosuximide	The interaction has not been investigated. Theoretically, a pharmacokinetic interaction would not be anticipated
Fenfluramine	The interaction has not been investigated. Theoretically, a pharmacokinetic interaction would not be anticipated
Felbamate	The interaction has not been investigated. Theoretically, a pharmacokinetic interaction would not be anticipated
Gabapentin	The interaction has not been investigated. Theoretically, a pharmacokinetic interaction would not be anticipated
Lacosamide	The interaction has not been investigated. Theoretically, a pharmacokinetic interaction would not be anticipated
Lamotrigine	Does not affect the pharmacokinetics of brivaracetam [3]
Levetiracetam	Does not affect the pharmacokinetics of brivaracetam [3]
	The efficacy of brivaracetam is decreased when co-administered with levetiracetam consequent to a pharmacodynamic interaction [4]
Methsuximide	The interaction has not been investigated. Theoretically, a pharmacokinetic interaction would not be anticipated
Oxcarbazepine	Does not affect the pharmacokinetics of brivaracetam [3]
Perampanel	The interaction has not been investigated. Theoretically, a pharmacokinetic interaction would not be anticipated
Phenobarbital	Enhances the metabolism of brivaracetam
Consequence	Mean plasma brivaracetam AUC values can decrease by 19% [5]
Phenytoin	Enhances the metabolism of brivaracetam
Consequence	Mean plasma brivaracetam levels can decrease by 23% [5]
Piracetam	The interaction has not been investigated. Theoretically, a pharmacokinetic interaction would not be anticipated
Pregabalin	The interaction has not been investigated. Theoretically, a pharmacokinetic interaction would not be anticipated
Primidone	Enhances the metabolism of brivaracetam
Consequence	Mean plasma brivaracetam AUC values can decrease by 19% [5]

Rufinamide	The interaction has not been investigated. Theoretically, a pharmacokinetic interaction would not be anticipated
Stiripentol	The interaction has not been investigated. Theoretically, a pharmacokinetic interaction could occur
Sulthiame	The interaction has not been investigated. Theoretically, a pharmacokinetic interaction could occur
Tiagabine	The interaction has not been investigated. Theoretically, a pharmacokinetic interaction would not be anticipated
Topiramate	Does not affect the pharmacokinetics of brivaracetam [3]
Valproic acid	Decreases the metabolism of brivaracetam
Consequence	Mean plasma brivaracetam AUC values can increase by 11% [6]
Vigabatrin	The interaction has not been investigated. Theoretically, a pharmacokinetic interaction would not be anticipated
Zonisamide	The interaction has not been investigated. Theoretically, a pharmacokinetic interaction would not be anticipated

References

1. Klotz KA, Hirsch M, Heers M, Schulze-Bonhage A, Jacobs J. Effects of cannabidiol on brivaracetam plasma levels. Epilepsia. 2019;60:e74–7.
2. Hagemann A, Klimpel D, Bien CG, Brandt C, May TW. Influence of dose and antiepileptic comedication on brivaracetam serum concentrations. Epilepsia. 2020;61:e43–8.
3. Summary of product characteristics: Brivaracetam (Briviact). UCB Pharma Ltd. Last update 27 Nov 2020.
4. Biton V, Berkovic SF, Abou-Khalil B, Sperling MR, Johnson ME, Lu S. Brivaracetam as adjunctive treatment for uncontrolled partial epilepsy in adults: a phase III randomized, double-blind, placebo-controlled trial. Epilepsia. 2014;55:57–66.
5. Moseley BD, Chanteux H, Nicolas JM, Laloyaux C, Gidal B. A review of the drug-drug interactions of the antiepileptic drug brivaracetam. Epilepsy Res. 2020;163:106327.
6. Schoemaker R, Wade JR, Stockis A. Brivaracetam population pharmacokinetics in children with epilepsy aged 1 month to 16 years. Eur J Clin Pharmacol. 2017;73:727–33.

Cannabidiol

Cannabidiol (Fig. 1) corresponds chemically to (2S)-2-[(4R)-2-oxo-4-propylpyrrolidinyl] butanamide with an empirical formula of $C_{21}H_{30}O_2$ and a molecular weight of 314.46.

Pharmacokinetic Characteristics

Absorption and Distribution

After oral ingestion, cannabidiol is rapidly absorbed (T_{max} = 1.5–2.0 h) with a bioavailability of ~6%. Its volume of distribution is 0.2–0.4 L/kg, and plasma protein binding is 94–99%.

Biotransformation

Cannabidiol is extensively metabolized in the liver, primarily by CYP2C19, to form 7-hydroxy-cannabidiol, the concentration of which represents 40% of that of cannabidiol in plasma. Subsequently, 7-hydroxy-cannabidiol, which is pharmacologically active, is further metabolized to inactive metabolites as carboxylic and

Fig. 1 Cannabidiol

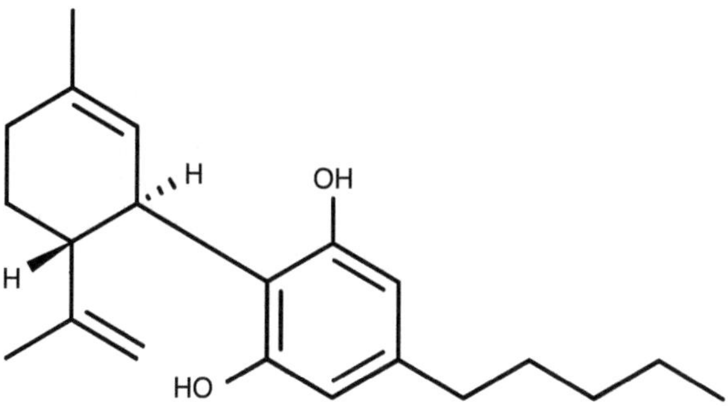

P. N. Patsalos, *Antiseizure Medication Interactions*,
https://doi.org/10.1007/978-3-030-82790-8_4

glucuronides (7-carboxylic-cannabidiol, 6-hydroxy-cannabidiol) via CYP3A4 and UGT1A7, UGT1A9 and UGT2B7. Both cannabidiol and hydroxylated metabolites of cannabidiol also undergo direct conjugation by UGTs.

Renal Excretion
The renal elimination of unchanged cannabidiol in urine is minor (12%).

Elimination
The plasma elimination half-life values for cannabinoid in healthy adults administered twice daily cannabinoid are 56–61 h.

Time to new steady-state blood levels consequent to an inhibition of metabolism interaction:

- Cannabinoid = 9–15 days later

Effects on Isoenzymes
In vitro, at clinically relevant concentrations, cannabidiol is an inhibitor of CYP1A2, CYP2B6, CYP2C8, CYP2C9, CYP2C19, UGT1A9, and UGT2B7 activity. The metabolite 7-carboxy-cannabidiol inhibits UGT1A1, UGT1A4, and UGT1A6 activity. Cannabidiol and its pharmacologically active metabolite 7-hydroxy cannabidiol do not interact with major transporters including: OAT1, OAT3, OCT1, OCT2, MATE1, MATE2-K, OATP1B1, and OATP1B3. Cannabidiol is not a substrate or inhibitor of the brain uptake transporters OATP1A2 and OATP2B1. Neither cannabidiol nor 7-carboxy-cannabidiol is a substrate or inhibitor of efflux transporters PgP/MDR1, BCRP, and BSEP. In contrast, the metabolite 7-carboxy-cannabidiol is a substrate of PgP/MDR1 and has the potential to inhibit BCRP, QATP1B3, and OAT3.

Therapeutic Drug Monitoring
There are no data relating plasma cannabidiol levels with that of seizure suppression or adverse effects.

Propensity to Be Associated with Pharmacokinetic Interactions

- Cannabidiol affects the pharmacokinetics of other drugs—moderate
- Other drugs affect the pharmacokinetics of cannabidiol—substantial

Interactions with ASMs

Acetazolamide	The interaction has not been investigated. Theoretically, a pharmacokinetic interaction would not be anticipated
Brivaracetam	The interaction has not been investigated. Theoretically, a pharmacokinetic interaction would not be anticipated
Carbamazepine	The interaction has not been investigated. Theoretically, a pharmacokinetic interaction could occur
Cenobamate	The interaction has not been investigated. Theoretically, a pharmacokinetic interaction could occur
Clobazam	Inhibits the metabolism of cannabidiol

Consequence	Mean plasma cannabidiol AUC values increase by 30% and mean plasma 7-hydroxy-cannabidiol, the pharmacologically active metabolite of cannabidiol, AUC values increase by 47% [1] An additive antiseizure effect may occur between clobazam and cannabidiol consequent to a bi-directional pharmacokinetic interaction resulting in increases of their respective pharmacologically active metabolites [2]
Clonazepam	The interaction has not been investigated. Theoretically, a pharmacokinetic interaction would not be anticipated
Eslicarbazepine acetate	The interaction has not been investigated. Theoretically, a pharmacokinetic interaction could occur
Ethosuximide	The interaction has not been investigated. Theoretically, a pharmacokinetic interaction would not be anticipated
Everolimus	The interaction has not been investigated. Theoretically, a pharmacokinetic interaction could occur
Felbamate	The interaction has not been investigated. Theoretically, a pharmacokinetic interaction could occur
Fenfluramine	The interaction has not been investigated. Theoretically, a pharmacokinetic interaction could occur
Gabapentin	The interaction has not been investigated. Theoretically, a pharmacokinetic interaction would not be anticipated
Lacosamide	The interaction has not been investigated. Theoretically, a pharmacokinetic interaction would not be anticipated
Lamotrigine	The interaction has not been investigated. Theoretically, a pharmacokinetic interaction could occur
Levetiracetam	The interaction has not been investigated. Theoretically, a pharmacokinetic interaction would not be anticipated
Methsuximide	The interaction has not been investigated. Theoretically, a pharmacokinetic interaction would not be anticipated
Oxcarbazepine	The interaction has not been investigated. Theoretically, a pharmacokinetic interaction could occur
Perampanel	The interaction has not been investigated. Theoretically, a pharmacokinetic interaction could occur
Phenobarbital	The interaction has not been investigated. Theoretically, a pharmacokinetic interaction could occur
Phenytoin	The interaction has not been investigated. Theoretically, a pharmacokinetic interaction could occur
Piracetam	The interaction has not been investigated. Theoretically, a pharmacokinetic interaction would not be anticipated
Pregabalin	The interaction has not been investigated. Theoretically, a pharmacokinetic interaction would not be anticipated
Primidone	The interaction has not been investigated. Theoretically, a pharmacokinetic interaction could occur
Rufinamide	The interaction has not been investigated. Theoretically, a pharmacokinetic interaction could occur
Stiripentol	Affects the pharmacokinetics of cannabidiol
Consequence	While stiripentol has no effect on plasma cannabidiol levels, it decreases mean plasma 7-hydroxy-cannabidiol AUC values, the pharmacologically active metabolite of cannabidiol, by 28% [3]

Sulthiame	The interaction has not been investigated. Theoretically, a pharmacokinetic interaction could occur
Tiagabine	The interaction has not been investigated. Theoretically, a pharmacokinetic interaction would not be anticipated
Topiramate	The interaction has not been investigated. Theoretically, a pharmacokinetic interaction could occur
Valproic acid	Affects the pharmacokinetic of cannabidiol
Consequence	While valproic acid has no effect on plasma cannabidiol levels, it inhibits the metabolism of the pharmacologically active metabolite 7-hydroxy-cannabinoid and increases mean plasma 7-hydroxy-cannabinoid AUC values by 22% [1] A synergistic increase in aspartate aminotransferase can occur consequent to a pharmacodynamic interaction [2]
Vigabatrin	The interaction has not been investigated. Theoretically, a pharmacokinetic interaction would not be anticipated
Zonisamide	The interaction has not been investigated. Theoretically, a pharmacokinetic interaction could occur

References

1. Patsalos PN, Szaflarski JP, Gidal B, VanLandingham K, Critchley D, Morrison G. Clinical implications of trials investigating drug-drug interactions between cannabidiol and enzyme inducers or inhibitors or common antiseizure drugs. Epilepsia. 2020;61:1854–68.
2. Summary of product characteristics: Cannabidiol (Epidyolex). GW Pharma Ltd. Last update 27 July 2020.
3. Morrison G, Crockett J, Blakey G, Sommerville K. A phase I, open-label, pharmacokinetic trial to investigate possible drug-drug interactions between clobazam, stiripentol, or valproate and cannabidiol in healthy subjects. Clin Pharmacol Drug Develop. 2019;8:1009–31.

Carbamazepine

Carbamazepine (Fig. 1) corresponds chemically to 5H-dibenz[b,f]azepine-5-carboxamide with an empirical formula of $C_{15}H_{12}N_2O$ and a molecular weight of 236.27.

Pharmacokinetic Characteristics

Absorption and Distribution

After oral ingestion, carbamazepine is rapidly absorbed (T_{max} is formulation-dependent) with a bioavailability of 75–85%. Its volume of distribution is 0.8–2.0 L/kg, and plasma protein binding is 75%. The protein binding of the pharmacologically active metabolite, carbamazepine-10,11-epoxide, is 50%.

Fig. 1 Carbamazepine

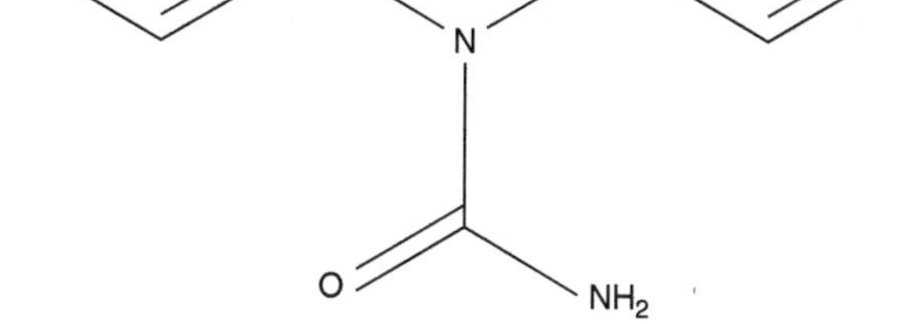

P. N. Patsalos, *Antiseizure Medication Interactions*,
https://doi.org/10.1007/978-3-030-82790-8_5

Biotransformation

Carbamazepine is extensively metabolized in the liver, primarily by CYP3A4, to carbamazepine-10,11-epoxide which is pharmacologically active. Additional isoenzymes that contribute to the metabolism of carbamazepine include CYP2C8, CYP2B6, CYP2E1, CYP1A2, and CYP2A6. Carbamazepine-10,11-epoxide is in turn metabolized, via epoxide hydrolase, to an inactive trans-carbamazepine diol. Carbamazepine is an enzyme inducer, and additionally, carbamazepine undergoes autoinduction so that its clearance can increase threefold within several weeks of starting therapy and this often requires an upward dosage adjustment.

Renal Excretion

Less than 2% of an administered dose is excreted as unchanged carbamazepine in urine.

Elimination

Following a single dose, plasma elimination half-life values in adults and children are 18–55 h and 3–32 h, respectively. During maintenance carbamazepine monotherapy, half-life values in adults and children are 8–20 h and 10–13 h, respectively, while in the elderly, carbamazepine half-life values are 30–50 h. The half-life of carbamazepine-10,11-epoxide is ~34 h.

Time to new steady-state blood levels consequent to an inhibition of metabolism interaction:

- Carbamazepine = 2–5 days later
- Carbamazepine-10,11-epoxide = 7 days later

Effects on Isoenzymes

No in vitro data on the induction or inhibition potential of carbamazepine on human CYP or UGT isoenzymes have been published.

Therapeutic Drug Monitoring

Optimum seizure control in patients on carbamazepine monotherapy is most likely to occur at plasma carbamazepine levels of 4–12 mg/L (17–51 μmol/L). The upper boundary of the reference range for carbamazepine-10,11-epoxide is 9 μmol/L. The conversion factor from mg/L to μmol/L for carbamazepine is 4.23 (i.e., 1 mg/L = 4.23 μmol/L), while that of carbamazepine-10,11-epoxide, it is 3.96 (i.e., 1 mg/L = 3.96 μmol/L).

Propensity to Be Associated with Pharmacokinetic Interactions

- Carbamazepine affects the pharmacokinetics of other drugs—substantial.
- Other drugs affect the pharmacokinetics of carbamazepine—substantial.

Interactions with ASMs

Acetazolamide	Affects the pharmacokinetics of carbamazepine
Consequence	Increases carbamazepine plasma levels via an unknown mechanism [1]
Brivaracetam	Enhances the metabolism of carbamazepine

Consequence	Mean carbamazepine plasma AUC values can decrease by 12%, and mean carbamazepine-10,11-epoxide plasma AUC values (the pharmacologically active metabolite of carbamazepine) can increase by 157%. The interaction may be the consequence of induction of carbamazepine metabolism through CYP3A4 and inhibition of the metabolism of carbamazepine-10,11-epoxide via an action on epoxide hydrolase [2]
Cannabidiol	Does not affect the pharmacokinetics of carbamazepine [3]
Cenobamate	Enhances the metabolism of carbamazepine
Consequence	Mean plasma carbamazepine levels can be decreased by 11–34% [4]
Clobazam	Inhibits the metabolism of carbamazepine
Consequence	Carbamazepine plasma levels can increase by 15%, and carbamazepine-10,11-epoxide plasma levels (the pharmacologically active metabolite of carbamazepine) can increase by 87% [5]
Clonazepam	Does not affect the pharmacokinetics of carbamazepine [6]
Eslicarbazepine acetate	Does not affect the pharmacokinetics of carbamazepine [7]
	During combination therapy, carbamazepine enhances eslicarbazepine adverse effects including diplopia, abnormal coordination, and dizziness. These effects are probably the consequence of a pharmacodynamic interaction [8]
Ethosuximide	Does not affect the pharmacokinetics of carbamazepine [9]
Everolimus	The interaction has not been investigated. Theoretically, a pharmacokinetic interaction could occur
Felbamate	Enhances the metabolism of carbamazepine
Consequence	Mean carbamazepine plasma levels can decrease by 19%, and mean carbamazepine-10,11-epoxide plasma levels (the pharmacologically active metabolite of carbamazepine) can increase by 33%. The interaction is the consequence of induction of carbamazepine metabolism through CYP3A4 and inhibition of the metabolism of carbamazepine-10,11-epoxide via an action on epoxide hydrolase [10]
Fenfluramine	The interaction has not been investigated. Theoretically, a pharmacokinetic interaction could occur
Gabapentin	Does not affect the pharmacokinetics of carbamazepine [11]
Lacosamide	Does not affect the pharmacokinetics of carbamazepine [12]
	Neurotoxicity may occur in combination with carbamazepine, and other voltage-gated sodium channel blocking antiseizure medications, consequent to a pharmacodynamic interaction [13]
Lamotrigine	Does not affect the pharmacokinetics of carbamazepine [14]
	The high frequency of neurotoxicity observed with this drug combination represents a pharmacodynamic rather than pharmacokinetic interaction [15]
Levetiracetam	Does not affect the pharmacokinetics of carbamazepine [16]
	A pharmacodynamic interaction may occur whereby symptoms of carbamazepine toxicity present [17]
Methsuximide	Enhances the metabolism of carbamazepine
Consequence	Plasma levels of carbamazepine can decrease by 23%. The interaction is the consequence of induction of carbamazepine metabolism through CYP3A4 [18]
Oxcarbazepine	Enhances the metabolism of carbamazepine

Consequence	Median carbamazepine plasma AUC values can decrease by 9%, and median carbamazepine-10,11-epoxide plasma AUC values (pharmacologically active metabolite of carbamazepine) can increase by 33%. The interaction is the consequence of induction of carbamazepine metabolism through CYP3A4 and inhibition of the metabolism of carbamazepine-10,11-epoxide via an action on epoxide hydrolase [19]
Perampanel	Enhances the metabolism of carbamazepine
Consequence	Mean carbamazepine clearance is increased by 4.3% [20]
	Perampanel in combination with carbamazepine is associated with increased sedation. This effect may be the consequence of a pharmacodynamic interaction [20]
Phenobarbital	Enhances the metabolism of carbamazepine
Consequence	Mean carbamazepine plasma levels can decrease by 33%, and mean carbamazepine-10, 11-epoxide plasma levels (the pharmacologically active metabolite of carbamazepine) can increase by 24%. The interaction is the consequence of induction of carbamazepine metabolism through CYP3A4 and inhibition of the metabolism of carbamazepine-10,11-epoxide via an action on epoxide hydrolase [21]
Phenytoin	Enhances the metabolism of carbamazepine
Consequence	Mean carbamazepine plasma levels can decrease by 44%. However, carbamazepine-10,11-epoxide levels (the pharmacologically active metabolite of carbamazepine) are unaffected. The interaction is the consequence of induction of carbamazepine metabolism through CYP3A4 [20]
Piracetam	Does not affect the pharmacokinetics of carbamazepine [22]
Pregabalin	Does not affect the pharmacokinetics of carbamazepine [23]
Primidone	Enhances the metabolism of carbamazepine
Consequence	Mean carbamazepine plasma levels can decrease by 25%, and mean carbamazepine-10,11-epoxide levels (the pharmacologically active metabolite of carbamazepine) can increase by 75%
	The interaction is the consequence of induction of carbamazepine metabolism through CYP3A4 and inhibition of the metabolism of carbamazepine-10,11-epoxide via an action on epoxide hydrolase [20]
Rufinamide	Increases the clearance of carbamazepine
Consequence	The clearance of carbamazepine is increased by 8–15% so that plasma carbamazepine levels are decreased by 7–13%. The action is probably the consequence of induction of CYP3A4 [24]
Stiripentol	Inhibits the metabolism of carbamazepine
Consequence	The clearance of carbamazepine is decreased by 27–70% so that plasma carbamazepine levels are increased, while plasma levels of carbamazepine-10,11-epoxide (the pharmacologically active metabolite carbamazepine) are decreased. The action is the consequence of inhibition, primarily of CYP3A4, but with a minor effect on CYP2C8. Epoxide hydrolase, the enzyme responsible for the metabolism of carbamazepine-10,11-epoxide, is unaffected [25]
Sulthiame	Enhances the metabolism of carbamazepine
Consequence	Plasma carbamazepine levels are decreased [26]
Tiagabine	Does not affect the pharmacokinetics of carbamazepine [27]

Topiramate	Does not affect the pharmacokinetics of carbamazepine [28]
	Carbamazepine toxicity has been described in patients co-prescribed with topiramate, and this is considered to be the consequence of a pharmacodynamic interaction [29]
Valproic acid	Inhibits the metabolism of the pharmacologically active metabolite carbamazepine-10,11-epoxide
Consequence	Mean plasma levels of carbamazepine-10,11-epoxide (the pharmacologically active metabolite carbamazepine), with either no change or a small decrease in plasma carbamazepine levels, can increase by 25%. This interaction is related to valproic acid inhibition of epoxide hydrolase, the enzyme responsible for the metabolism of the epoxide metabolite [30, 31]
	During combination therapy, valproic acid can synergistically enhance the antiseizure efficacy (partial seizures) of carbamazepine. This effect is the consequence of a pharmacodynamic interaction [32]
Vigabatrin	The effect of vigabatrin on the pharmacokinetics of carbamazepine is controversial
Consequence	There is a suggestion that in patients with low carbamazepine levels (<9 mg/L), the plasma carbamazepine levels can be significantly increased (20–132%), through an unknown mechanism, during concomitant administration with vigabatrin. Another study reports that mean carbamazepine levels are decreased by 18% and that mean carbamazepine clearance increases by 35% [33, 34]
	During combination therapy, vigabatrin may synergistically enhance the antiseizure efficacy (partial seizures) of carbamazepine. This effect is probably the consequence of a pharmacodynamic interaction [32]
Zonisamide	Inhibits the metabolism of the pharmacologically active metabolite carbamazepine-10,11-epoxide
Consequence	Mean plasma carbamazepine-10,11-epoxide C_{max} and AUC values can increase by 38% and 17%, respectively. Carbamazepine is not affected. The interaction is the consequence of a decrease in the renal clearance of carbamazepine-10,11-epoxide [35]

References

1. Forsythe WI, Owens JR, Toothill C. Effectiveness of acetazolamide in the treatment of carbamazepine-resistant epilepsy in children. Dev Med Child Neurol. 1981;23:761–9.
2. Stockis A, Chanteux H, Rosa M, Rolan P. Brivaracetam and carbamazepine interaction in healthy subjects and in vitro. Epilepsy Res. 2015;113:19–27.
3. Gaston TE, Bekib EM, Cutter GR, Liu Y, Szaflarski JP, UAB CBD Program. Interactions between cannabidiol and commonly used antiepileptic drugs. Epilepsia. 2017;58:1586–92.
4. Bialer M, Johannessen SI, Koepp MJ, Levy RH, Perucca E, Perucca P, Tomson T, White HS. Progress report on new antiepileptic drugs: a summary of the fifteenth Eilat conference on new antiepileptic drugs and devices (EILAT XV). II. Drugs in more advanced clinical development. Epilepsia. 2020;61:2365–85.
5. Genton P, Nguyen VH, Mesdjian E. Carbamazepine intoxication and negative myoclonus after the addition of clobazam. Epilepsia. 1998;39:1115–8.

6. Johannessen SI, Strandjord RE, Munthe-Kaas AW. Lack of effect of clonazepam on serum levels of diphenylhydantoin, phenobarbital and carbamazepine. Acta Neurol Scand. 1977;55:506–12.
7. Elger C, Halasz P, Maia J, Almeidas L, Soares-da-Silva P, on behalf of the BIA-2093-301 Investigators Study Group. Efficacy and safety of eslicarbazepine acetate as adjunctive treatment in adults with refractory partial seizures: a randomized, double-blind, placebo-controlled, parallel-group phase III study. Epilepsia. 2009;50:454–63.
8. Almeida L, Bialer M, Soares-da-Silva P. Eslicarbazepine acetate. In: Shorvon SD, Perucca E, Engel J, editors. The treatment of epilepsy. 3rd ed. Oxford: Blackwell; 2009. p. 485–98.
9. Altafullah I, Talwar D, Loewenson R, Olson K, Lockman LA. Factors influencing serum levels of carbamazepine and carbamazepine-10,11-epoxide in children. Epilepsy Res. 1989;4:72–80.
10. Wagner ML, Remmel RP, Graves NM, Leppik IE. Effect of felbamate on carbamazepine and its metabolites. Clin Pharmacol Ther. 1993;53:536–43.
11. Radulovic LL, Wilder BJ, Leppik IE, Bockbrader HN, Chang T, Posvar EL, Sedman AJ, Uthman BM, Erdman GR. Lack of interaction of gabapentin with carbamazepine and valproate. Epilepsia. 1994;35:155–61.
12. Cawello W, Nickel B, Eggert-Formella A. No pharmacokinetic interaction between lacosamide and carbamazepine in healthy volunteers. J Clin Pharmacol. 2010;50:459–71.
13. Novy J, Patsalos PN, Sander JW, Sisodiya SM. Lacosamide neurotoxicity associated with concomitant use of sodium-blocking antiepileptic drugs: a pharmacodynamic interaction? Epilepsy Behav. 2011;20:20–3.
14. Malminiemi K, Keranen T, Kerttula T, Moilanen E, Ylitalo P. Effects of short-term lamotrigine on pharmacokinetics of carbamazepine. Int J Clin Pharmacol Ther. 2000;38:540–5.
15. Besag FM, Berry DJ, Pool F, Newbery JE, Subel B. Carbamazepine toxicity with lamotrigine: pharmacokinetic or pharmacodynamic interaction? Epilepsia. 1998;39:183–7.
16. Gidal BE, Baltes E, Otoul C, Perucca E. Effect of levetiracetam on the pharmacokinetics of adjunctive antiepileptic drugs: a pooled analysis of data from the randomized clinical trials. Epilepsy Res. 2005;64:1–11.
17. Sisodiya SM, Sander JW, Patsalos PN. Carbamazepine toxicity during combination therapy with levetiracetam: a pharmacodynamic interaction. Epilepsy Res. 2002;48:217–9.
18. Browne TR, Feldman RG, Buchanan RA, Allen CA, Fawcett-Vickers L, Szabo GK, Mattson GF, Norman SE, Greenblatt DJ. Methsuximide for complex partial seizures: efficacy, toxicity, clinical pharmacology, and drug interactions. Neurology. 1983;33:414–8.
19. McKee PJW, Blacklaw J, Forrest G, Gillham RA, Walker SM, Connelly D, Brodie MJ. A double-blind, placebo-controlled interaction study between oxcarbazepine and carbamazepine, sodium valproate and phenytoin in epileptic patients. Br J Clin Pharmacol. 1994;37:27–32.
20. Majid O, Laurenza A, Ferry J, Hussein Z. Impact of perampanel on pharmacokinetics of concomitant antiepileptics in patients with partial-onset seizures: pooled analysis of clinical trials. Br J Clin Pharmacol. 2016;82:422–30.
21. Rambeck B, May T, Juergens U. Serum concentrations of carbamazepine and its epoxide and diol metabolites in epileptic patients: the influence of dose and comedication. Ther Drug Monit. 1987;9:298–303.
22. Summary of product characteristics: Piracetam (Nootropil). UCB Pharma Ltd. Last update 9 Feb 2017.
23. Brodie MJ, Wilson EA, Wesche DL, Alvey CW, Randinitis EJ, Posvar EL, Hounslow NJ, Bron NJ, Gibson GL, Bockbrader HN. Pregabalin drug interaction studies: lack of effect on the pharmacokinetics of carbamazepine, phenytoin, lamotrigine, and valproate in patients with partial epilepsy. Epilepsia. 2005;46:1407–13.
24. Perucca E, Cloyd J, Critchley D, Fuseau E. Rufinamide: clinical pharmacokinetics and concentration-response relationships in patients with epilepsy. Epilepsia. 2008;49:1123–41.
25. Cazali N, Tran A, Treluyer JM, Rey E, d'Athis P, Vincent J, Pons G. Inhibitory effect of stiripentol on carbamazepine and saquinavir metabolism in human. Br J Clin Pharmacol. 2003;56:526–36.

26. Summary of product characteristics: Sulthiame (Ospolot). Phebra Pty, Ltd. Last update 21 Nov 2013.
27. Gustavson LE, Cato A, Boellner SW, Cao GX, Quian JX, Guenther HJ, Sommerville KW. Lack of pharmacokinetic drug interactions between tiagabine and carbamazepine or phenytoin. Am J Ther. 1998;5:9–16.
28. Sachdeo RC, Sachdeo SK, Walker SA, Kramer LD, Nayak RK, Doose DR. Steady-state pharmacokinetics of topiramate and carbamazepine in patients with epilepsy during monotherapy and concomitant therapy. Epilepsia. 1996;37:774–80.
29. Mack CJ, Kuc S, Mulcrone SA, Pilley A, Grunewald RA. Interaction between topiramate and carbamazepine: two case reports and a review of clinical experience. Seizure. 2002;11:464–7.
30. Pisani F, Caputo M, Fazio A, Oteri G, Russo M, Spina E, Perucca E, Bertilsson L. Interaction of carbamazepine-10,11-epoxide, an active metabolite of carbamazepine, with valproate: a pharmacokinetic interaction. Epilepsia. 1990;31:339–42.
31. McKee PJW, Blacklaw J, Butler E, Gillham RA, Brodie MJ. Variability and clinical relevance of the interaction between sodium valproate and carbamazepine in epileptic patients. Epilepsy Res. 1992;11:193–8.
32. Brodie MJ, Mumford JP. Double-blind substitution of vigabatrin and valproate in carbamazepine-resistant partial epilepsy. 012 Study group. Epilepsy Res. 1999;34:199–205.
33. Sanchez-Alcaraz A, Quintana MB, Lopez E, Rodriguez I, Llopis P. Effect of vigabatrin on the pharmacokinetics of carbamazepine. J Clin Pharm Ther. 2002;27:427–30.
34. Jedrzejczak J, Dlawichowska E, Owczarek K, Majkowski J. Effect of vigabatrin addition on carbamazepine serum levels in patients with epilepsy. Epilepsy Res. 2000;39:115–20.
35. Ragueneau-Majlessi I, Levy RH, Bergen D, Garnet W, Rosenfeld W, Mather G, Shah J, Grundy JS. Carbamazepine pharmacokinetics are not affected by zonisamide: in vitro mechanistic study and in vivo clinical study in epileptic patients. Epilepsy Res. 2004;62:1–11.

Cenobamate

Cenobamate (Fig. 1) corresponds chemically to ([(IR)-1-(2-Chlorophenyl)-2-(tetrazol-2-yl) ethyl] carbamate with an empirical formula of $C_{10}H_{10}Cl_5O_2$ and a molecular weight of 267.67.

Pharmacokinetic Characteristics

Absorption and Distribution

After oral ingestion, cenobamate is rapidly absorbed (T_{max} = 1–4 h) with a bioavailability of >88%. Its volume of distribution is 0.4–0.5 L/kg, and plasma protein binding is 60%.

Fig. 1 Cenobamate

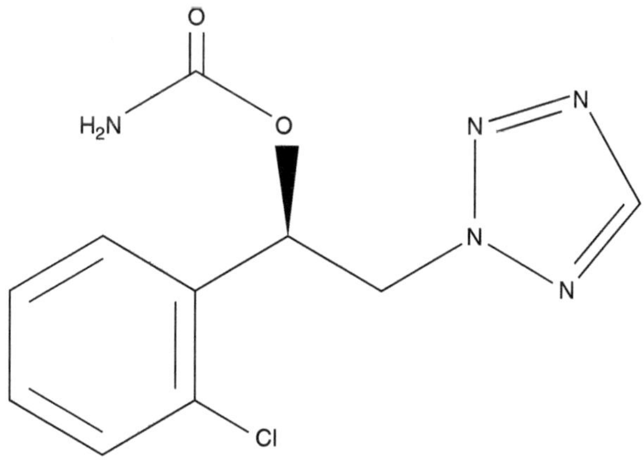

P. N. Patsalos, *Antiseizure Medication Interactions*,
https://doi.org/10.1007/978-3-030-82790-8_6

Biotransformation

Cenobamate is extensively metabolized in the liver, primarily by glucuronidation via UGT2B7 and to a lesser extent by UGT2B4, and by oxidation via CYP2E1, CYP2A6, and CYP2B6 and to a lesser extent via CYP2C19 and CYP3A4/5.

Renal Excretion

Approximately 6.8% of an administered dose is excreted as unchanged cenobamate in urine.

Elimination

Plasma elimination half-life values for cenobamate in adults are 50–60 h.

Time to new steady-state blood levels consequent to an inhibition of metabolism interaction:

- Cenobamate = 8–15 h later

Effects on Isoenzymes

In vitro, at clinically relevant concentrations, cenobamate is an inducer of CYP2B6, CYP2C8, and CYP3A4, and an inhibitor of CYP2B6, CYP2C19, and CYP3A. It does not induce CYP1A2, CYP2C9, or CYP2C19 activity nor does it inhibit CYP1A2, CYP2C8, CYP2C9, or CYP2D6 activity. Consequently, pharmacokinetic interactions of metabolic origin with other antiseizure medications and other medicines can be expected.

Cenobamate does not inhibit P-gp, OAT1, OCT1, OCT2, OATP1B3, BSEP, OAT3, or OATP1B1, and cenobamate is not a substrate of P-gP, BCRP, OAT1, OAT3, OCT2, MATE1, or MATE2-K.

Therapeutic Drug Monitoring

There are no data relating plasma cenobamate levels with that of seizure suppression or adverse effects.

Propensity to Be Associated with Pharmacokinetic Interactions

- Cenobamate affects the pharmacokinetics of other drugs—substantial.
- Other drugs affect the pharmacokinetics of cenobamate—moderate.

Interactions with ASMs

Acetazolamide	The interaction has not been investigated. Theoretically, a pharmacokinetic interaction would not be anticipated
Brivaracetam	The interaction has not been investigated. Theoretically, a pharmacokinetic interaction would not be anticipated
Cannabidiol	The interaction has not been investigated. Theoretically, a pharmacokinetic interaction could occur
Carbamazepine	Does not affect the pharmacokinetics of cenobamate [1]
Clobazam	Inhibits the metabolism of cenobamate
Consequence	Mean plasma cenobamate AUC values, based on population pharmacokinetic analysis, are increased by 24% during comedication with clobazam [2]
Clonazepam	The interaction has not been investigated. Theoretically, a pharmacokinetic interaction would not be anticipated

Eslicarbazepine acetate	The interaction has not been investigated. Theoretically, a pharmacokinetic interaction could occur
Ethosuximide	The interaction has not been investigated. Theoretically, a pharmacokinetic interaction would not be anticipated
Everolimus	The interaction has not been investigated. Theoretically, a pharmacokinetic interaction could occur
Felbamate	The interaction has not been investigated. Theoretically, a pharmacokinetic interaction could occur
Fenfluramine	The interaction has not been investigated. Theoretically, a pharmacokinetic interaction could occur
Gabapentin	The interaction has not been investigated. Theoretically, a pharmacokinetic interaction would not be anticipated
Lacosamide	The interaction has not been investigated. Theoretically, a pharmacokinetic interaction would not be anticipated
Lamotrigine	The interaction has not been investigated. Theoretically, a pharmacokinetic interaction would not be anticipated
Levetiracetam	The interaction has not been investigated. Theoretically, a pharmacokinetic interaction would not be anticipated
Methsuximide	The interaction has not been investigated. Theoretically, a pharmacokinetic interaction would not be anticipated
Oxcarbazepine	Does not affect the pharmacokinetics of cenobamate [1]
Perampanel	The interaction has not been investigated. Theoretically, a pharmacokinetic interaction could occur
Phenobarbital	Does not affect the pharmacokinetics of cenobamate [1]
Phenytoin	Enhances the metabolism of cenobamate
Consequence	Mean plasma cenobamate AUC values are decreased by 28% during co-medication with phenytoin [2]
Piracetam	The interaction has not been investigated. Theoretically, a pharmacokinetic interaction would not be anticipated
Pregabalin	The interaction has not been investigated. Theoretically, a pharmacokinetic interaction would not be anticipated
Primidone	The interaction has not been investigated. Theoretically, a pharmacokinetic interaction could occur
Rufinamide	The interaction has not been investigated. Theoretically, a pharmacokinetic interaction would not be anticipated
Stiripentol	The interaction has not been investigated. Theoretically, a pharmacokinetic interaction could occur
Sulthiame	The interaction has not been investigated. Theoretically, a pharmacokinetic interaction could occur
Tiagabine	The interaction has not been investigated. Theoretically, a pharmacokinetic interaction would not be anticipated
Topiramate	The interaction has not been investigated. Theoretically, a pharmacokinetic interaction could occur
Valproic acid	Does not affect the pharmacokinetics of cenobamate [1]
Vigabatrin	The interaction has not been investigated. Theoretically, a pharmacokinetic interaction would not be anticipated
Zonisamide	The interaction has not been investigated. Theoretically, a pharmacokinetic interaction could occur

References

1. Summary of product characteristics: Cenobamate (XCopri). SK Life Science Inc. Last update Aug 2020.
2. Bialer M, Johannessen SI, Koepp MJ, Levy RH, Perucca E, Perucca P, Tomson T, White HS. Progress report on new antiepileptic drugs: a summary of the fifteenth EILAT conference on new antiepileptic drugs and devices (EILAT XV). II. Drugs in more advanced clinical development. Epilepsia. 2020;61:2365–85.

Clobazam

Clobazam (Fig. 1) corresponds chemically to 7-chloro-1-methyl-5-phenyl-1,5-benzodiazepine-2,4-dione with an empirical formula of $C_{16}H_{13}Cl_2O_2$ and a molecular weight of 300.74.

Fig. 1 Clobazam

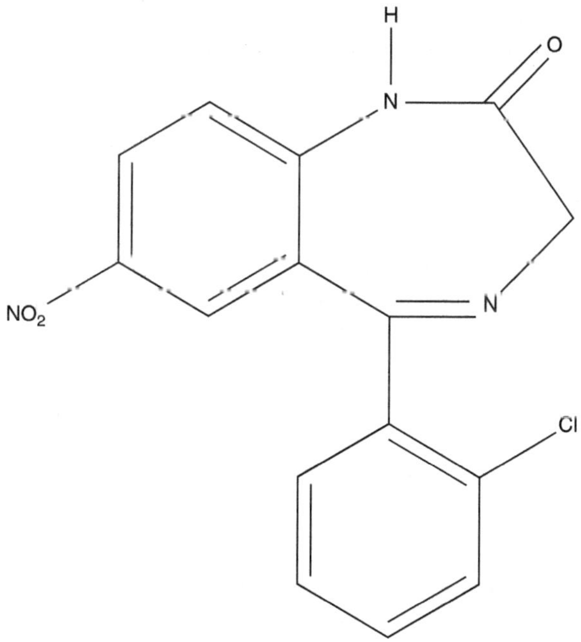

P. N. Patsalos, *Antiseizure Medication Interactions*,
https://doi.org/10.1007/978-3-030-82790-8_7

Pharmacokinetic Characteristics

Absorption and Distribution

After oral ingestion, clobazam is rapidly absorbed (T_{max} = 1–3 h) with a bioavailability of >95%. Its volume of distribution is 0.87–1.83 L/kg, and plasma protein binding is 85%. The plasma protein binding of the pharmacologically active metabolite, *N*-desmethylclobazam, is 89%.

Biotransformation

Clobazam is extensively metabolized in the liver, primarily by demethylation, to *N*-desmethylclobazam, which is pharmacologically active and contributes significantly to the efficacy of clobazam. Clobazam also undergoes metabolism by hydroxylation to form other metabolites, namely, 4-hydroxyclobazam and 4-hydroxy desmethylclobazam. *N*-desmethylclobazam is subsequently metabolized by CYP2C19.

Renal Excretion

Less than 1% of an administered dose is excreted as unchanged clobazam in urine.

Elimination

Plasma elimination half-life values for clobazam and *N*-desmethylclobazam in adults are 10–30 h and 36–46 h, respectively. In children, clobazam half-life values are ~16 h, while in the elderly, clobazam half-life values are 30–48 h.

Time to new steady-state blood levels consequent to an inhibition of metabolism interaction:

- Clobazam = 2–8 days later
- *N*-desmethylclobazam = 7–10 days later

Effects on Isoenzymes

No in vitro data on the induction or inhibition potential of clobazam on human CYP or UGT isoenzymes have been published.

Therapeutic Drug Monitoring

Optimum seizure control in patients on clobazam monotherapy is most likely to occur at plasma clobazam levels of 0.03–0.30 mg/L (0.1–1.0 μmol/L). The reference range for *N*-desmethylclobazam is 0.30–3.00 mg/L (1–10 μmol/L). The conversion factor from mg/L to μmol/L for clobazam is 3.33 (i.e., 1 mg/L = 3.33 μmol/L), while that for *N*-desmethylclobazam it is 3.49 (i.e., 1 mg/L = 3.49 μmol/L).

Propensity to Be Associated with Pharmacokinetic Interactions

- Clobazam affects the pharmacokinetics of other drugs—minimal.
- Other drugs affect the pharmacokinetics of clobazam—minimal.

Interactions with ASMs

Acetazolamide	The interaction has not been investigated. Theoretically, a pharmacokinetic interaction would not be anticipated
Brivaracetam	Does not affect the pharmacokinetics of clobazam [1]
Cannabidiol	Inhibits the metabolism of clobazam
Consequence	Mean plasma clobazam AUC values increase by 21%, while mean plasma AUC values of the pharmacologically active metabolite of clobazam, *N*-desmethylclobazam, are increased by 238% [2] An additive antiseizure effect may occur between clobazam and cannabidiol consequent to a bi-directional pharmacokinetic interaction resulting in increases of their respective pharmacologically active metabolites [3]
Carbamazepine	Enhances the metabolism of clobazam
Consequence	Plasma levels of the pharmacologically active metabolite of clobazam, *N*-desmethylclobazam, are increased during comedication with carbamazepine. The mean plasma *N*-desmethylclobazam/clobazam ratio is increased by 117% [4]
Cenobamate	The interaction has not been investigated. Theoretically, a pharmacokinetic interaction could occur
Clonazepam	The interaction has not been investigated. Theoretically, a pharmacokinetic interaction would not be anticipated
Eslicarbazepine acetate	Does not affect the pharmacokinetics of clobazam [5]
Ethosuximide	The interaction has not been investigated. Theoretically, a pharmacokinetic interaction would not be anticipated
Everolimus	The interaction has not been investigated. Theoretically, a pharmacokinetic interaction could occur
Felbamate	Inhibits the metabolism of clobazam
Consequence	Plasma levels of the pharmacologically active metabolite of clobazam, *N*-desmethylclobazam, are increased during comedication with felbamate. Typically, the plasma level to weight-adjusted dose ratio of *N*-desmethylclobazam can be expected to be fivefold higher, while the ratio for clobazam decreases by 57%. The interaction may be the consequence of inhibition of *N*-desmethylclobazam metabolism through CYP2C19 [6]
Fenfluramine	Does not affect the pharmacokinetics of clobazam [7]
Gabapentin	The interaction has not been investigated. Theoretically, a pharmacokinetic interaction would not be anticipated
Lacosamide	The interaction has not been investigated. Theoretically, a pharmacokinetic interaction would not be anticipated
Lamotrigine	Does not affect the pharmacokinetics of clobazam [6]
Levetiracetam	Does not affect the pharmacokinetics of clobazam [8]
Methsuximide	The interaction has not been investigated. Theoretically, a pharmacokinetic interaction could occur
Oxcarbazepine	The interaction has not been investigated. Theoretically, a pharmacokinetic interaction could occur
Perampanel	Enhances the metabolism of clobazam
Consequence	Mean clobazam clearance is increased by 3.4% [9]
Phenobarbital	Enhances the metabolism of clobazam

Consequence	Plasma levels of the pharmacologically active metabolite of clobazam, *N*-desmethylclobazam, are increased during comedication with phenobarbital. The mean plasma *N*-desmethylclobazam/clobazam ratio is increased by 90% [4]
Phenytoin	Enhances the metabolism of clobazam
Consequence	Plasma levels of the pharmacologically active metabolite of clobazam, *N*-desmethylclobazam, are increased during comedication with phenytoin. The mean plasma *N*-desmethylclobazam/clobazam ratio is increased by 294% [4]
Piracetam	The interaction has not been investigated. Theoretically, a pharmacokinetic interaction would not be anticipated
Pregabalin	The interaction has not been investigated. Theoretically, a pharmacokinetic interaction would not be anticipated
Primidone	The interaction has not been investigated. Theoretically, a pharmacokinetic interaction could occur
Rufinamide	Does not affect the pharmacokinetics of clobazam [10]
Stiripentol	Inhibits the metabolism of clobazam
Consequence	Plasma levels of clobazam and the pharmacologically active metabolite of clobazam, *N*-desmethylclobazam, are increased during comedication with stiripentol. Typically, the plasma levels of clobazam and *N*-desmethylclobazam can be expected to be twofold higher and threefold higher, respectively. The interaction is the consequence of inhibition of *N*-demethylation of clobazam through CYP3A4 and the inhibition of the hydroxylation of *N*-desmethylclobazam by CYP2C19 [11]
Sulthiame	Plasma levels of the pharmacologically active metabolite of clobazam, *N*-desmethylclobazam, are increased during comedication with sulthiame. Plasma levels of clobazam are unaffected. The mean plasma *N*-desmethylclobazam/clobazam ratio is increased by 83–248% [12]
Tiagabine	The interaction has not been investigated. Theoretically, a pharmacokinetic interaction would not be anticipated
Topiramate	The interaction has not been investigated. Theoretically, a pharmacokinetic interaction could occur
Valproic acid	Does not affect the pharmacokinetics of clobazam [4]
Vigabatrin	The interaction has not been investigated. Theoretically, a pharmacokinetic interaction would not be anticipated
Zonisamide	The interaction has not been investigated. Theoretically, a pharmacokinetic interaction could occur

References

1. Moseley BD, Otoul C, Staelens L, Stockis A. Pharmacokinetic interaction of brivaracetam on other antiepileptic drugs in adults with focal seizures: pooled analysis of data from randomized clinical trials. Epilepsy Res. 2019;158:106218.
2. Patsalos PN, Szaflarski JP, Gidal B, VanLandingham K, Critchley D, Morrison G. Clinical implications of trials investigating drug-drug interactions between cannabidiol and enzyme inducers or inhibitors or common antiseizure drugs. Epilepsia. 2020;61:1854–68.
3. Summary of product characteristics: Cannabidiol (Epidyolex). GW Pharma Ltd. Last update 27 July 2020.

4. Sennoune S, Mesdjian E, Bonneton J, Genton P, Dravet C, Roger J. Interactions between clobazam and standard antiepileptic drugs in patients with epilepsy. Ther Drug Monit. 1992;14:269–74.
5. Falcao A, Fuseau E, Nunes T, Almeida L, Soares-da-Silva P. Pharmacokinetics, drug interactions and exposure-response relationships of eslicarbazepine acetate in adult patients with partial-onset seizures: population pharmacokinetic and pharmacokinetic/pharmacodynamic analysis. CNS Drugs. 2012;26:79–91.
6. Contin M, Riva R, Albani F, Baruzzi A. Effect of felbamate on clobazam and its metabolite kinetics in patients with epilepsy. Ther Drug Monit. 1999;21:604–8.
7. Boyd B, Smith S, Gammaitoni A, Galer BS, Farfel GM. A phase 1, randomized, open-label, single dose, 3 period crossover study to evaluate the drug-drug interaction between ZX008 (fenfluramine HCl oral solution) and a regimen of stiripentol, clobazam, and valproate in healthy subjects. Int J Clin Pharmacol Therapeut. 2019;57:11–9.
8. Perucca E, Baltes E, Ledent E. Levetiracetam: absence of pharmacokinetic interactions with other antiepileptic drugs (AEDs). Epilepsia. 2000;41(Suppl):150.
9. Majid O, Laurenza A, Ferry J, Hussein Z. Impact of perampanel on pharmacokinetics of concomitant antiepileptics in patients with partial-onset seizures: pooled analysis of clinical trials. Br J Clin Pharmacol. 2016;82:422–30.
10. Perucca E, Cloyd J, Critchley D, Fuseau E. Rufinamide: clinical pharmacokinetics and concentration-response relationships in patients with epilepsy. Epilepsia. 2008;49:1123–41.
11. Giraud C, Treluyer JM, Rey E, Chiron C, Vincent J, Pons G, Tran A. In vitro and in vivo inhibitory effect of stiripentol on clobazam metabolism. Drug Metab Dispos. 2006;34:608–11.
12. Yamamoto Y, Takahashi Y, Imai K, Mogami Y, Matsusa K, Nakai M, Kagawa Y, Inoue Y. Interaction between sulthiame and clobazam; sulthiame inhibits the metabolism of clobazam, possibly via an action on CYP2C19. Epilepsy Behav. 2014;34:124–6.

Clonazepam

Clonazepam (Fig. 1) corresponds chemically to 5-(2-chlorophenol)-1,3-dihydro-7-nitro-2H-1,4 benzodiazepine-2-one with an empirical formula of $C_{15}H_{10}ClN_3O_3$ and a molecular weight of 315.71.

Fig. 1 Clonazepam

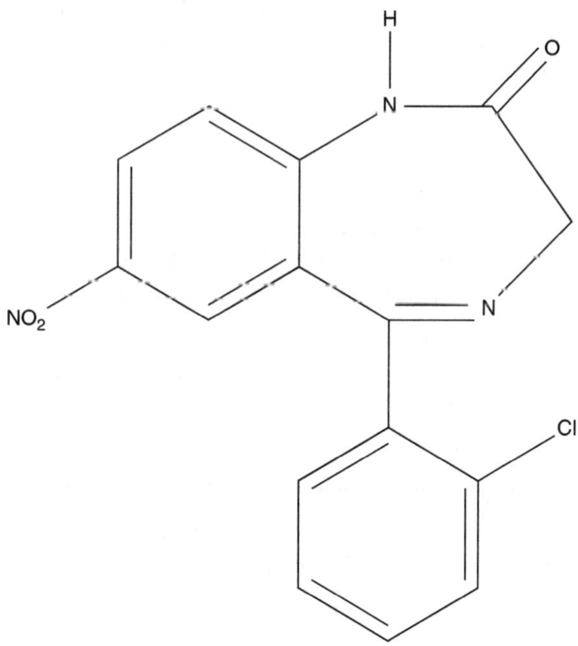

P. N. Patsalos, *Antiseizure Medication Interactions*,
https://doi.org/10.1007/978-3-030-82790-8_8

Pharmacokinetic Characteristics

Absorption and Distribution

After oral ingestion, clonazepam is rapidly absorbed (T_{max} = 1–4 h) with a bioavailability of >80%. Its volume of distribution is 1.5–4.4 L/kg, and plasma protein binding is 86%.

Biotransformation

Clonazepam is extensively metabolized in the liver by reduction (via CYP3A4) to produce 7-amino-clonazepam, which is subsequently metabolized by acetylation (via *N*-acetyl-transferase) to form 7-acetamido-clonazepam. Clonazepam is also hydroxylated (isoenzyme not identified) to form 3-hydroxyclonazepam. None of the metabolites of clonazepam are pharmacologically active.

Renal Excretion

Less than 1% of an administered dose is excreted as unchanged clonazepam in urine.

Elimination

In healthy adult subjects, plasma elimination half-life values are 17–56 h, while in adult patients with enzyme-inducing antiseizure medications, half-life values are 12–46 h. In neonates and children, half-life values are 22–81 h and 22–33 h, respectively.

Time to new steady-state blood levels consequent to inhibition of metabolism interaction:

- Adults = 2–10 days later
- Children = 5–7 days later

Effects on Isoenzymes

No in vitro data on the induction or inhibition potential of clonazepam on human CYP or UGT isoenzymes have been published.

Therapeutic Drug Monitoring

Optimum seizure control in patients on clonazepam monotherapy is most likely to occur at plasma clonazepam levels of 13–70 μg/L (41–222 nmol/L). The conversion factor from μg/L to nmol/L is 3.17 (i.e., 1 μg/L = 3.17 nmol/L).

Propensity to Be Associated with Pharmacokinetic Interactions

- Clonazepam affects the pharmacokinetics of other drugs—minimal.
- Other drugs affect the pharmacokinetics of clonazepam—minimal.

Interactions with ASMs

Acetazolamide	The interaction has not been investigated. Theoretically, a pharmacokinetic interaction would not be anticipated
Brivaracetam	Does not affect the pharmacokinetics of clonazepam [1]
Cannabidiol	Does not affect the pharmacokinetics of clonazepam [2]
Carbamazepine	Enhances the metabolism of clonazepam
Consequence	Plasma clonazepam levels can decrease by 19–37% [3]

Cenobamate	The interaction has not been investigated. Theoretically, a pharmacokinetic interaction could occur
Clobazam	The interaction has not been investigated. Theoretically, a pharmacokinetic interaction would not be anticipated
Eslicarbazepine acetate	The interaction has not been investigated. Theoretically, a pharmacokinetic interaction would not be anticipated
Ethosuximide	The interaction has not been investigated. Theoretically, a pharmacokinetic interaction would not be anticipated
Everolimus	The interaction has not been investigated. Theoretically, a pharmacokinetic interaction would not be anticipated
Felbamate	Inhibits the metabolism of clonazepam
Consequence	Mean plasma clonazepam levels and AUC values can be increased by 17% and 14%, respectively [4]
Fenfluramine	The interaction has not been investigated. Theoretically, a pharmacokinetic interaction would not be anticipated
Gabapentin	The interaction has not been investigated. Theoretically, a pharmacokinetic interaction would not be anticipated
Lacosamide	Does not affect the pharmacokinetics of clonazepam [5]
Lamotrigine	Enhances the metabolism of clonazepam
Consequence	Plasma clonazepam levels can decrease by 20–38% [6]
Levetiracetam	Does not affect the pharmacokinetics of clonazepam [7]
Methsuximide	The interaction has not been investigated. Theoretically, a pharmacokinetic interaction could occur
Oxcarbazepine	The interaction has not been investigated. Theoretically, a pharmacokinetic interaction could occur
Perampanel	Does not affect the pharmacokinetics of clonazepam [8]
Phenobarbital	Enhances the metabolism of clonazepam
Consequence	Mean plasma clonazepam clearance is increased by 19–24%, and mean plasma clonazepam levels can decrease by 11% [9]
Phenytoin	Enhances the metabolism of clonazepam
Consequence	Mean plasma clonazepam clearance can increase by 46–58%, and mean plasma clonazepam levels can decrease by 28% [9]
Piracetam	The interaction has not been investigated. Theoretically, a pharmacokinetic interaction would not be anticipated
Pregabalin	The interaction has not been investigated. Theoretically, a pharmacokinetic interaction would not be anticipated
Primidone	Enhances the metabolism of clonazepam
Consequence	Plasma clonazepam levels can be decreased [10]
Rufinamide	The interaction has not been investigated. Theoretically, a pharmacokinetic interaction would not be anticipated
Stiripentol	The interaction has not been investigated. Theoretically, a pharmacokinetic interaction could occur
Sulthiame	The interaction has not been investigated. Theoretically, a pharmacokinetic interaction could occur
Tiagabine	The interaction has not been investigated. Theoretically, a pharmacokinetic interaction would not be anticipated
Topiramate	The interaction has not been investigated. Theoretically, a pharmacokinetic interaction could occur

Valproic acid	The interaction has not been investigated. Theoretically, a pharmacokinetic interaction could occur
Vigabatrin	The interaction has not been investigated. Theoretically, a pharmacokinetic interaction would not be anticipated
Zonisamide	The interaction has not been investigated. Theoretically, a pharmacokinetic interaction could occur

References

1. Moseley BD, Otoul C, Staelens L, Stockis A. Pharmacokinetic interaction of brivaracetam on other antiepileptic drugs in adults with focal seizures: pooled analysis of data from randomized clinical trials. Epilepsy Res. 2019;158:106218.
2. Gaston TE, Bekib EM, Cutter GR, Liu Y, Szaflarski JP, UAB CBD Program. Interactions between cannabidiol and commonly used antiepileptic drugs. Epilepsia. 2017;58:1586–92.
3. Lai AA, Levy RH, Cutler RE. Time-course of interaction between carbamazepine and clonazepam in normal man. Clin Pharmacol Ther. 1978;24:316–23.
4. Colucci R, Glue P, Banfield C, Reidenberg P, Meehan J, Radwanski E, Korduba C, Lin C, Dogterom P, Ebels T, Hendriks G, Jonkman JHG, Affrime M. Effect of felbamate on the pharmacokinetics of clonazepam. Am J Ther. 1996;3:294–7.
5. Halasz P, Kalviainen R, Mazurkiewicz-Beldzinska M, Rosenow F, Doty P, Hebert D, Sullivan T. Adjunctive lacosamide for partialonset seizures: efficacy and safety results from a randomized controlled trial. Epilepsia. 2009;50:443–53.
6. Eriksson AS, Hoppu K, Nergardh A, Boreu L. Pharmacokinetic interactions between lamotrigine and other antiepileptic drugs in children with intractable epilepsy. Epilepsia. 1996;37:769–73.
7. Perucca E, Baltes E, Ledent E. Levetiracetam: absence of pharmacokinetic interactions with other antiepileptic drugs (AEDs). Epilepsia. 2000;41(Suppl):150.
8. Patsalos PN. The clinical pharmacology profile of the new antiepileptic drug perampanel: a novel noncompetitive AMPA receptor antagonist. Epilepsia. 2015;56:12–27.
9. Khoo KC, Mendels J, Rothbart M, Garland WA, Colburn WA, Min BH, Lucek R, Carbone JJ, Boxenbaum HG, Kaplan SA. Influence of phenytoin and phenobarbital on the disposition of a single oral dose of clonazepam. Clin Pharmacol Ther. 1980;28:368–75.
10. Nanda RN, Johnson RH, Keogh HJ, Lambie DG, Melville ID. Treatment of epilepsy with clonazepam and its effect on other anticonvulsants. J Neurol Neurosurg Psychiatry. 1977;40:538–43.

Eslicarbazepine Acetate

Eslicarbazepine (Fig. 1) acetate corresponds chemically to (S)-10-acetoxy-10,11-dihydro-5H-dibenz[b,f]azepine-5-carboxamide with an empirical formula of $C_{17}H_{16}N_2O_3$ and a molecular weight of 296.32.

Fig. 1 Eslicarbazepine

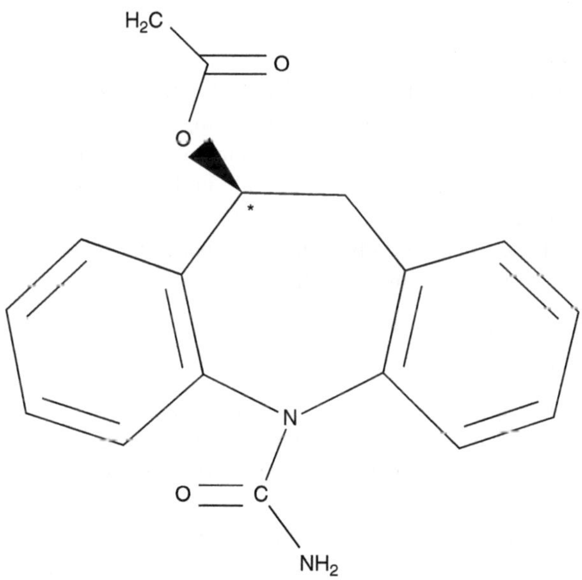

P. N. Patsalos, *Antiseizure Medication Interactions*,
https://doi.org/10.1007/978-3-030-82790-8_9

Pharmacokinetic Characteristics

Absorption and Distribution

After oral ingestion, eslicarbazepine acetate is rapidly absorbed (T_{max} = 2–3 h) with a bioavailability of >90%. Its volume of distribution is 2.7 L/kg, and plasma protein binding is 30%. These values relate to eslicarbazepine, the pharmacologically active metabolite of eslicarbazepine acetate.

Biotransformation

Eslicarbazepine acetate is rapidly metabolized (hydrolysis) in the liver to its pharmacologically active metabolite, eslicarbazepine (also known as *S*-licarbazepine and 10-hydroxycarbazepine), by esterases (91%). Eslicarbazepine (33%) is subsequently metabolized by conjugation with glucuronic acid. Other minor metabolites, which are pharmacologically active, include *S*-licarbazepine (~5%) and oxcarbazepine (~1%). UGT1A4, UGT1A9, UGT2B4, UGT2B7, and (particularly) UGT2B17 are all involved in the conjugation of eslicarbazepine with glucuronic acid.

Renal Excretion

Less than 1% of an administered dose is excreted as unchanged eslicarbazepine in urine.

Elimination

The plasma elimination half-life of eslicarbazepine acetate is <2 h; thus, eslicarbazepine acetate is a prodrug that is rapidly converted to its eslicarbazepine metabolite. In the absence of enzyme-inducing antiseizure medications, half-life values for eslicarbazepine are 10–20 h, while in the presence of enzyme-inducing antiseizure medications, half-life values are 13–20 h.

Time to new steady-state eslicarbazepine blood levels consequent to an inhibition of metabolism interaction:

- Adults = 2–4 days later

Effects on Isoenzymes

At therapeutic concentrations, eslicarbazepine in vitro is a weak inducer of CYP3A4, a moderate inducer of UGT1A1, and a moderate inhibitor of CYP2C9 and CYP2C19 activities. Consequently, pharmacokinetic interactions of metabolic origin with other antiseizure medications and other medicines can be expected.

Eslicarbazepine has no in vitro inhibitory effect on the activity of CYP1A2, CYP2A6, CYP2B6, CYP2D, CYP2E1, CYP3A4, and CYP4A9/11; UGT1A1 and UGT1A6; and epoxide hydrolase. Furthermore, eslicarbazepine has no in vitro induction effects on CYP1A2 or CYP3A4.

Therapeutic Drug Monitoring

The current reference range for eslicarbazepine in plasma is 3–35 mg/L (12–139 μmol/L) which is based on that for racemic 10-hydroxycarbazepine derived from oxcarbazepine. The conversion factor from mg/L to μmol/L for eslicarbazepine is 3.96 (i.e., 1 mg/L = 3.96 μmol/L).

Propensity to Be Associated with Pharmacokinetic Interactions

- Eslicarbazepine acetate affects the pharmacokinetics of other drugs—minimal.
- Other drugs affect the pharmacokinetics of eslicarbazepine acetate—minimal.

Interactions with ASMs

Acetazolamide	The interaction has not been investigated. Theoretically, a pharmacokinetic interaction would not be anticipated
Brivaracetam	The interaction has not been investigated. Theoretically, a pharmacokinetic interaction would not be anticipated
Cannabidiol	Inhibits the metabolism of eslicarbazepine
Consequence	Increases mean plasma eslicarbazepine levels by 24% [1]
Carbamazepine	Enhances the clearance of eslicarbazepine
Consequence	Mean eslicarbazepine clearance values can be increased by 12%, while mean eslicarbazepine plasma levels can be decreased by 12% [2]
	During combination therapy, carbamazepine enhances eslicarbazepine adverse effects, including diplopia, abnormal coordination, and dizziness. These effects are probably the consequence of a pharmacodynamic interaction [3]
Cenobamate	The interaction has not been investigated. Theoretically, a pharmacokinetic interaction could occur
Clobazam	Clobazam does not affect the pharmacokinetics of eslicarbazepine [2]
Clonazepam	The interaction has not been investigated. Theoretically, a pharmacokinetic interaction would not be anticipated
Ethosuximide	The interaction has not been investigated. Theoretically, a pharmacokinetic interaction would not be anticipated
Everolimus	The interaction has not been investigated. Theoretically, a pharmacokinetic interaction could occur
Felbamate	The interaction has not been investigated. Theoretically, a pharmacokinetic interaction could occur
Fenfluramine	The interaction has not been investigated. Theoretically, a pharmacokinetic interaction could occur
Gabapentin	Gabapentin does not affect the pharmacokinetics of eslicarbazepine [2]
Lacosamide	The interaction has not been investigated. Theoretically, a pharmacokinetic interaction would not be anticipated
Lamotrigine	Does not affect the pharmacokinetics of eslicarbazepine [4]
Levetiracetam	Does not affect the pharmacokinetics of eslicarbazepine [2]
Methsuximide	The interaction has not been investigated. Theoretically, a pharmacokinetic interaction would not be anticipated
Perampanel	The interaction has not been investigated. Theoretically, a pharmacokinetic interaction could occur
Oxcarbazepine	Oxcarbazepine and eslicarbazepine acetate in combination are contraindicated
Phenobarbital	The interaction has not been investigated. Theoretically, a pharmacokinetic interaction could occur
Phenytoin	Enhances the metabolism of eslicarbazepine
Consequence	Plasma eslicarbazepine AUC values can decrease by 31–33%. The interaction is considered to be the consequence of induction of eslicarbazepine metabolism, most likely of glucuronidation [2]
Piracetam	The interaction has not been investigated. Theoretically, a pharmacokinetic interaction would not be anticipated

Pregabalin	The interaction has not been investigated. Theoretically, a pharmacokinetic interaction would not be anticipated
Primidone	The interaction has not been investigated. Theoretically, a pharmacokinetic interaction could occur
Rufinamide	The interaction has not been investigated. Theoretically, a pharmacokinetic interaction would not be anticipated
Stiripentol	The interaction has not been investigated. Theoretically, a pharmacokinetic interaction could occur
Sulthiame	The interaction has not been investigated. Theoretically, a pharmacokinetic interaction could occur
Tiagabine	The interaction has not been investigated. Theoretically, a pharmacokinetic interaction would not be anticipated
Topiramate	Enhances the metabolism of eslicarbazepine
Consequence	In healthy volunteers, eslicarbazepine mean plasma C_{max} and AUC values are decreased by 13% and 7%, respectively [5]
	In contrast, population pharmacokinetic data indicate that topiramate does not affect the pharmacokinetics of eslicarbazepine [6]
Valproic acid	Does not affect the pharmacokinetics of eslicarbazepine [2]
Vigabatrin	The interaction has not been investigated. Theoretically, a pharmacokinetic interaction would not be anticipated
Zonisamide	The interaction has not been investigated. Theoretically, a pharmacokinetic interaction would not be anticipated

References

1. Gaston TE, Bekib EM, Cutter GR, Liu Y, Szaflarski JP, UAB CBD Program. Interactions between cannabidiol and commonly used antiepileptic drugs. Epilepsia. 2017;58:1586–92.
2. Falcao A, Fuseau E, Nunes T, Almeida L, Soares-da-Silva P. Pharmacokinetics, drug interactions and exposure-response relationships of eslicarbazepine acetate in adult patients with partial-onset seizures: population pharmacokinetic and pharmacokinetic/pharmacodynamic analysis. CNS Drugs. 2012;26:79–91.
3. Almeida L, Bialer M, Soares-da-Silva P. Eslicarbazepine acetate. In: Shorvon SD, Perucca E, Engel J, editors. The treatment of epilepsy. 3rd ed. Oxford: Blackwell; 2009. p. 485–98.
4. Almeida L, Nunes T, Sicard E, Rocha JF, Falcao A, Brunet JS, Lefebvre M, Soares-da-Silva P. Pharmacokinetic interaction study between eslicarbazepine acetate and lamotrigine in healthy subjects. Acta Neurol Scand. 2010;121:257–64.
5. Nunes T, Sicard E, Almeida L, Falcao A, Rocha JF, Brunet JS, Lefebvre M, Soares-da-Silva P. Pharmacokinetic interaction study between eslicarbazepine acetate and topiramate in healthy subjects. Curr Med Res Opin. 2010;26:1355–62.
6. Bialer M, Soares-da-Siva P. Pharmacokinetics and drug interactions of eslicarbazepine acetate. Epilepsia. 2012;53:935–46.

Ethosuximide

Ethosuximide (Fig. 1) corresponds chemically to 2-ethyl-2-methylsuccinimide with an empirical formula of $C_7H_{11}NO_2$ and a molecular weight of 141.7.

Fig. 1 Ethosuximide

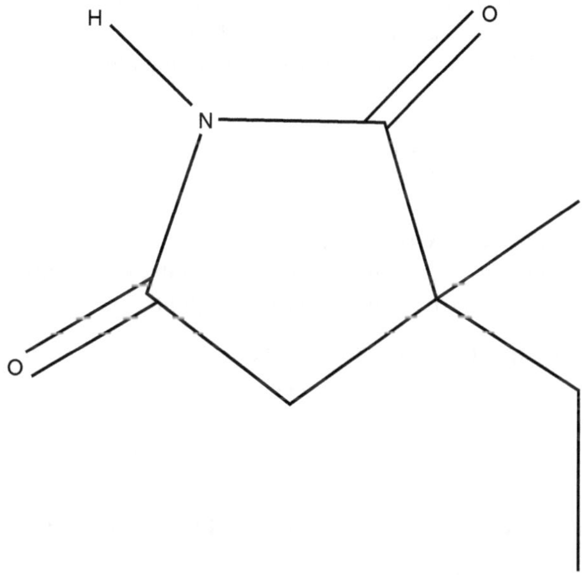

P. N. Patsalos, *Antiseizure Medication Interactions*,
https://doi.org/10.1007/978-3-030-82790-8_10

Pharmacokinetic Characteristics

Absorption and Distribution

After oral ingestion, ethosuximide is rapidly absorbed (T_{max} = 1–4 h) with a bioavailability of >90%. Its volume of distribution is 0.7 L/kg, and plasma protein binding is 0%.

Biotransformation

Ethosuximide is extensively metabolized in the liver by hydroxylation (primarily by CYP3A and to a lesser extent by CYP2E and CYP2B/C) to form isomers of 2-(1-hydroxyethyl)-2-methylsuccinimide, of which at least 40% are glucuronide conjugates.

Renal Excretion

Approximately 20% of an administered dose is excreted as unchanged ethosuximide in urine.

Elimination

Plasma elimination half-life values of ethosuximide are 40–60 h in adults and 30–40 h in children. In patients co-prescribed with enzyme-inducing antiseizure medications, half-life values are 20–40 h.

Time to new steady-state ethosuximide blood levels consequent to inhibition of metabolism interaction:

- Adults = 8–12 days later
- Children = 6–8 days later

Effects on Isoenzymes

No in vitro data on the induction or inhibition potential of ethosuximide on human CYP or UGT isoenzymes have been published.

Therapeutic Drug Monitoring

Optimum seizure control in patients on ethosuximide monotherapy is most likely to occur at ethosuximide plasma levels of 40–100 mg/L (300–700 μmol/L). The conversion factor from mg/L to μmol/L for ethosuximide is 7.06 (i.e., 1 mg/L = 7.06 μmol/L).

Propensity to Be Associated with Pharmacokinetic Interactions

- Ethosuximide affects the pharmacokinetics of other drugs—minimal.
- Other drugs affect the pharmacokinetics of ethosuximide—minimal.

Interactions with ASMs

Acetazolamide	The interaction has not been investigated. Theoretically, a pharmacokinetic interaction would not be anticipated
Brivaracetam	The interaction has not been investigated. Theoretically, a pharmacokinetic interaction would not be anticipated
Cannabidiol	Does not affect the pharmacokinetics of ethosuximide [1]

Carbamazepine	Enhances the metabolism of ethosuximide
Consequence	Mean plasma ethosuximide AUC values can be decreased by 49%. The interaction is the consequence of the induction of ethosuximide metabolism through CYP3A [2]
Cenobamate	The interaction has not been investigated. Theoretically, a pharmacokinetic interaction could occur
Clobazam	The interaction has not been investigated. Theoretically, a pharmacokinetic interaction would not be anticipated
Clonazepam	The interaction has not been investigated. Theoretically, a pharmacokinetic interaction would not be anticipated
Eslicarbazepine acetate	The interaction has not been investigated. Theoretically, a pharmacokinetic interaction would not be anticipated
Everolimus	The interaction has not been investigated. Theoretically, a pharmacokinetic interaction could occur
Felbamate	The interaction has not been investigated. Theoretically, a pharmacokinetic interaction could occur
Fenfluramine	The interaction has not been investigated. Theoretically, a pharmacokinetic interaction could occur
Gabapentin	The interaction has not been investigated. Theoretically, a pharmacokinetic interaction would not be anticipated
Lacosamide	The interaction has not been investigated. Theoretically, a pharmacokinetic interaction would not be anticipated
Lamotrigine	Does not affect the pharmacokinetics of ethosuximide [3]
Levetiracetam	Does not affect the pharmacokinetics of ethosuximide [4]
Methsuximide	The interaction has not been investigated. Theoretically, a pharmacokinetic interaction could occur
Oxcarbazepine	The interaction has not been investigated. Theoretically, a pharmacokinetic interaction could occur
Perampanel	The interaction has not been investigated. Theoretically, a pharmacokinetic interaction would not be anticipated
Phenobarbital	Enhances the metabolism of ethosuximide
Consequence	Mean plasma ethosuximide AUC values can be decreased by 49%. The interaction is the consequence of the induction of ethosuximide metabolism through CYP3A [2]
Phenytoin	Enhances the metabolism of ethosuximide
Consequence	Mean plasma ethosuximide AUC values can be decreased by 49%. The interaction is the consequence of the induction of ethosuximide metabolism through CYP3A [2]
Piracetam	The interaction has not been investigated. Theoretically, a pharmacokinetic interaction would not be anticipated
Pregabalin	The interaction has not been investigated. Theoretically, a pharmacokinetic interaction would not be anticipated
Primidone	Enhances the metabolism of ethosuximide
Consequence	The mean level/dose ratio for ethosuximide is decreased by 33% [5]
Rufinamide	The interaction has not been investigated. Theoretically, a pharmacokinetic interaction would not be anticipated
Stiripentol	Inhibits the metabolism of ethosuximide
Consequence	Ethosuximide blood levels will increase [6]

Sulthiame	The interaction has not been investigated. Theoretically, a pharmacokinetic interaction could occur
Tiagabine	The interaction has not been investigated. Theoretically, a pharmacokinetic interaction would not be anticipated
Topiramate	The interaction has not been investigated. Theoretically, a pharmacokinetic interaction would not be anticipated
Valproic acid	Conflicting effects have been reported
Consequence	Plasma ethosuximide levels are reported to decrease, increase, and not change during co-administration with valproic acid [5, 7]
	During combination therapy, valproic acid synergistically enhances the antiseizure efficacy (absence seizures) and toxicity of ethosuximide. These effects are probably the consequence of a pharmacodynamic interaction [8]
Vigabatrin	The interaction has not been investigated. Theoretically, a pharmacokinetic interaction would not be anticipated
Zonisamide	The interaction has not been investigated. Theoretically, a pharmacokinetic interaction could occur

References

1. Gaston TE, Bekib EM, Cutter GR, Liu Y, Szaflarski JP, UAB CBD Program. Interactions between cannabidiol and commonly used antiepileptic drugs. Epilepsia. 2017;58:1586–92.
2. Giaccone M, Bartoli A, Gatti G, Marchiselli R, Pisani F, Latella MA, Perucca E. Effect of enzyme inducing anticonvulsants on ethosuximide pharmacokinetics in epileptic patients. Br J Clin Pharmacol. 1996;41:575–9.
3. Eriksson AS, Hoppu K, Nergardh A, Boreu L. Pharmacokinetic interactions between lamotrigine and other antiepileptic drugs in children with intractable epilepsy. Epilepsia. 1996;37:769–73.
4. Kasteleijn-Nolst Trenite DGA, Marescaux C, Stodieck S, Edelbroek PM, Oosting J. Evaluation of the piracetam analogue, levetiracetam. Epilepsy Res. 1996;25:225–30.
5. Battino D, Cusi C, Franceschetti S, Moise A, Spina S, Avanzini G. Ethosuximide plasma concentrations: influence of age and associated concomitant therapy. Clin Pharmacokinet. 1982;7:176–80.
6. Loiseau P, Duché B. Rolandic paroxysmal epilepsy or partial benign epilepsy in children. Rev Prat. 1988;38:1194–6.
7. Pisani F, Narbone MC, Trunfio C, Fazio A, La Rosa G, Oteri G, Di Perri R. Valproic acid-ethosuximide interaction: a pharmacokinetic study. Epilepsia. 1984;25:229–33.
8. Rowan AJ, Meijer JW, de Beer-Pawlikowski N, van der Geest P, Meinardi H. Valproate-ethosuximide combination therapy for refractory seizures. Arch Neurol. 1983;40:797–802.

Everolimus

Everolimus (Fig. 1) corresponds chemically to 40-O-(2-hydroxyethyl) derivative of rapamycin with an empirical formula of $C_{53}H_{83}NO_{14}$ and a molecular weight of 958.2.

Pharmacokinetic Characteristics

Absorption and Distribution

After oral ingestion, everolimus is rapidly absorbed (T_{max} = 1–2 h), and its plasma protein binding is ~74%. The bioavailability and volume of distribution of everolimus are not known.

Fig. 1 Everolimus

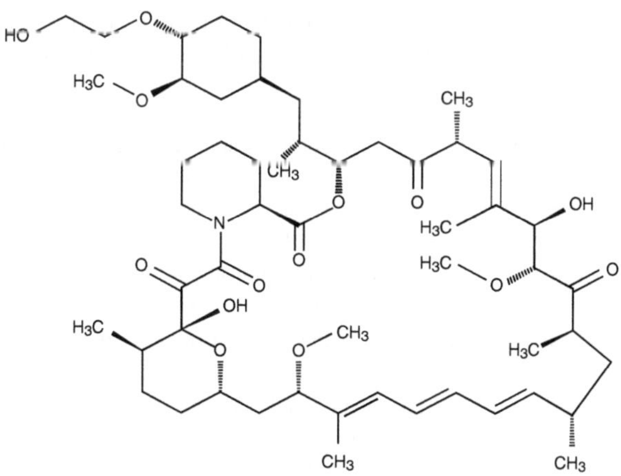

P. N. Patsalos, *Antiseizure Medication Interactions*,
https://doi.org/10.1007/978-3-030-82790-8_11

Biotransformation
Everolimus undergoes extensive hepatic metabolism by CYP3A4, resulting in six metabolites, including three monohydroxylated metabolites, two hydrolytic ring-opened products, and a phosphatidylcholine conjugate of everolimus. All metabolites exhibit weak pharmacological activity.

Renal Excretion
No unchanged everolimus is detected in urine.

Elimination
The plasma elimination half-life value of everolimus is ~30 h.

Time to new steady-state everolimus blood levels consequent to an inhibition of metabolism interaction:

- Adults = 5–8 days later

Effects on Isoenzymes
In vitro, at clinically relevant concentrations, everolimus inhibits the activity of CYP3A4 and is a mixed inhibitor of CYP2D6 and a moderate inhibitor of PgP. It is a substrate of both CYP3A4 and PgP. Consequently, pharmacokinetic interactions of metabolic origin with other antiseizure medications and other medicines can be expected.

No in vitro data on the induction potential of everolimus on human CYP enzymes have been published.

Therapeutic Drug Monitoring
There are no data relating plasma everolimus levels with that of seizure suppression or adverse effects.

Propensity to Be Associated with Pharmacokinetic Interactions

- Everolimus affects the pharmacokinetics of other drugs—substantial.
- Other drugs affect the pharmacokinetics of everolimus—substantial.

Interactions with ASMs

Acetazolamide	The interaction has not been investigated. Theoretically, a pharmacokinetic interaction would not be anticipated
Brivaracetam	The interaction has not been investigated. Theoretically, a pharmacokinetic interaction would not be anticipated
Cannabidiol	Inhibits the metabolism of everolimus
Consequence	Plasma everolimus levels are increased [1, 2]
Carbamazepine	Enhances the metabolism of everolimus
Consequence	Plasma everolimus levels are decreased [3]
Cenobamate	The interaction has not been investigated. Theoretically, a pharmacokinetic interaction could occur
Clobazam	The interaction has not been investigated. Theoretically, a pharmacokinetic interaction would not be anticipated
Clonazepam	The interaction has not been investigated. Theoretically, a pharmacokinetic interaction would not be anticipated

Eslicarbazepine acetate	The interaction has not been investigated. Theoretically, a pharmacokinetic interaction could occur
Ethosuximide	The interaction has not been investigated. Theoretically, a pharmacokinetic interaction would not be anticipated
Felbamate	The interaction has not been investigated. Theoretically, a pharmacokinetic interaction could occur
Fenfluramine	The interaction has not been investigated. Theoretically, a pharmacokinetic interaction could occur
Gabapentin	The interaction has not been investigated. Theoretically, a pharmacokinetic interaction would not be anticipated
Lacosamide	The interaction has not been investigated. Theoretically, a pharmacokinetic interaction would not be anticipated
Lamotrigine	The interaction has not been investigated. Theoretically, a pharmacokinetic interaction could occur
Levetiracetam	The interaction has not been investigated. Theoretically, a pharmacokinetic interaction would not be anticipated
Methsuximide	The interaction has not been investigated. Theoretically, a pharmacokinetic interaction would not be anticipated
Perampanel	The interaction has not been investigated. Theoretically, a pharmacokinetic interaction would not be anticipated
Oxcarbazepine	Enhances the metabolism of everolimus
Consequence	Plasma everolimus levels are decreased [3]
Phenobarbital	Enhances the metabolism of everolimus
Consequence	Plasma everolimus levels are decreased [3]
Phenytoin	Enhances the metabolism of everolimus
Consequence	Plasma everolimus levels are decreased [3]
Piracetam	The interaction has not been investigated. Theoretically, a pharmacokinetic interaction would not be anticipated
Pregabalin	The interaction has not been investigated. Theoretically, a pharmacokinetic interaction would not be anticipated
Primidone	The interaction has not been investigated. Theoretically, a pharmacokinetic interaction similar to that seen with phenobarbital can be expected
Rufinamide	The interaction has not been investigated. Theoretically, a pharmacokinetic interaction would not be anticipated
Stiripentol	Inhibits the metabolism of everolimus
Consequence	Plasma everolimus levels are increased [3]
Sulthiame	The interaction has not been investigated. Theoretically, a pharmacokinetic interaction could occur
Tiagabine	The interaction has not been investigated. Theoretically, a pharmacokinetic interaction would not be anticipated
Topiramate	The interaction has not been investigated. Theoretically, a pharmacokinetic interaction could occur
Valproic acid	The interaction has not been investigated. Theoretically, a pharmacokinetic interaction could occur
Vigabatrin	The interaction has not been investigated. Theoretically, a pharmacokinetic interaction would not be anticipated
Zonisamide	The interaction has not been investigated. Theoretically, a pharmacokinetic interaction would not be anticipated

References

1. Ebrahim-Fakhari D, Agricola KD, Tudor C, Krueger D, Franz DN. Cannabidiol elevates mechanistic target of rapamycin inhibitor levels in patients with tuberous sclerosis complex. Pediatr Neurol. 2020;105:59–61.
2. Wiemer-Kruel A, Stiller B, Bast T. Cannabidiol interacts significantly with everolimus – report of a patient with tuberous sclerosis complex. Neuropediatrics. 2019;50:400–3.
3. Bialer M, Johannessen SI, Levy RH, Levy RH, Perucca E, Tomson T, White HS. Progress report on new antiepileptic drugs: a summary of the thirteenth Eilat conference on new antiepileptic drugs and devices (EILAT XII). Epiepsia. 2017;58:181–221.

Felbamate

Felbamate (Fig. 1) corresponds chemically to 2-phenyl-1,3-propanediol dicarbamate with an empirical formula of $C_{11}H_{14}N_2O_4$ and a molecular weight of 238.24.

Pharmacokinetic Characteristics

Absorption and Distribution

After oral ingestion, felbamate is rapidly absorbed (T_{max} = 2–6 h) with a bioavailability of >90%. Its volume of distribution is 0.7–0.91 L/kg, and plasma protein binding is 25%.

Fig. 1 Felbamate

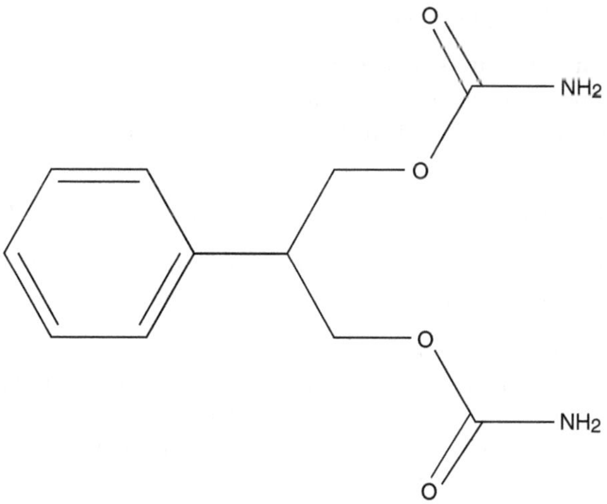

P. N. Patsalos, *Antiseizure Medication Interactions*,
https://doi.org/10.1007/978-3-030-82790-8_12

Biotransformation

Only 50% of an administered dose is metabolized in the liver, by CYP3A4 and CYP2E1, to form two hydroxylated metabolites (*para*-hydroxyfelbamate and 2-hydroxyfelbamate—10–15%) and a variety of other unidentified polar metabolites, some of them being glucuronides or sulfate esters. The atropaldehyde (2-phenylpropenal) metabolite may contribute to the cytotoxicity seen in some patients treated with felbamate.

Renal Excretion

Approximately 50% of an administered dose is excreted as unchanged felbamate in urine.

Elimination

In adult volunteers, plasma elimination half-life values are 16–22 h, while in patients co-prescribed with enzyme-inducing antiseizure medications, half-life values are 10–18 h.

Time to new steady-state felbamate blood levels consequent to an inhibition of metabolism interaction:

- Adults = 3–5 days later

Effects on Isoenzymes

At therapeutic concentrations, felbamate in vitro inhibits the activity of CYP2C19. Consequently, pharmacokinetic interactions of metabolic origin with other antiseizure medications and other medicines can be expected.

Felbamate has no in vitro inhibitory effect on the activity of CYP1A2, CYP2A6, CYP2C9, CYP2D6, CYP2E1, and CYP3A4.

No in vitro data on the induction potential of felbamate on human CYP enzymes have been published.

Therapeutic Drug Monitoring

Optimum seizure control in patients on felbamate monotherapy is most likely to occur at plasma felbamate levels of 30–60 mg/L (125–250 μmol/L). The conversion factor from mg/L to μmol/L for felbamate is 4.20 (i.e., 1 mg/L = 4.20 μmol/L).

Propensity to Be Associated with Pharmacokinetic Interactions

- Felbamate affects the pharmacokinetics of other drugs—minimal.
- Other drugs affect the pharmacokinetics of felbamate—minimal.

Interactions with ASMs

Acetazolamide	The interaction has not been investigated. Theoretically, a pharmacokinetic interaction would not be anticipated
Brivaracetam	The interaction has not been investigated. Theoretically, a pharmacokinetic interaction would not be anticipated
Cannabidiol	The interaction has not been investigated. Theoretically, a pharmacokinetic interaction would not be anticipated
Carbamazepine	Enhances the metabolism of felbamate

Consequence	Mean plasma felbamate levels can decrease by 17%. The interaction is the consequence of the induction of felbamate metabolism through CYP3A4 [1]
Cenobamate	The interaction has not been investigated. Theoretically, a pharmacokinetic interaction could occur
Clobazam	The interaction has not been investigated. Theoretically, a pharmacokinetic interaction would not be anticipated
Clonazepam	Does not affect the pharmacokinetics of felbamate [2]
Eslicarbazepine acetate	The interaction has not been investigated. Theoretically, a pharmacokinetic interaction would not be anticipated
Ethosuximide	The interaction has not been investigated. Theoretically, a pharmacokinetic interaction would not be anticipated
Everolimus	The interaction has not been investigated. Theoretically, a pharmacokinetic interaction could occur
Fenfluramine	The interaction has not been investigated. Theoretically, a pharmacokinetic interaction could occur
Gabapentin	Decreases the elimination of felbamate
Consequence	The mean plasma elimination half-life of felbamate can be increased by 46%, and mean plasma clearance decreased by 37%. This interaction is considered to occur at the level of renal excretion [3]
Lacosamide	The interaction has not been investigated. Theoretically, a pharmacokinetic interaction would not be anticipated
Lamotrigine	Does not affect the pharmacokinetics of felbamate [4]
Levetiracetam	The interaction has not been investigated. Theoretically, a pharmacokinetic interaction would not be anticipated
Methsuximide	The interaction has not been investigated. Theoretically, a pharmacokinetic interaction would not be anticipated
Perampanel	The interaction has not been investigated. Theoretically, a pharmacokinetic interaction would not be anticipated
Oxcarbazepine	Does not affect the pharmacokinetics of felbamate [5]
Phenobarbital	Does not affect the pharmacokinetics of felbamate [6]
Phenytoin	Enhances the metabolism of felbamate
Consequence	Mean plasma felbamate levels can decrease by 51%. The interaction is the consequence of the induction of felbamate metabolism through CYP3A4 [2]
Piracetam	The interaction has not been investigated. Theoretically, a pharmacokinetic interaction would not be anticipated
Pregabalin	The interaction has not been investigated. Theoretically, a pharmacokinetic interaction would not be anticipated
Primidone	The interaction has not been investigated. Theoretically, a pharmacokinetic interaction similar to that seen with phenobarbital can be expected
Rufinamide	The interaction has not been investigated. Theoretically, a pharmacokinetic interaction would not be anticipated
Stiripentol	The interaction has not been investigated. Theoretically, a pharmacokinetic interaction could occur
Sulthiame	The interaction has not been investigated. Theoretically, a pharmacokinetic interaction could occur
Tiagabine	The interaction has not been investigated. Theoretically, a pharmacokinetic interaction would not be anticipated

Topiramate	The interaction has not been investigated. Theoretically, a pharmacokinetic interaction could occur
Valproic acid	Inhibits the metabolism of felbamate
Consequence	Mean plasma felbamate clearance values are decreased by 21%, and mean plasma felbamate levels can increase by 53% [7]
Vigabatrin	Does not affect the pharmacokinetics of felbamate [8]
Zonisamide	The interaction has not been investigated. Theoretically, a pharmacokinetic interaction could occur

References

1. Wagner ML, Graves NM, Marienau K, Holmes GB, Remmel RP, Leppik IE. Discontinuation of phenytoin and carbamazepine in patients receiving felbamate. Epilepsia. 1991;32:398–406.
2. Glue P, Banfield CR, Perhach JL, Mather GG, Racha JK, Levy RH. Pharmacokinetic interactions with felbamate. In vitro-in vivo correlation. Clin Pharmacokinet. 1997;33:214–24.
3. Hussein G, Troupin AS, Montouris G. Gabapentin interaction with felbamate. Neurology. 1996;47:1106.
4. Colucci R, Glue P, Holt B, Babfield C, Reidenberg P, Meechan JW, Pai S, Nomeir A, Lim J, Lin CC, Affrime MB. Effect of felbamate on the pharmacokinetics of lamotrigine. J Clin Pharmacol. 1996;36:634–8.
5. Hulsman JARJ, Rentmeester TW, Banfield CR, Reidenberg P, Colucci RD, Meehan JW, Radwanski E, Mojavarian P, Lin CC, Nezamis J, Affrime MB, Glue P. Effects of felbamate on the pharmacokinetics of the monohydroxy and dihydroxy metabolites of oxcarbazepine. Clin Pharmacol Ther. 1995;58:383–9.
6. Kelley MT, Walson PD, Cox S, Dusci LJ. Population pharmacokinetics of felbamate in children. Ther Drug Monit. 1997;19:29–36.
7. Wagner ML, Graves NM, Leppik IE, Remmel RP, Shmaker RC, Ward D, Perhach JL. The effect of felbamate on valproic acid disposition. Clin Pharmacol Ther. 1994;56:494–502.
8. Reidenberg P, Glue P, Banfield C, Colucci R, Meehan J, Rey E, Radwanski E, Nomeir A, Lim J, Lin C, Guillaume M, Affrime MB. Pharmacokinetic interaction studies between felbamate and vigabatrin. Br J Clin Pharmacol. 1995;40:157–60.

Fenfluramine

Fenfluramine (Fig. 1) corresponds chemically to 3-trifluoromethyl-N-ethylamphetamine with an empirical formula of $C_{12}H_{16}F_3N$ and a molecular weight of 231.26.

Pharmacokinetic Characteristics

Absorption and Distribution

After oral ingestion in healthy volunteers, fenfluramine is rapidly absorbed (T_{max} = ~3 h) with a bioavailability of 75–83%. Its volume of distribution is 11.9 L/kg, and plasma protein binding is 50%. The plasma protein binding of the pharmacologically active metabolite, norfenfluramine, is not known.

Biotransformation

Fenfluramine is extensively (75%) metabolized primarily by CYP1A2, CYP2B6 and CYP2D6, with additional metabolism via CYP2C9, CYP2C19 and CYP3A4. Norfenfluramine, which is pharmacologically active, is subsequently metabolized, via deamination and oxidation and possibly glucuronidation, to various pharmacologically inactive metabolites.

Fig. 1 Fenfluramine

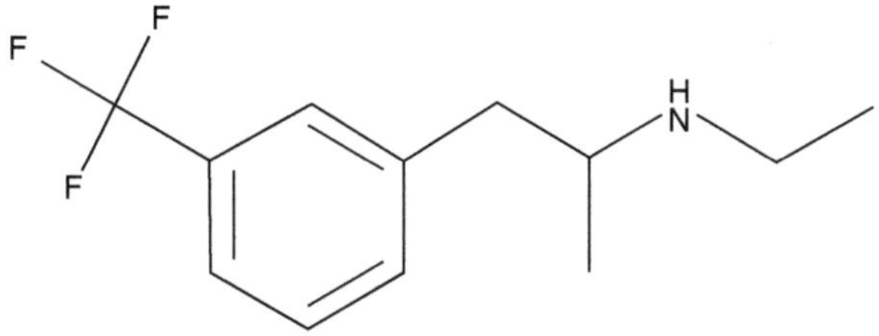

P. N. Patsalos, *Antiseizure Medication Interactions*,
https://doi.org/10.1007/978-3-030-82790-8_13

Renal Excretion

Approximately >90% of an administered dose is excreted in the urine primarily as metabolites.

Elimination

Plasma elimination half-life values for fenfluramine and norfenfluramine in normal adult volunteers are 20 h and 23 h, respectively.

Time to new steady-state blood levels consequent to an inhibition of metabolism interaction:

- Fenfluramine = 3–5 days later
- Norfenfluramine = 4–6 days later

Effects on Isoenzymes

In vitro, at clinically relevant concentrations, fenfluramine is an inhibitor of CYP2D6 and an inducer of CYP2B6 and CYP3A4. The transporter MATE-1 can be inhibited by norfenfluramine (the primary and pharmacologically active metabolite of fenfluramine) at clinically relevant concentrations. Neither fenfluramine nor norfenfluramine are substrates of PgP, BCRP, OATP1B, OATP1B3, OATP1A2, OATP2B1, OCT1, OAT1, OAT3, OCT2, MATE1 and MATE2-K.

Therapeutic Drug Monitoring

There are no data relating plasma fenfluramine levels with that of seizure suppression or adverse effects.

Propensity to Be Associated with Pharmacokinetic Interactions

- Fenfluramine affects the pharmacokinetics of other drugs—minimal.
- Other drugs affect the pharmacokinetics of fenfluramine—moderate.

Interactions with ASMs

Acetazolamide	The interaction has not been investigated. Theoretically, a pharmacokinetic interaction would not be anticipated
Brivaracetam	The interaction has not been investigated. Theoretically, a pharmacokinetic interaction would not be anticipated
Cannabidiol	Inhibits the metabolism of fenfluramine
Consequence	Fenfluramine AUC values can increase by 59% while norfenfluramine AUC values, the pharmacologically active metabolite of fenfluramine can decrease by 22% [1]
Carbamazepine	The interaction has not been investigated. Theoretically, a pharmacokinetic interaction could occur
Cenobamate	The interaction has not been investigated. Theoretically, a pharmacokinetic interaction would not be anticipated
Clobazam	Inhibits the metabolism of fenfluramine
Consequence	Fenfluramine AUC values can increase by a mean of 69% while norfenfluramine mean AUC values, the pharmacologically active metabolite of fenfluramine, can decrease by 59% [2]
Clonazepam	The interaction has not been investigated. Theoretically, a pharmacokinetic interaction would not be anticipated
Eslicarbazepine acetate	The interaction has not been investigated. Theoretically, a pharmacokinetic interaction would not be anticipated

Ethosuximide	The interaction has not been investigated. Theoretically, a pharmacokinetic interaction would not be anticipated
Everolimus	The interaction has not been investigated. Theoretically, a pharmacokinetic interaction could occur
Felbamate	The interaction has not been investigated. Theoretically, a pharmacokinetic interaction could occur
Gabapentin	The interaction has not been investigated. Theoretically, a pharmacokinetic interaction would not be anticipated
Lacosamide	The interaction has not been investigated. Theoretically, a pharmacokinetic interaction would not be anticipated
Lamotrigine	The interaction has not been investigated. Theoretically, a pharmacokinetic interaction would not be anticipated
Levetiracetam	The interaction has not been investigated. Theoretically, a pharmacokinetic interaction would not be anticipated
Methsuximide	The interaction has not been investigated. Theoretically, a pharmacokinetic interaction would not be anticipated
Oxcarbazepine	The interaction has not been investigated. Theoretically, a pharmacokinetic interaction could occur
Perampanel	The interaction has not been investigated. Theoretically, a pharmacokinetic interaction would not be anticipated
Phenobarbital	The interaction has not been investigated. Theoretically, a pharmacokinetic interaction could occur
Phenytoin	The interaction has not been investigated. Theoretically, a pharmacokinetic interaction could occur
Piracetam	The interaction has not been investigated. Theoretically, a pharmacokinetic interaction would not be anticipated
Pregabalin	The interaction has not been investigated. Theoretically, a pharmacokinetic interaction would not be anticipated
Primidone	The interaction has not been investigated. Theoretically, a pharmacokinetic interaction could occur
Rufinamide	The interaction has not been investigated. Theoretically, a pharmacokinetic interaction would not be anticipated
Stiripentol	Inhibits the metabolism of fenfluramine
Consequence	Fenfluramine AUC values can increase by a mean of 69% while norfenfluramine mean AUC values, the pharmacologically active metabolite of fenfluramine, can decrease by 59% [2]
Sulthiame	The interaction has not been investigated. Theoretically, a pharmacokinetic interaction would not be anticipated
Tiagabine	The interaction has not been investigated. Theoretically, a pharmacokinetic interaction would not be anticipated
Topiramate	The interaction has not been investigated. Theoretically, a pharmacokinetic interaction could occur
Valproic acid	Inhibits the metabolism of fenfluramine
Consequence	Fenfluramine AUC values can increase by a mean of 69% while norfenfluramine mean AUC values can decrease by 59% [2]
Vigabatrin	The interaction has not been investigated. Theoretically, a pharmacokinetic interaction would not be anticipated
Zonisamide	The interaction has not been investigated. Theoretically, a pharmacokinetic interaction would not be anticipated

References

1. Summary of product characteristics: Fenfluramine (Fintepla). ZogenIix Int. Ltd. Last update 6 Jan 2021.
2. Boyd B, Smith S, Gammaitoni A, Galer BS, Farfel GM. A phase 1, randomized, open-label, single dose, 3 period crossover study to evaluate the drug-drug interaction between ZX008 (fenfluramine HCl oral solution) and a regimen of stiripentol, clobazam, and valproate in healthy subjects. Int J Clin Pharmaol Therapeut. 2019;57:11–9.

Gabapentin

Gabapentin (Fig. 1) corresponds chemically to 1-(aminomethyl)-cyclohexane acetic acid with an empirical formula of $C_9H_{17}NO_2$ and a molecular weight of 171.23.

Pharmacokinetic Characteristics

Absorption and Distribution

After oral ingestion, gabapentin is rapidly absorbed (T_{max} = 2–3 h) with a bioavailability of <60%. Its volume of distribution is 0.65–1.04 L/kg, and plasma protein binding is 0%.

Biotransformation

Gabapentin is not metabolized.

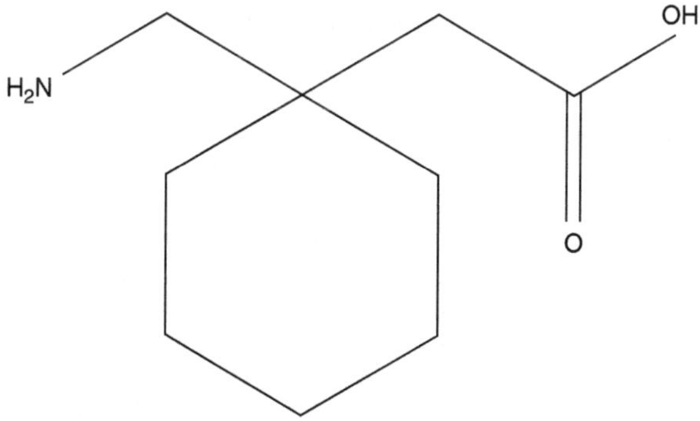

Fig. 1 Gabapentin

P. N. Patsalos, *Antiseizure Medication Interactions*, https://doi.org/10.1007/978-3-030-82790-8_14

Renal Excretion
Approximately 100% of an administered dose is excreted as unchanged gabapentin in urine.

Elimination
Following a single dose, plasma elimination half-life values in adults is 5–9 h.

Effects on Isoenzymes
No in vitro data on the induction or inhibition potential of gabapentin on human CYP or UGT isoenzymes have been published.

Therapeutic Drug Monitoring
Optimum seizure control in patients on gabapentin monotherapy is most likely to occur at plasma levels of 2–20 mg/L (12–117 μmol/L). The conversion factor from mg/L to μmol/L for gabapentin is 5.84 (i.e., 1 mg/L = 5.84 μmol/L).

Propensity to Be Associated with Pharmacokinetic Interactions
- Gabapentin affects the pharmacokinetics of other drugs—does not interact.
- Other drugs affect the pharmacokinetics of gabapentin—does not interact.

Interactions with ASMs

Acetazolamide	The interaction has not been investigated. Theoretically, a pharmacokinetic interaction would not be anticipated
Brivaracetam	The interaction has not been investigated. Theoretically, a pharmacokinetic interaction would not be anticipated
Cannabidiol	The interaction has not been investigated. Theoretically, a pharmacokinetic interaction would not be anticipated
Carbamazepine	Does not affect the pharmacokinetics of gabapentin [1]
Clobazam	The interaction has not been investigated. Theoretically, a pharmacokinetic interaction would not be anticipated
Cenobamate	The interaction has not been investigated. Theoretically, a pharmacokinetic interaction would not be anticipated
Clonazepam	The interaction has not been investigated. Theoretically, a pharmacokinetic interaction would not be anticipated
Eslicarbazepine acetate	Does not affect the pharmacokinetics of gabapentin [2]
Ethosuximide	The interaction has not been investigated. Theoretically, a pharmacokinetic interaction would not be anticipated
Everolimus	The interaction has not been investigated. Theoretically, a pharmacokinetic interaction would not be anticipated
Felbamate	The interaction has not been investigated. Theoretically, a pharmacokinetic interaction would not be anticipated
Fenfluramine	The interaction has not been investigated. Theoretically, a pharmacokinetic interaction would not be anticipated
Lacosamide	Does not affect the pharmacokinetics of gabapentin [3]
Lamotrigine	The interaction has not been investigated. Theoretically, a pharmacokinetic interaction would not be anticipated
Levetiracetam	Does not affect the pharmacokinetics of gabapentin [4]
Methsuximide	The interaction has not been investigated. Theoretically, a pharmacokinetic interaction would not be anticipated

Oxcarbazepine	The interaction has not been investigated. Theoretically, a pharmacokinetic interaction would not be anticipated
Perampanel	The interaction has not been investigated. Theoretically, a pharmacokinetic interaction would not be anticipated
Phenobarbital	Does not affect the pharmacokinetics of gabapentin [5]
Phenytoin	Does not affect the pharmacokinetics of gabapentin [6]
Piracetam	The interaction has not been investigated. Theoretically, a pharmacokinetic interaction would not be anticipated
Pregabalin	Does not affect the pharmacokinetics of gabapentin [7]
Primidone	The interaction has not been investigated. Theoretically, a pharmacokinetic interaction would not be anticipated
Rufinamide	The interaction has not been investigated. Theoretically, a pharmacokinetic interaction would not be anticipated
Stiripentol	The interaction has not been investigated. Theoretically, a pharmacokinetic interaction would not be anticipated
Sulthiame	The interaction has not been investigated. Theoretically, a pharmacokinetic interaction would not be anticipated
Tiagabine	The interaction has not been investigated. Theoretically, a pharmacokinetic interaction would not be anticipated
Topiramate	The interaction has not been investigated. Theoretically, a pharmacokinetic interaction would not be anticipated
Valproic acid	Does not affect the pharmacokinetics of gabapentin [1]
Vigabatrin	The interaction has not been investigated. Theoretically, a pharmacokinetic interaction would not be anticipated
Zonisamide	The interaction has not been investigated. Theoretically, a pharmacokinetic interaction would not be anticipated

References

1. Radulovic LL, Wilder BJ, Leppik IE, Bockbrader HN, Chang T, Posvar EL, Sedman AJ, Uthman BM, Erdman GR. Lack of interaction of gabapentin with carbamazepine and valproate. Epilepsia. 1994;35:155–61.
2. Falcao A, Fuseau E, Nunes T, Almeida L, Soares-da-Silva P. Pharmacokinetics, drug interactions and exposure-response relationships of eslicarbazepine acetate in adult patients with partial-onset seizures: population pharmacokinetic and pharmacokinetic/pharmacodynamic analysis. CNS Drugs. 2012;26:79–91.
3. Sachdeo R. Lacosamide. In: Shorvon SD, Perucca E, Engel J, editors. The treatment of epilepsy. 3rd ed. Oxford: Blackwell; 2009. p. 527–34.
4. Perucca E, Baltes E, Ledent E. Levetiracetam: absence of pharmacokinetic interactions with other antiepileptic drugs (AEDs). Epilepsia. 2000;41(Suppl):150.
5. Hooper WD, Kavanagh MC, Herkes GK, Eadie MJ. Lack of a pharmacokinetic interaction between phenobarbitone and gabapentin. Br J Clin Pharmacol. 1991;31:171–4.
6. Graves NM, Holmes GB, Leppik IE, et al. Pharmacokinetics of gabapentin in patients treated with phenytoin. Pharmacotherapy. 1989;9:196.
7. Ben-Menachem E. Pregabalin pharmacology and its relevance to clinical practice. Epilepsia. 2004;45(Suppl 6):13–8.

Lacosamide

Lacosamide (Fig. 1) corresponds chemically to (R)-2acetamido-*N*-benzyl-3-methoxypropanamide with an empirical formula of $C_{13}H_{18}N_2O_3$ and a molecular weight of 250.29.

Pharmacokinetic Characteristics

Absorption and Distribution

After oral ingestion, lacosamide is rapidly absorbed (T_{max} = 1–2 h) with a bioavailability of 100%. Its volume of distribution is 0.6–0.7 L/kg, and plasma protein binding is <30%.

Biotransformation

Lacosamide is moderately metabolized in the liver, by demethylation, to *O*-desmethyl lacosamide (30%) and to other unidentified metabolites (30%). The formation of *O*-desmethyl lacosamide is due to CYP2C19.

Fig. 1 Lacosamide

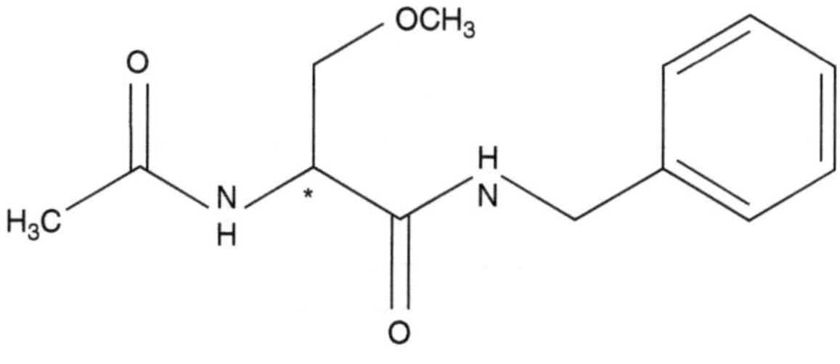

P. N. Patsalos, *Antiseizure Medication Interactions*,
https://doi.org/10.1007/978-3-030-82790-8_15

Renal Excretion
Approximately 40% of an administered dose is excreted as unchanged lacosamide in urine.

Elimination
The plasma elimination half-life in healthy volunteers and in patients with epilepsy is 13 h.

Time to new steady-state lacosamide blood levels consequent to an inhibition of metabolism interaction:

- Adults = 2–3 days later

Effects on Isoenzymes
At therapeutic concentrations, lacosamide in vitro does not inhibit or induce the activities of CYP1A1, CYP1A2, CYP2A6, CYP2B6, CYP2C8, CYP2C9, CYP2D6, CYP2E1, and CYP3A4/5. Consequently, pharmacokinetic interactions of metabolic origin with other antiseizure medications and other medicines are not expected.

Therapeutic Drug Monitoring
Optimum seizure control in patients on lacosamide monotherapy is most likely to occur at plasma lacosamide levels of 10–20 mg/L (40–80 μmol/L). The conversion factor from mg/L to μmol/L for lacosamide is 3.99 (i.e., 1 mg/L = 3.99 μmol/L).

Propensity to Be Associated with Pharmacokinetic Interactions

- Lacosamide affects the pharmacokinetics of other drugs—does not interact.
- Other drugs affect the pharmacokinetics of lacosamide—minimal.

Interactions with ASMs

Acetazolamide	The interaction has not been investigated. Theoretically, a pharmacokinetic interaction would not be anticipated
Brivaracetam	Does not affect the pharmacokinetics of lacosamide [1]
Cannabidiol	Does not affect the pharmacokinetics of lacosamide [2]
Carbamazepine	Enhances the metabolism of lacosamide
Consequence	Mean plasma lacosamide levels can decrease by 26% [3, 4]
	Neurotoxicity may occur in combination with carbamazepine and other voltage-gated sodium channel blocking antiseizure medications, consequent to a pharmacodynamic interaction [5]
Cenobamate	Does not affect the pharmacokinetics of lacosamide [6]
Clobazam	The interaction has not been investigated. Theoretically, a pharmacokinetic interaction would not be anticipated
Clonazepam	The interaction has not been investigated. Theoretically, a pharmacokinetic interaction would not be anticipated
Eslicarbazepine acetate	The interaction has not been investigated. Theoretically, a pharmacokinetic interaction would not be anticipated
Ethosuximide	The interaction has not been investigated. Theoretically, a pharmacokinetic interaction would not be anticipated
Everolimus	The interaction has not been investigated. Theoretically, a pharmacokinetic interaction could occur

Felbamate	The interaction has not been investigated. Theoretically, a pharmacokinetic interaction would not be anticipated
Fenfluramine	The interaction has not been investigated. Theoretically, a pharmacokinetic interaction could occur
Gabapentin	The interaction has not been investigated. Theoretically, a pharmacokinetic interaction would not be anticipated
Lamotrigine	Does not affect the pharmacokinetics of lacosamide [7]
	Neurotoxicity may occur in combination with lamotrigine and other voltage-gated sodium channel blocking antiseizure medications, consequent to a pharmacodynamic interaction [5]
Levetiracetam	Does not affect the pharmacokinetics of lacosamide [7]
Methsuximide	Enhances the metabolism of lacosamide
Consequence	Mean plasma lacosamide levels can decrease by 41% [8]
Oxcarbazepine	Does not affect the pharmacokinetics of lacosamide [7]
	Neurotoxicity may occur in combination with oxcarbazepine and other voltage-gated sodium channel blocking antiseizure medications, consequent to a pharmacodynamic interaction [4]
Perampanel	The interaction has not been investigated. Theoretically, a pharmacokinetic interaction would not be anticipated
Phenobarbital	Enhances the metabolism of lacosamide
Consequence	Mean plasma lacosamide AUC values are decreased by ~30% [9]
Phenytoin	Enhances the metabolism of lacosamide
Consequence	Mean plasma lacosamide levels can decrease by 25% [3]
	Neurotoxicity may occur in combination with phenytoin and other voltage-gated sodium channel blocking antiseizure medications, consequent to a pharmacodynamic interaction [5]
Piracetam	The interaction has not been investigated. Theoretically, a pharmacokinetic interaction would not be anticipated
Pregabalin	The interaction has not been investigated. Theoretically, a pharmacokinetic interaction would not be anticipated
Primidone	Enhances the metabolism of lacosamide
Consequence	Mean plasma lacosamide levels can decrease by 34% [8]
Rufinamide	The interaction has not been investigated. Theoretically, a pharmacokinetic interaction would not be anticipated
Stiripentol	The interaction has not been investigated. Theoretically, a pharmacokinetic interaction would not be anticipated
Sulthiame	The interaction has not been investigated. Theoretically, a pharmacokinetic interaction would not be anticipated
Tiagabine	The interaction has not been investigated. Theoretically, a pharmacokinetic interaction would not be anticipated
Topiramate	Does not affect the pharmacokinetics of lacosamide [7]
Valproic acid	Does not affect the pharmacokinetics of lacosamide [10]
	Hyperammonemic encephalopathy may occur in combination with valproic acid consequent to a pharmacodynamic interaction [11]
Vigabatrin	The interaction has not been investigated. Theoretically, a pharmacokinetic interaction would not be anticipated
Zonisamide	The interaction has not been investigated. Theoretically, a pharmacokinetic interaction would not be anticipated

References

1. Moseley BD, Otoul C, Staelens L, Stockis A. Pharmacokinetic interaction of brivaracetam on other antiepileptic drugs in adults with focal seizures: pooled analysis of data from randomized clinical trials. Epilepsy Res. 2019;158:106218.
2. Gaston TE, Bekib EM, Cutter GR, Liu Y, Szaflarski JP, UAB CBD Program. Interactions between cannabidiol and commonly used antiepileptic drugs. Epilepsia. 2017;58:1586–92.
3. Markoula S, Teotonio R, Ratnaraj N, Duncan JS, Sander JW, Patsalos PN. Lacosamide serum concentrations in adult patients with epilepsy: the influence of gender, age, dose, and concomitant antiepileptic drugs. Ther Drug Monit. 2014;36:494–8.
4. Contin M, Albani F, Riva R, Candela C, Mohamed S, Baruzzi A. Lacosamide therapeutic monitoring in patients with epilepsy: effect of concomitant antiepileptic drugs. Ther Drug Monit. 2013;35:849–52.
5. Novy J, Patsalos PN, Sander JW, Sisodiya SM. Lacosamide neurotoxicity associated with concomitant use of sodium-blocking antiepileptic drugs: a pharmacodynamic interaction? Epilepsy Behav. 2011;20:20–3.
6. Bialer M, Johannessen SI, Koepp MJ, Levy RH, Perucca E, Perucca P, Tomson T, White HS. Progress report on new antiepiletis drugs: a summary of the fifteenth Eilat conference on new antiepileptic drugs and devices (EILAT XV). II. Drugs in more advanced clinical development. Epilepsia. 2020;61:2365–85.
7. Thomas D, Scharfenecker U, Schiltmeyer B, Doty P, Cawello W, Horstmann R. Low potential for drug-drug interactions of lacosamide. Epilepsia. 2006;47(Suppl 4):200.
8. May TW, Helmer R, Bien CG, Brandt C. Influence of dose and antiepileptic comedication on lacosamide serum concentrations in patients with epilepsy of different ages. Ther Drug Monit. 2018;40:620–7.
9. Nickel B, Zisowsky J, Cawello W, Lovern M, Sargentini-Maier ML. Population pharmacokinetics of LCM in subjects with partial onset seizures: results from two phase III trials. J Clin Pharmacol. 2008;48:1129.
10. Cawello W, Bonn R. No pharmacokinetic interaction between lacosamide and valproic acid in healthy volunteers. J Clin Pharmacol. 2012;52:1739–48.
11. Jones GL, Popli GS, Silvia MT. Lacosamide-induced valproic acid toxicity. Pediatr Neurol. 2013;48:308–10.

Lamotrigine

Lamotrigine (Fig. 1) corresponds chemically to 3,5-diamino-6[2,3-dichlorophenyl]-1,2,4-triazine with an empirical formula of $C_9H_7Cl_2N_5$ and a molecular weight of 256.09.

Pharmacokinetic Characteristics

Absorption and Distribution

After oral ingestion, lamotrigine is rapidly absorbed (T_{max} = 1–3 h) with a bioavailability of ≥95%. Its volume of distribution is 0.9–1.3 L/kg, and plasma protein binding is 55%.

Biotransformation

Lamotrigine undergoes extensive metabolism in the liver, by conjugation with glucuronic acid, to various metabolites including 2-*N*-glucuronide (76% of dose) and

Fig. 1 Lamotrigine

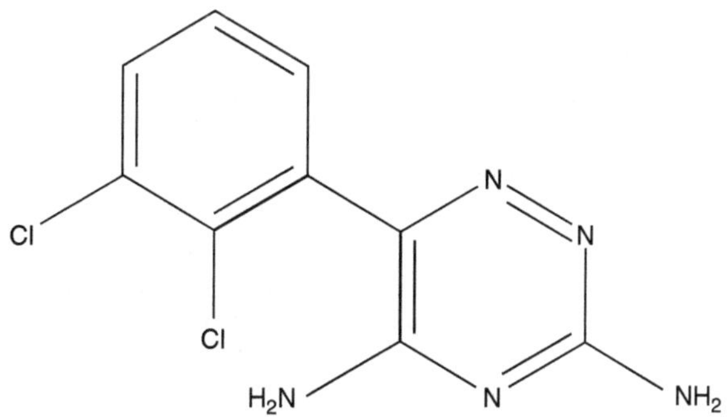

P. N. Patsalos, *Antiseizure Medication Interactions*,
https://doi.org/10.1007/978-3-030-82790-8_16

5-*N*-glucuronide (10% of dose), a 2-*N*-methyl metabolite (0.14% of dose), and other unidentified minor metabolites (4% of dose). Glucuronidation is primarily via UGT1A4, but UGT1A1 and UGT2B7 also contribute. Lamotrigine undergoes autoinduction so that clearance can increase by 17–37%, and this may require an upward dosage adjustment, particularly when prescribed as monotherapy.

Renal Excretion
Approximately 10% of an administered dose is excreted as unchanged lamotrigine in urine.

Elimination
In the absence of enzyme-inducing antiseizure medications, plasma elimination half-life values in adults are 15–35 h while in the presence of enzyme-inducing antiseizure medications, half-life values are 8–20 h. In the absence of enzyme-inducing antiseizure medications, but with valproic acid comedication, half-life values are 30–90 h. In the presence of enzyme-inducing antiseizure medications, and also with valproic acid comedication, half-life values are 15–35 h.

Time to new steady-state lamotrigine blood levels consequent to an inhibition of metabolism interaction:

- Adults = 3–7 days later

Effects on Isoenzymes
No in vitro data on the induction or inhibition potential of lamotrigine on human CYP or UGT isoenzymes have been published.

Therapeutic Drug Monitoring
Optimum seizure control in patients on lamotrigine monotherapy is most likely to occur at plasma lamotrigine levels of 3–15 mg/L (12–58 µmol/L). The conversion factor from mg/L to µmol/L for lamotrigine is 3.90 (i.e., 1 mg/L = 3.90 µmol/L).

Propensity to Be Associated with Pharmacokinetic Interactions
- Lamotrigine affects the pharmacokinetics of other drugs—minimal.
- Other drugs affect the pharmacokinetics of lamotrigine—moderate.

Interactions with ASMs

Acetazolamide	The interaction has not been investigated. Theoretically, a pharmacokinetic interaction would not be anticipated
Brivaracetam	Does not affect the pharmacokinetics of lamotrigine [1]
Cannabidiol	Does not affect the pharmacokinetics of lamotrigine [2]
Carbamazepine	Enhances the metabolism of lamotrigine
Consequence	Mean plasma lamotrigine clearance is increased by 30–50%, resulting in decreased plasma lamotrigine levels. The interaction is the consequence of the induction of lamotrigine metabolism through UGT1A4 glucuronidation [3]
	The high frequency of neurotoxicity observed with this drug combination represents a pharmacodynamic rather than pharmacokinetic interaction [4]
Cenobamate	Enhances the metabolism of lamotrigine

Consequence	Mean plasma lamotrigine concentrations, based on population pharmacokinetic analysis, are decreased by 21–52% during comedication with lamotrigine [5]
Clobazam	Does not affect the pharmacokinetics of lamotrigine [6]
Clonazepam	Does not affect the pharmacokinetics of lamotrigine [6]
Eslicarbazepine acetate	Enhances the metabolism of lamotrigine
Consequence	Mean plasma lamotrigine Cmax and AUC values can decrease by 13% and 14%, respectively [7]
Ethosuximide	Does not affect the pharmacokinetics of lamotrigine [6]
Everolimus	The interaction has not been investigated. Theoretically, a pharmacokinetic interaction could occur
Felbamate	Inhibits the metabolism of lamotrigine
Consequence	Mean plasma lamotrigine Cmax and AUC values can be increased by 13% and 14%, respectively [8]
Fenfluramine	The interaction has not been investigated. Theoretically, a pharmacokinetic interaction could occur
Gabapentin	Does not affect the pharmacokinetics of lamotrigine [6]
Lacosamide	Does not affect the pharmacokinetics of lamotrigine [9]
	Neurotoxicity may occur in combination with lamotrigine and other voltage-gated sodium channel blocking antiseizure medications, consequent to a pharmacodynamic interaction [10]
Levetiracetam	Does not affect the pharmacokinetics of lamotrigine [3]
Methsuximide	Enhances the metabolism of lamotrigine
Consequence	Mean plasma lamotrigine levels can be decreased by 36–72%. The interaction is the consequence of the induction of lamotrigine metabolism through UGT1A4 glucuronidation [11]
Oxcarbazepine	Enhances the metabolism of lamotrigine
Consequence	Mean plasma lamotrigine levels can be decreased by 34%. The interaction is the consequence of induction of lamotrigine metabolism, probably through UGT1A4 glucuronidation [12]
Perampanel	Enhances the metabolism of lamotrigine
Consequence	Mean lamotrigine clearance is increased by 9.3% [13]
Phenobarbital	Enhances the metabolism of lamotrigine
Consequence	Clearance can be increased by 100%, and mean plasma lamotrigine levels can be decreased [14]
Phenytoin	Enhances the metabolism of lamotrigine
Consequence	Mean plasma lamotrigine clearance is increased by 125%, resulting in decreased plasma lamotrigine levels. The interaction is the consequence of the induction of lamotrigine metabolism through UGT1A4 glucuronidation [3]
	During combination therapy with phenytoin, drug-induced chorea can occur. This is considered to be the consequence of a pharmacodynamic interaction [15]
Piracetam	The interaction has not been investigated. Theoretically, a pharmacokinetic interaction would not be anticipated
Pregabalin	Does not affect the pharmacokinetics of lamotrigine [16]
Primidone	Enhances the metabolism of lamotrigine

Consequence	Mean plasma lamotrigine clearance can be increased by 100%, and mean plasma lamotrigine levels can be decreased [3, 14]
Rufinamide	Enhances the metabolism of lamotrigine
Consequence	Plasma lamotrigine clearance is increased by 8–16% so that plasma lamotrigine levels are decreased by 7–13%. The interaction is probably the consequence of the induction of UGT1A4 [17]
Stiripentol	The interaction has not been investigated. Theoretically, a pharmacokinetic interaction could occur
Sulthiame	Inhibits the metabolism of lamotrigine
Consequence	Plasma lamotrigine levels can be increased [18]
Tiagabine	Does not affect the pharmacokinetics of lamotrigine [6]
Topiramate	Does not affect the pharmacokinetics of lamotrigine [19]
	Topiramate and lamotrigine can have a synergistic anticonvulsant effect consequent to a pharmacodynamic interaction [20]
Valproic acid	Inhibits the metabolism of lamotrigine
Consequence	Mean plasma lamotrigine clearance is decreased by 60%, resulting in increased plasma lamotrigine levels. The interaction is the consequence of inhibition of lamotrigine metabolism through UGT1A4 glucuronidation [3]
	Concurrent valproic acid therapy is a risk factor for the development of skin rash with lamotrigine. The introduction of lamotrigine to patients already taking valproic acid should be undertaken with caution, using a low starting dose and a slow-dose escalation rate. However, there is no risk of the rash if valproic acid is introduced to patients already stabilized on lamotrigine [21]
	During combination therapy, valproic acid synergistically enhances the antiseizure efficacy (partial and generalized seizures) and toxicity of lamotrigine. This is considered to be the consequence of a pharmacodynamic interaction [22–24]
	A case of delirium has been reported when valproic acid was added to lamotrigine. This effect is probably the consequence of a pharmacodynamic interaction [25]
Vigabatrin	Does not affect the pharmacokinetics of lamotrigine [3]
	Lamotrigine and vigabatrin in combination may be associated with synergistic efficacy in patients with partial and secondary generalized tonic-clonic seizures consequent to a pharmacodynamic interaction [26]
Zonisamide	Does not affect the pharmacokinetics of lamotrigine [27]

References

1. Moseley BD, Otoul C, Staelens L, Stockis A. Pharmacokinetic interaction of brivaracetam on other antiepileptic drugs in adults with focal seizures: pooled analysis of data from randomized clinical trials. Epilepsy Res. 2019;158:106218.
2. Gaston TE, Bekib EM, Cutter GR, Liu Y, Szaflarski JP, UAB CBD Program. Interactions between cannabidiol and commonly used antiepileptic drugs. Epilepsia. 2017;58:1586–92.
3. Weintraub D, Buchsbaum R, Resor SR, Hirsch LJ. Effect of antiepileptic drug comedication on lamotrigine clearance. Arch Neurol. 2005;62:1432–6.
4. Besag FM, Berry DJ, Pool F, Newbery JE, Subel B. Carbamazepine toxicity with lamotrigine: pharmacokinetic or pharmacodynamic interaction? Epilepsia. 1998;39:183–7.
5. Summary of product characteristics: Cenobamate (XCopri). SK Life Science Inc. Last update Aug 2020.

6. Armijo JA, Bravo J, Cuadrado A, Herranz JL. Lamotrigine serum concentration-to-dose ratio: influence of age and concomitant antiepileptic drugs and dosage implications. Ther Drug Monit. 1999;21:182–90.
7. Almeida L, Nunes T, Sicard E, Rocha JF, Falcao A, Brunet JS, Lefebvre M, Soares-da-Silva P. Pharmacokinetic interaction study between eslicarbazepine acetate and lamotrigine in healthy subjects. Acta Neurol Scand. 2010;121:257–64.
8. Colucci R, Glue P, Holt B, Banfield C, Reidenberg P, Meehan JW, Pai S, Nomeir A, Lim J, Lin CC, Affrime MB. Effect of felbamate on the pharmacokinetics of lamotrigine. J Clin Pharmacol. 1996;36:634–8.
9. Halasz P, Kalviainen R, Mazurkiewicz-Beldzinska M, Rosenow F, Doty P, Hebert D, Sullivan T. Adjunctive lacosamide for partial onset seizures: efficacy and safety results from a randomized controlled trial. Epilepsia. 2009;50:443–53.
10. Novy J, Patsalos PN, Sander JW, Sisodiya SM. Lacosamide neurotoxicity associated with concomitant use of sodium-blocking antiepileptic drugs: a pharmacodynamic interaction? Epilepsy Behav. 2011;20:20–3.
11. Besag FM, Berry DJ, Pool F. Methsuximide lowers lamotrigine blood levels: a pharmacokinetic antiepileptic drug interaction. Epilepsia. 2000;41:624–7.
12. May TW, Rambeck B, Jurgens U. Serum concentrations of lamotrigine in epileptic patients: the influence of dose and comedication. Ther Drug Monit. 1996;18:523–31.
13. Majid O, Laurenza A, Ferry J, Hussein Z. Impact of perampanel on pharmacokinetics of concomitant antiepileptics in patients with partial-onset seizures: pooled analysis of clinical trials. Br J Clin Pharmacol. 2016;82:422–30.
14. Rivas N, Buelga DS, Elger CE, Santos-Borbujo J, Otero MJ, Dominguez-Gil A, Garcia MJ. Population pharmacokinetics of lamotrigine with data from therapeutic drug monitoring in German and Spanish patients with epilepsy. Ther Drug Monit. 2008;30:483–9.
15. Zatreeh M, Tennison M, D'Cruz O, Beach RL. Anticonvulsant induced chorea: a role for pharmacodynamic drug interaction? Seizure. 2001;10:596–9.
16. Bockbrader HN, Burger P, Knapp L. Pregabalin effect on steady state pharmacokinetics of carbamazepine, lamotrigine, phenobarbital, phenytoin, topiramate, valproate, and tiagabine. Epilepsia. 2011;52:405–9.
17. Perucca E, Cloyd J, Critchley D, Fuseau E. Rufinamide: clinical pharmacokinetics and concentration-response relationships in patients with epilepsy. Epilepsia. 2008;49:1123–41.
18. Summary of product characteristics: Sulthiame (Ospolot). Phebra Pty, Ltd. Last update 21 Nov 2013.
19. Berry DJ, Besag FMC, Pool F, Natarajan J, Doose D. Lack of effect of topiramate on lamotrigine serum concentrations. Epilepsia. 2002;43:818–23.
20. Stephen LJ, Sills GJ, Brodie MJ. Lamotrigine and topiramate may be a useful combination. Lancet. 1998;351:958–9.
21. Kanner AM. When thinking of lamotrigine and valproic acid, think "pharmacokinetically". Epilepsy Curr. 2004;4:206–7.
22. Brodie MJ, Yuen AW. Lamotrigine substitution study: evidence for synergism with sodium valproate? 105 Study Group. Epilepsy Res. 1997;26:423–32.
23. Reutens DC, Duncan JS, Patsalos PN. Disabling tremor after lamotrigine with sodium valproate. Lancet. 1993;342:185–6.
24. Pisani F, Oteri G, Russo MF, Di Perri R, Perucca E, Richens A. The efficacy of valproate-lamotrigine comedication in refractory complex partial seizures: evidence for a pharmacodynamic interaction. Epilepsia. 1999;40:1141–6.
25. Mueller TH, Beeber AR. Delirium from valproic acid with lamotrigine. Am J Psychiatry. 2004;161:1128–9.
26. Stolarek I, Blacklaw J, Forrest G, Brodie MJ. Vigabatrin and lamotrigine in refractory epilepsy. J Neurol Neurosurg Psychiatry. 1994;57:921–4.
27. Levy RH, Ragueneau-Majlessi I, Brodie MJ, Smith DF, Shah J, Pan WJ. Lack of clinically significant pharmacokinetic interactions between zonisamide and lamotrigine at steady state in patients with epilepsy. Ther Drug Monit. 2005;27:193–8.

Levetiracetam

Levetiracetam (Fig. 1) corresponds chemically to (S)-alpha ethyl-2 oxo-1-pyrrolidine acetamide with an empirical formula of $C_8H_{14}N_2O_2$ and a molecular weight of 170.21.

Fig. 1 Levetiracetam

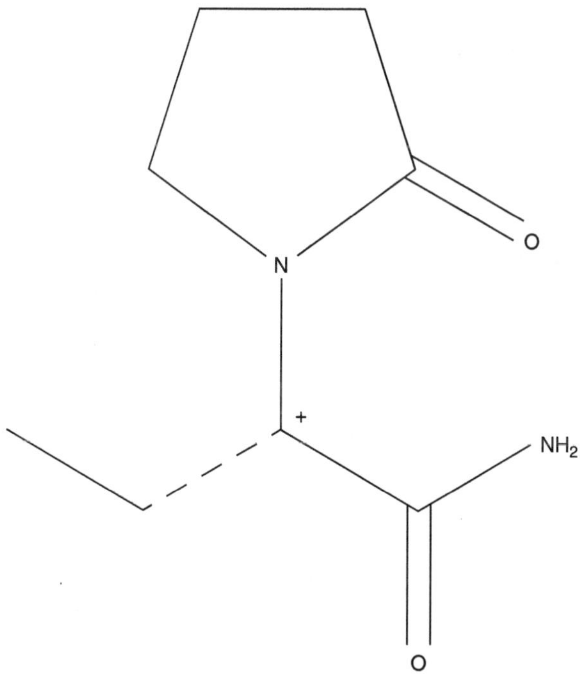

P. N. Patsalos, *Antiseizure Medication Interactions*,
https://doi.org/10.1007/978-3-030-82790-8_17

Pharmacokinetic Characteristics

Absorption and Distribution
After oral ingestion, levetiracetam is rapidly absorbed (T_{max} = 1–2 h) with a bioavailability of ≥95%. Its volume of distribution is 0.5–0.7 L/kg, and plasma protein binding is 0%.

Biotransformation
Levetiracetam undergoes minimal metabolism with ~30% of the dose metabolized by hydrolysis to a deaminated metabolite. This metabolism is independent of the hepatic cytochrome P450 system and is via a type-B esterase enzyme located in whole blood.

Renal Excretion
Approximately 66% of an administered dose is excreted as unchanged levetiracetam in urine.

Elimination
Plasma elimination half-life values are 6–8 h in adults, 5–6 h in children, and 10–11 h in the elderly.

Effects on Isoenzymes
At therapeutic concentrations, levetiracetam has no in vitro inhibitory or induction effects on the activity of CYP1A2, CYP2C9, CYP2D6, CYP2E1, CYP3A4, CYP2A6, epoxide hydrolase, UGT1*6, UGT1*1, UGT (pl6.2), and UDT glucuro-conjugating valproic acid. Consequently, pharmacokinetic interactions of metabolic origin with other antiseizure medications and other medicines are not expected.

Therapeutic Drug Monitoring
Optimum seizure control in patients on levetiracetam monotherapy is most likely to occur at plasma levetiracetam levels of 12–46 mg/L (70–270 μmol/L). The conversion factor from mg/L to μmol/L for levetiracetam is 5.88 (i.e., 1 mg/L = 5.88 μmol/L).

Propensity to Be Associated with Pharmacokinetic Interactions
- Levetiracetam affects the pharmacokinetics of other drugs—does not interact.
- Other drugs affect the pharmacokinetics of levetiracetam—minimal.

Interactions with ASMs

Acetazolamide	The interaction has not been investigated. Theoretically, a pharmacokinetic interaction would not be anticipated
Brivaracetam	Does not affect the pharmacokinetics of levetiracetam [1]
	The efficacy of brivaracetam is decreased when co-administered with levetiracetam consequent to a pharmacodynamic interaction [2]
Cannabidiol	Does not affect the pharmacokinetics of levetiracetam [3]
Carbamazepine	Enhances the metabolism of levetiracetam
Consequence	The mean plasma clearance of levetiracetam is increased by 81% [4]
	A pharmacodynamic interaction may occur whereby symptoms of carbamazepine toxicity present [5]

Cenobamate	Enhances the metabolism of levetiracetam
Consequence	Mean plasma levetiracetam concentrations, based on population pharmacokinetic analysis, are decreased by 2–13% during co-medication with cenobamate [6]
Clobazam	Does not affect the pharmacokinetics of levetiracetam [7]
Clonazepam	Does not affect the pharmacokinetics of levetiracetam [7]
Eslicarbazepine acetate	Does not affect the pharmacokinetics of levetiracetam [8]
Ethosuximide	Does not affect the pharmacokinetics of levetiracetam [7]
Everolimus	The interaction has not been investigated. Theoretically, a pharmacokinetic interaction would not be anticipated
Felbamate	Does not affect the pharmacokinetics of levetiracetam [9]
Fenfluramine	The interaction has not been investigated. Theoretically, a pharmacokinetic interaction would not be anticipated
Gabapentin	Does not affect the pharmacokinetics of levetiracetam [7]
Lacosamide	Enhances the metabolism of levetiracetam
Consequence	Plasma levetiracetam levels are decreased [10]
Lamotrigine	Enhances the metabolism of levetiracetam
Consequence	Levetiracetam plasma levels are decreased so that the median level to dose ratio for levetiracetam is decreased by 14% [11]
Methsuximide	Enhances the metabolism of levetiracetam
Consequence	Levetiracetam plasma levels are decreased so that the median level to dose ratio for levetiracetam is decreased by 27% [11]
Oxcarbazepine	Enhances the metabolism of levetiracetam
Consequence	The mean plasma clearance of levetiracetam is increased by 64% [4]
Perampanel	Does not affect the pharmacokinetics of levetiracetam [12]
	Perampanel, in combination with levetiracetam, is associated with an increased likelihood of developing fatigue. This effect may be the consequence of a pharmacodynamic interaction [13]
Phenobarbital	Enhances the metabolism of levetiracetam
Consequence	The mean plasma clearance of levetiracetam is increased by 44% [4]
Phenytoin	Enhances the metabolism of levetiracetam
Consequence	The mean plasma clearance of levetiracetam is increased by 26%, so that mean plasma AUC values are decreased by 21%. The mean plasma elimination half-life of levetiracetam can be decreased by 16% [4]
Piracetam	The interaction has not been investigated. Theoretically, a pharmacokinetic interaction would not be anticipated
Pregabalin	Does not affect the pharmacokinetics of levetiracetam [14]
Primidone	Does not affect the pharmacokinetics of levetiracetam [14]
Rufinamide	The interaction has not been investigated. Theoretically, a pharmacokinetic interaction would not be anticipated
Stiripentol	Does not affect the pharmacokinetics of levetiracetam [15]
Sulthiame	The interaction has not been investigated. Theoretically, a pharmacokinetic interaction would not be anticipated
Tiagabine	Does not affect the pharmacokinetics of levetiracetam [16]
Topiramate	Does not affect the pharmacokinetics of levetiracetam [16]
	A pharmacodynamic interaction may occur whereby symptoms of decreased appetite, weight loss, and nervousness present [8]

Valproic acid	Does not affect the pharmacokinetics of levetiracetam [17]
Vigabatrin	Does not affect the pharmacokinetics of levetiracetam [16]
Zonisamide	The interaction has not been investigated. Theoretically, a pharmacokinetic interaction would not be anticipated

References

1. Moseley BD, Otoul C, Staelens L, Stockis A. Pharmacokinetic interaction of brivaracetam on other antiepileptic drugs in adults with focal seizures: pooled analysis of data from randomized clinical trials. Epilepsy Res. 2019;158:106218.
2. Biton V, Berkovic SF, Abou-Khalil B, Sperling MR, Johnson ME, Lu S. Brivaracetam as adjunctive treatment for uncontrolled partial epilepsy in adults: a phase III randomized, double-blind, placebo-controlled trial. Epilepsia. 2014;55:57–66.
3. Gaston TE, Bekib EM, Cutter GR, Liu Y, Szaflarski JP, UAB CBD Program. Interactions between cannabidiol and commonly used antiepileptic drugs. Epilepsia. 2017;58:1586–92.
4. Aldaz A, Alzueta N, Viteri C. Influence of comedication on levetiracetam pharmacokinetics. Ther Drug Monit. 2018;40:130–4.
5. Sisodiya SM, Sander JW, Patsalos PN. Carbamazepine toxicity during combination therapy with levetiracetam: a pharmacodynamic interaction. Epilepsy Res. 2002;48:217–9.
6. Summary of product characteristics: Cenobamate (XCopri). SK Life Science Inc. Last update Aug 2020.
7. Patsalos PN. Clinical pharmacokinetics of levetiracetam. Clin Pharmacokinet. 2004;43:707–24.
8. Falcao A, Fuseau E, Nunes T, Almeida L, Soares-da-Silva P. Pharmacokinetics, drug interactions and exposure-response relationships of eslicarbazepine acetate in adult patients with partialonset seizures: population pharmacokinetic and pharmacokinetic/pharmacodynamic analysis. CNS Drugs. 2012;26:79–91.
9. Glauser TA, Pellock JM, Bebin EM, Fountain NB, Ritter FJ, Jensen CB, Shields WD. Efficacy and safety of levetiracetam in children with partial seizures: an open-label trial. Epilepsia. 2002;43:518–24.
10. Toutopoulou M, Weshke B, Kaindl AM. Lacsamide lowers valproate and levetiracetam levels. Neuropediatrics. 2017;48:188–9.
11. May TW, Rambeck B, Jurgens U. Serum concentrations of levetiracetam in epileptic patients: the influence of dose and co-medication. Ther Drug Monit. 2003;25:690–9.
12. Majid O, Laurenza A, Ferry J, Hussein Z. Impact of perampanel on pharmacokinetics of concomitant antiepileptics in patients with partial-onset: pooled analysis of clinical trials. Br J Clin Pharmacol. 2016;82:422–30.
13. Gidal BE, Ferry J, Majid O, Hussein Z. Concentration-effect relationships with perampanel in patients with pharmacoresistant partial-onset seizures. Epilepsia. 2013;54:1490–7.
14. Patsalos PN. Pharmacokinetic profile of levetiracetam: toward ideal characteristics. Pharmacol Ther. 2000;85:77–85.
15. Summary of product characteristics: Stiripentol (Diacomit). Alan Pharmceuticals. Last update 20 Sept 2018.
16. Patsalos PN. Levetiracetam: pharmacology and therapeutics in the treatment of epilepsy and other neurological conditions. Rev Contemp Pharmacother. 2004;13:1–168.
17. Coupez R, Nicolas JM, Browne TR. Levetiracetam, a new antiepileptic agent: lack of in vitro and in vivo pharmacokinetic interaction with valproic acid. Epilepsia. 2003;44:171–8.

Methsuximide

Methsuximide (Fig. 1) corresponds chemically to *N*-2-dimethyl-2-phenyl-succinimide with an empirical formula of $C_{12}H_{13}NO_2$ and a molecular weight of 203.23.

Pharmacokinetic Characteristics

Absorption and Distribution

After oral ingestion, methsuximide is rapidly absorbed with T_{max} values of 1–4 h for the pharmacologically active metabolite *N*-desmethylmethsuximide. Neither its oral bioavailability nor its volume of distribution has been established, but the plasma protein binding of *N*-desmethylmethsuximide is 45–60%.

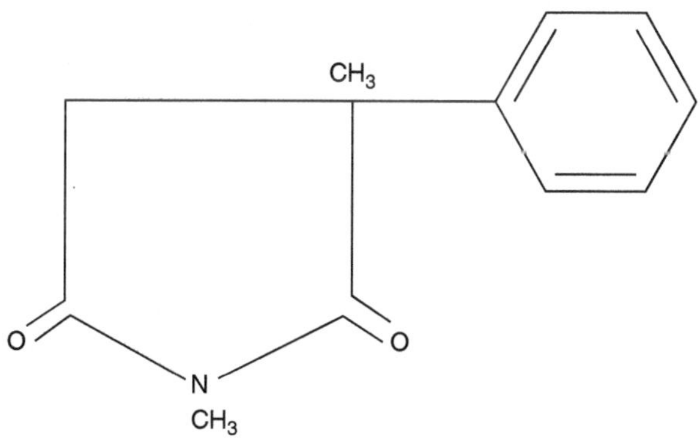

Fig. 1 Methsuximide

P. N. Patsalos, *Antiseizure Medication Interactions*,
https://doi.org/10.1007/978-3-030-82790-8_18

Biotransformation

Methsuximide is rapidly metabolized in the liver to its primary pharmacologically active metabolite *N*-desmethylmethsuximide, which is subsequently hydroxylated by CYP2C19.

Renal Excretion

Less than 1% of an administered dose is excreted as unchanged methsuximide in urine.

Elimination

Plasma elimination half-life values for methsuximide in adults are 1.0–2.6 h. Plasma elimination half-life values for *N*-desmethylmethsuximide are 34–80 h in adults and 16–45 h in children.

Effects on Isoenzymes

No in vitro data on the induction or inhibition potential of methsuximide on human CYP or UGT isoenzymes have been published.

Therapeutic Drug Monitoring

Optimum seizure control in patients on methsuximide monotherapy is most likely to occur at plasma *N*-desmethylmethsuximide levels of 10–40 mg/L (50–200 μmol/L). The conversion factor from mg/L to μmol/L for *N*-desmethylmethsuximide is 4.92 (i.e., 1 mg/L = 4.92 μmol/L).

Propensity to Be Associated with Pharmacokinetic Interactions

- Methsuximide affects the pharmacokinetics of other drugs—minimal.
- Other drugs affect the pharmacokinetics of methsuximide—minimal.

Interactions with ASMs

Acetazolamide	The interaction has not been investigated. Theoretically, a pharmacokinetic interaction would not be anticipated
Brivaracetam	The interaction has not been investigated. Theoretically, a pharmacokinetic interaction would not be anticipated
Cannabidiol	The interaction has not been investigated. Theoretically, a pharmacokinetic interaction would not be anticipated
Carbamazepine	The interaction has not been investigated. Theoretically, a pharmacokinetic interaction could occur
Cenobamate	The interaction has not been investigated. Theoretically, a pharmacokinetic interaction could occur
Clobazam	The interaction has not been investigated. Theoretically, a pharmacokinetic interaction would not be anticipated
Clonazepam	The interaction has not been investigated. Theoretically, a pharmacokinetic interaction would not be anticipated
Eslicarbazepine acetate	The interaction has not been investigated. Theoretically, a pharmacokinetic interaction would not be anticipated
Ethosuximide	The interaction has not been investigated. Theoretically, a pharmacokinetic interaction would not be anticipated
Everolimus	The interaction has not been investigated. Theoretically, a pharmacokinetic interaction could occur

Felbamate	Inhibits the metabolism of methsuximide
Consequence	*N*-desmethylmethsuximide (the pharmacologically active metabolite of methsuximide) plasma levels are increased by 26–46% [1]
Fenfluramine	The interaction has not been investigated. Theoretically, a pharmacokinetic interaction would not be anticipated
Gabapentin	The interaction has not been investigated. Theoretically, a pharmacokinetic interaction would not be anticipated
Lacosamide	The interaction has not been investigated. Theoretically, a pharmacokinetic interaction would not be anticipated
Lamotrigine	The interaction has not been investigated. Theoretically, a pharmacokinetic interaction would not be anticipated
Levetiracetam	The interaction has not been investigated. Theoretically, a pharmacokinetic interaction would not be anticipated
Oxcarbazepine	The interaction has not been investigated. Theoretically, a pharmacokinetic interaction could occur
Perampanel	The interaction has not been investigated. Theoretically, a pharmacokinetic interaction would not be anticipated
Phenobarbital	Enhances the metabolism of methsuximide
Consequence	The plasma clearance of methsuximide is increased so that *N*-desmethylmethsuximide/methsuximide plasma ratios are increased [2]
Phenytoin	Enhances the metabolism of methsuximide
Consequence	The plasma clearance of methsuximide is increased so that *N*-desmethylmethsuximide/methsuximide plasma ratios are increased [2]
Piracetam	The interaction has not been investigated. Theoretically, a pharmacokinetic interaction would not be anticipated
Pregabalin	The interaction has not been investigated. Theoretically, a pharmacokinetic interaction would not be anticipated
Primidone	The interaction has not been investigated. Theoretically, a pharmacokinetic interaction could occur
Rufinamide	The interaction has not been investigated. Theoretically, a pharmacokinetic interaction would not be anticipated
Stiripentol	The interaction has not been investigated. Theoretically, a pharmacokinetic interaction could occur
Sulthiame	The interaction has not been investigated. Theoretically, a pharmacokinetic interaction could occur
Tiagabine	The interaction has not been investigated. Theoretically, a pharmacokinetic interaction would not be anticipated
Topiramate	The interaction has not been investigated. Theoretically, a pharmacokinetic interaction could occur
Valproic acid	The interaction has not been investigated. Theoretically, a pharmacokinetic interaction could occur
Vigabatrin	The interaction has not been investigated. Theoretically, a pharmacokinetic interaction would not be anticipated
Zonisamide	The interaction has not been investigated. Theoretically, a pharmacokinetic interaction could occur

References

1. Patrias J, Espe-Lillo J, Ritter FJ. Felbamate-methsuximide interaction. Epilepsia. 1992;33(Suppl 3):84.
2. Rambeck B. Pharmacological interactions of methsuximide with phenobarbital and phenytoin in hospitalized epileptic patients. Epilepsia. 1979;20:147–56.

Oxcarbazepine

Oxcarbazepine (Fig. 1) corresponds chemically to 10,11-dihydro-10-oxo-5H--dibenz(b,f)azepine-4-carboxamide with an empirical formula of $C_{15}H_{12}N_2O_2$ and a molecular weight of 254.29.

Pharmacokinetic Characteristics

Absorption and Distribution

After oral ingestion, oxcarbazepine is rapidly absorbed with T_{max} values of 3–6 h and with a bioavailability of 100%. The volume of distribution of its pharmacologically active metabolite, 10-hydroxycarbazepine, is 0.75 L/kg. The protein binding of 10-hydroxycarbazepine is 40%, while that of oxcarbazepine it is 60%.

Fig. 1 Oxcarbazepine

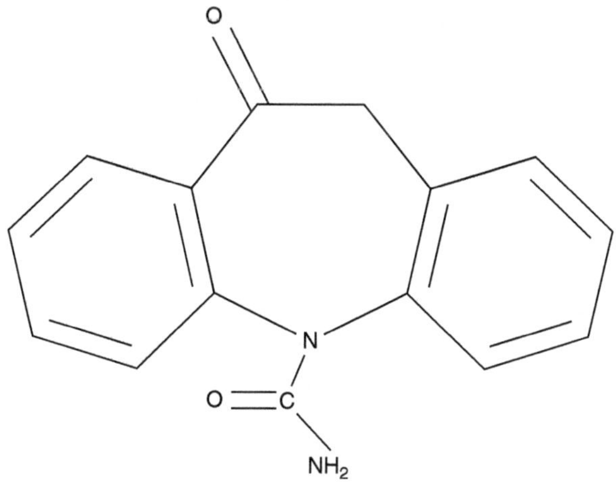

P. N. Patsalos, *Antiseizure Medication Interactions*,
https://doi.org/10.1007/978-3-030-82790-8_19

Biotransformation

Oxcarbazepine undergoes rapid and extensive metabolism to its pharmacologically active metabolite, 10-hydroxycarbazepine (also known as licarbazepine), by stereoselective biotransformation mediated by a cytosolic, non-microsomal, and non-inducible arylketone reductase. 10-hydroxycarbazepine subsequently undergoes glucuronidation (51%) or undergoes hydroxylation to form a dihydrodiol metabolite (28%). Minor amounts (4% of dose) of 10-hydroxycarbazepine are oxidized to an inactive 10,11-dihydroxy metabolite. Only the latter reaction depends on CYP isoenzymes.

Renal Excretion

Less than 1% of an administered dose is excreted as unchanged oxcarbazepine in urine.

Elimination

The plasma elimination half-life of oxcarbazepine is ~2 h; thus, oxcarbazepine is essentially a prodrug which is rapidly converted to its pharmacologically active 10-hydroxycarbazepine metabolite. In the absence of enzyme-inducing antiseizure medications, plasma half-life values for 10-hydroxycarbazepine are 8–15 h, while in the presence of enzyme-inducing antiseizure medications half-life values are 7–12 h.

Time to new steady-state blood levels consequent to an inhibition of metabolism interaction:

- Adults = 2–3 days later (10-hydroxycarbazepine)

Effects on Isoenzymes

No in vitro data on the induction or inhibition potential of 10-hydroxycarbazepine on human CYP or UGT isoenzymes have been published.

Therapeutic Drug Monitoring

Optimum seizure control in patients on oxcarbazepine monotherapy is most likely to occur at plasma 10-hydroxycarbazepine levels of 3–35 mg/L (12–137 µmol/L). The conversion factor from mg/L to µmol/L for 10-hydroxycarbazepine is 3.96 (i.e., 1 mg/L = 3.96 µmol/L).

During treatment with oxcarbazepine, only the pharmacologically active metabolite, 10-hydroxycarbazepine, is monitored because oxcarbazepine is very rapidly metabolized to its metabolite, and therefore, oxcarbazepine is essentially not detectable in blood by 1 h post-ingestion.

Propensity to Be Associated with Pharmacokinetic Interactions

- Oxcarbazepine affects the pharmacokinetics of other drugs—minimal.
- Other drugs affect the pharmacokinetics of oxcarbazepine—minimal.

Interactions with ASMs

Acetazolamide	The interaction has not been investigated. Theoretically, a pharmacokinetic interaction would not be anticipated
Brivaracetam	Does not affect the pharmacokinetics of 10-hydroxycarbazepine [1]
Cannabidiol	Does not affect the pharmacokinetics of 10-hydroxycarbazepine [2]

Carbamazepine	Enhances the metabolism of 10-hydroxycarbazepine
Consequence	Median plasma 10-hydroxycarbazepine AUC values can be decreased by 35% [3]
Cenobamate	Does not affect the pharmacokinetics of 10-hydroxycarbazepine [4]
Clobazam	Does not affect the pharmacokinetics of 10-hydroxycarbazepine [5]
Clonazepam	The interaction has not been investigated. Theoretically, a pharmacokinetic interaction would not be anticipated
Eslicarbazepine acetate	Eslicarbazepine acetate and oxcarbazepine in combination are contraindicated
Ethosuximide	The interaction has not been investigated. Theoretically, a pharmacokinetic interaction would not be anticipated
Everolimus	The interaction has not been investigated. Theoretically, a pharmacokinetic interaction could occur
Felbamate	Does not affect the pharmacokinetics of 10-hydroxycarbazepine [6]
Fenfluramine	The interaction has not been investigated. Theoretically, a pharmacokinetic interaction could occur
Gabapentin	The interaction has not been investigated. Theoretically, a pharmacokinetic interaction would not be anticipated
Lacosamide	Enhances the metabolism of 10-hydroxycarbazepine
Consequence	Mean plasma 10-hydroxycarbazepine levels can be decreased by 15% [7]
	Neurotoxicity may occur in combination with oxcarbazepine, and other voltage-gated sodium channel blocking antiseizure medications, consequent to a pharmacodynamic interaction [8]
Lamotrigine	Does not affect the pharmacokinetics of 10-hydroxycarbazepine [9]
Levetiracetam	The interaction has not been investigated. Theoretically, a pharmacokinetic interaction would not be anticipated
Methsuximide	The interaction has not been investigated. Theoretically, a pharmacokinetic interaction would not be anticipated
Perampanel	Inhibits the metabolism of oxcarbazepine
Consequence	Mean oxcarbazepine clearance can increase by 26% and mean oxcarbazepine plasma concentrations can decrease by 35%. The effect of perampanel on the metabolism of 10-hydroxycarbazepine has not been investigated [10]
	Perampanel in combination with oxcarbazepine is associated with an increased risk of decreased appetite. This effect may be the consequence of a pharmacodynamic interaction [11]
Phenobarbital	Enhances the metabolism of 10-hydroxycarbazepine
Consequence	Mean plasma 10-hydroxycarbazepine AUC values can decrease by 25% [12]
Phenytoin	Enhances the metabolism of 10-hydroxycarbazepine
Consequence	Mean plasma 10-hydroxycarbazepine AUC values can decrease by 32% [3]
Piracetam	The interaction has not been investigated. Theoretically, a pharmacokinetic interaction would not be anticipated
Pregabalin	The interaction has not been investigated. Theoretically, a pharmacokinetic interaction would not be anticipated
Primidone	The interaction has not been investigated. Theoretically, an interaction similar to that seen with phenobarbital can be expected
Rufinamide	The interaction has not been investigated. Theoretically, a pharmacokinetic interaction would not be anticipated
Stiripentol	The interaction has not been investigated. Theoretically, a pharmacokinetic interaction could occur

Sulthiame	The interaction has not been investigated. Theoretically, a pharmacokinetic interaction could occur
Tiagabine	The interaction has not been investigated. Theoretically, a pharmacokinetic interaction would not be anticipated
Topiramate	Does not affect the pharmacokinetics of 10-hydroxycarbazepine [9]
Valproic acid	Does not affect the pharmacokinetics of 10-hydroxycarbazepine [12]
	Valproic acid displaces 10-hydroxycarbazepine from its plasma protein binding sites [13]
Consequence	During combination therapy with valproic acid, 10-hydroxycarbazepine binding is 36% vs 47% for monotherapy oxcarbazepine. Clinical management may best be guided by monitoring free blood levels of 10-hydroxycarbazepine [13]
Vigabatrin	The interaction has not been investigated. Theoretically, a pharmacokinetic interaction would not be anticipated
Zonisamide	The interaction has not been investigated. Theoretically, a pharmacokinetic interaction could occur

References

1. Moseley BD, Otoul C, Staelens L, Stockis A. Pharmacokinetic interaction of brivaracetam on other antiepileptic drugs in adults with focal seizures: pooled analysis of data from randomized clinical trials. Epilepsy Res. 2019;158:106218.
2. Gaston TE, Bekib EM, Cutter GR, Liu Y, Szaflarski JP, UAB CBD Program. Interactions between cannabidiol and commonly used antiepileptic drugs. Epilepsia. 2017;58:1586–92.
3. McKee PJW, Blacklaw J, Forrest G, Gillham RA, Walker SM, Connelly D, Brodie MJ. A double-blind, placebo-controlled interaction study between oxcarbazepine and carbamazepine, sodium valproate and phenytoin in epileptic patients. Br J Clin Pharmacol. 1994;37:27–32.
4. Bialer M, Johannessen SI, Koepp MJ, Levy RH, Perucca E, Perucca P, Tomson T, White HS. Progress report on new antiepileptic drugs: a summary of the fifteenth Eilat conference on new antiepileptic drugs and devices (EILAT XV). II. Drugs in more advanced clinical development. Epilepsia. 2020;61:2365–85.
5. Arnoldussen W, Hulsman J, Rentmeester T. The interaction of valproate and clobazam on the metabolism of oxcarbazepine. Epilepsia. 1993;34(Suppl 2):160.
6. Hulsman JARJ, Rentmeester TW, Banfield CR, Reidenberg P, Colucci RD, Meehan JW, Radwanski E, Mojavarian P, Lin CC, Nezamis J, Affrime MB, Glue P. Effects of felbamate on the pharmacokinetics of the monohydroxy and dihydroxy metabolites of oxcarbazepine. Clin Pharmacol Ther. 1995;58:383–9.
7. Halasz P, Kalviainen R, Mazurkiewicz-Beldzinska M, Rosenow F, Doty P, Hebert D, Sullivan T. Adjunctive lacosamide for partial-onset seizures: efficacy and safety results from a randomized controlled trial. Epilepsia. 2009;50:443–53.
8. Novy J, Patsalos PN, Sander JW, Sisodiya SM. Lacosamide neurotoxicity associated with concomitant use of sodium-blocking antiepileptic drugs: a pharmacodynamic interaction? Epilepsy Behav. 2011;20:20–3.
9. Armijo JA, Vega-Gil N, Shushtarian M, Adin J, Herranz JL. 10-Hydroxycarbazepine serum concentration-to-oxcarbazepine dose ratio. Influence of age and concomitant antiepileptic drugs. Ther Drug Monit. 2005;27:199–204.
10. Patsalos PN. The clinical pharmacology profile of the new antiepileptic drug perampanel: a novel noncompetitive AMPA receptor antagonist. Epilepsia. 2015;56:12–27.

11. Gidal BE, Ferry J, Majid O, Hussein Z. Concentration-effect relationships with perampanel in patients with pharmacoresistant partial-onset seizures. Epilepsia. 2013;54:1490–7.
12. Tartara A, Galimberti CA, Manni R, Morino R, Limido G, Gatti G, Bartoli A, Strada G, Perucca E. The pharmacokinetics of oxcarbazepine and its active metabolite 10-hydroxy-carbazepine in healthy subjects and in epileptic patients treated with phenobarbital and valproic acid. Br J Clin Pharmacol. 1993;36:366–8.
13. May TW, Rambeck B, Salke-Kellermann A. Fluctuations of 10-hydroxy-carbazepine during the day in epileptic patients. Acta Neurol Scand. 1996;93:393–7.

Perampanel

Perampanel (Fig. 1) corresponds chemically to 2-(2-oxo-1-phenyl-5-pyridin-2-yl-1,2-dihydropyridin-3-yl) benzonitrile, with an empirical formula of $C_{23}H_{15}N_3O$ and a molecular weight of 349.4.

Fig. 1 Perampanel

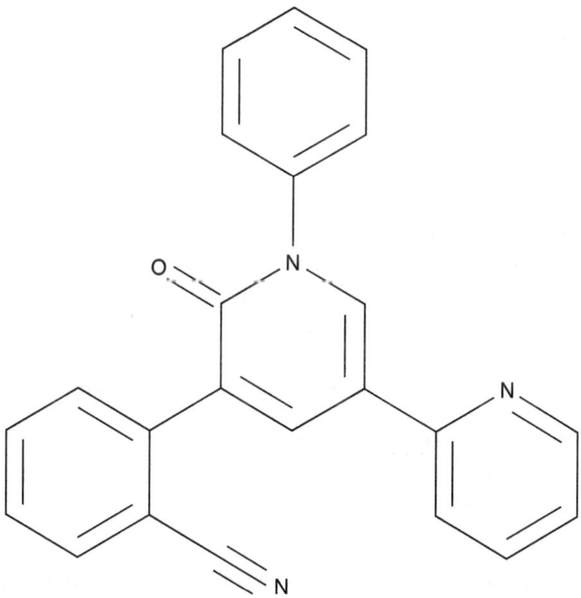

P. N. Patsalos, *Antiseizure Medication Interactions*,
https://doi.org/10.1007/978-3-030-82790-8_20

Pharmacokinetic Characteristics

Absorption and Distribution

After oral ingestion, perampanel is rapidly absorbed with T_{max} values of 0.5–2.5 h and with a bioavailability of 100%. The volume of distribution is 1.1 L/kg and protein binding is 95%.

Biotransformation

Perampanel undergoes extensive metabolism in the liver, via primary oxidation and sequential glucuronidation, to form various metabolites none of which are pharmacologically active. The primary oxidative route of metabolism entails CYP3A4 although CYP3A5 may also contribute.

Renal Excretion

Less than 0.12% of an administered dose is excreted as unchanged perampanel in urine.

Elimination

In the absence of enzyme-inducing antiseizure medications, plasma elimination half-life values in adults are 48 h, while in the presence of the enzyme-inducing antiseizure medication carbamazepine, half-life values are 25 h. In the presence of other enzyme-inducing antiseizure medications (phenytoin, oxcarbazepine, and topiramate) perampanel half-life values are also decreased.

Time to new steady-state blood levels consequent to an inhibition of metabolism interaction:

- Adults = 10–19 days later

Effects on Isoenzymes

At therapeutic concentrations, perampanel has no in vitro inhibitory or induction effects on the activity of CYP1A2, CYP2A6, CYP2C8.CYP2C9, CYP2C19, CYP2D6, CYP2E1, CYP3A4, UGT1A1, UGT1A9, UGT1A4, UGT1A6, or UGT2B7. Consequently, pharmacokinetic interactions of metabolic origin with other antiseizure medications and other medicines are not expected.

Therapeutic Drug Monitoring

Optimum seizure control in patients on perampanel monotherapy is most likely to occur at plasma perampanel levels of 200–1000 μg/L (573–2860 nmol/L). The conversion factor from μg/L to nmol/L for perampanel is 2.86 (i.e., 1 μg/L = 2.86 nmol/L).

Propensity to Be Associated with Pharmacokinetic Interactions

- Perampanel affects the pharmacokinetics of other drugs—minimal.
- Other drugs affect the pharmacokinetics of perampanel—substantial.

Interactions with ASMs

Acetazolamide	The interaction has not been investigated. Theoretically, a pharmacokinetic interaction would not be anticipated
Brivaracetam	The interaction has not been investigated. Theoretically, a pharmacokinetic interaction would not be anticipated
Cannabidiol	Does not affect the pharmacokinetics of perampanel [1]

Carbamazepine	Enhances the metabolism of perampanel
Consequence	Mean plasma perampanel Cmax and AUC values can be decreased by 26% and 67%, respectively. The interaction is the consequence of induction of perampanel metabolism through CYP3A4 [2]
	Carbamazepine in combination with perampanel is associated with increased sedation. This effect may be the consequence of a pharmacodynamic interaction [3]
Cenobamate	The interaction has not been investigated. Theoretically, a pharmacokinetic interaction could occur
Clobazam	Does not affect the pharmacokinetics of perampanel [2]
Clonazepam	Does not affect the pharmacokinetics of perampanel [2]
Eslicarbazepine acetate	The interaction has not been investigated. Theoretically, a pharmacokinetic interaction could occur
Ethosuximide	The interaction has not been investigated. Theoretically, a pharmacokinetic interaction would not be anticipated
Everolimus	The interaction has not been investigated. Theoretically, a pharmacokinetic interaction could occur
Felbamate	The interaction has not been investigated. Theoretically, a pharmacokinetic interaction could occur
Fenfluramine	The interaction has not been investigated. Theoretically, a pharmacokinetic interaction could occur
Gabapentin	The interaction has not been investigated. Theoretically, a pharmacokinetic interaction would not be anticipated
Lacosamide	The interaction has not been investigated. Theoretically, a pharmacokinetic interaction would not be anticipated
Lamotrigine	Does not affect the pharmacokinetics of perampanel [2]
Levetiracetam	Does not affect the pharmacokinetics of perampanel [4]
	Levetiracetam in combination with perampanel is associated with an increased likelihood of developing fatigue. This effect may be the consequence of a pharmacodynamic interaction [4]
Methsuximide	The interaction has not been investigated. Theoretically, a pharmacokinetic interaction would not be anticipated
Oxcarbazepine	Enhances the metabolism of perampanel
Consequence	Mean plasma perampanel AUC values can decrease by 50% [2]. The interaction is the consequence of induction of perampanel metabolism via CYP3A4
	Oxcarbazepine in combination with perampanel is associated with an increased risk of decreased appetite. This effect may be the consequence of a pharmacodynamic interaction [4]
Phenobarbital	Enhances the metabolism of perampanel
Consequence	Plasma perampanel concentrations are decreased [5]
	Phenobarbital in combination with perampanel is associated with increased irritability. This effect may be the consequence of a pharmacodynamic interaction [4]
Phenytoin	Enhances the metabolism of perampanel
Consequence	Mean plasma perampanel AUC values can decrease by 50% [2]. The interaction is the consequence of induction of perampanel metabolism through CYP3A4 Phenytoin plasma protein binding is not affected by perampanel [6]

Piracetam	The interaction has not been investigated. Theoretically, a pharmacokinetic interaction would not be anticipated
Pregabalin	The interaction has not been investigated. Theoretically, a pharmacokinetic interaction would not be anticipated
Primidone	The interaction has not been investigated. Theoretically, an interaction similar to that seen with phenobarbital can be expected
	Primidone in combination with perampanel is associated with an increased risk of decreased appetite. This effect may be the consequence of a pharmacodynamic interaction [4]
Rufinamide	The interaction has not been investigated. Theoretically, a pharmacokinetic interaction would not be anticipated
Stiripentol	The interaction has not been investigated. Theoretically, a pharmacokinetic interaction could occur
Sulthiame	The interaction has not been investigated. Theoretically, a pharmacokinetic interaction could occur
Tiagabine	The interaction has not been investigated. Theoretically, a pharmacokinetic interaction would not be anticipated
Topiramate	Enhances the metabolism of perampanel
Consequence	Mean plasma perampanel AUC values can decrease by 20% [2]. The interaction is the consequence of induction of perampanel metabolism via CYP3A4
Valproic acid	Inhibits the metabolism of perampanel
Consequence	Mean plasma perampanel concentration/dose ratios can increase by 66% [7] Valproic acid plasma protein binding is not affected by perampanel [6]
Vigabatrin	The interaction has not been investigated. Theoretically, a pharmacokinetic interaction would not be anticipated
Zonisamide	Does not affect the pharmacokinetics of perampanel [7]

References

1. Gaston TE, Bekib EM, Cutter GR, Liu Y, Szaflarski JP, UAB CBD Program. Interactions between cannabidiol and commonly used antiepileptic drugs. Epilepsia. 2017;58:1586–92.
2. Patsalos PN. The clinical pharmacology profile of the new antiepileptic drug perampanel: a novel noncompetitive AMPA receptor antagonist. Epilepsia. 2015;56:12–27.
3. Patsalos PN, Gougoulaki N, Sander JW. Perampanel serum concentrations in adults with epilepsy: effect of dose, age, sex and concomitant anti-epileptic drugs. Ther Drug Monit. 2016;38:358–64.
4. Gidal BE, Ferry J, Majid O, Hussein Z. Concentration-effect relationships with perampanel in patients with pharmacoresistant partial-onset seizures. Epilepsia. 2013;54:1490–7.
5. Yamamoto Y, Usui N, Nishida T, Takahashi Y, Imai K, Kagawa Y, Inoue Y. Therapeutic drug monitoring for perampanel in Japanese epilepsy patients: influence of concomitant antiepileptic drugs. Ther Drug Monit. 2017;39:446–9.
6. Gidal BE, Ferry J, Laurenza A, Ueno T. Potential protein-binding displacement interactions with perampanel: an in vitro analysis. Epilepsy Res. 2019;149:102–6.
7. Contin M, Bisulli F, Santucci M, Riva R, Tonon F, Ferri L, Stipa C, Tinuper P, on behalf of the Perampanel Study Group. Effect of valproic acid on perampanel pharmacokinetics in patients with epilepsy. Epilepsia. 2018;59:e103–8.

Phenobarbital

Phenobarbital (Fig. 1) corresponds chemically to 5-ethyl-5-phenylbarbituric acid with an empirical formula of $C_{12}H_{12}N_2O_3$ and a molecular weight of 232.23.

Pharmacokinetic Characteristics

Absorption and Distribution

After oral ingestion, phenobarbital is rapidly absorbed (T_{max} = 2–4 h) with a bioavailability of >90%. Its volume of distribution is 0.61 L/kg in adult and ~1.0 L/kg in newborns, and plasma protein binding is 55%.

Biotransformation

Phenobarbital is extensively metabolized in the liver to two major metabolites, *p*-hydroxyphenobarbital, which partially undergoes sequential metabolism to a

Fig. 1 Phenobarbital

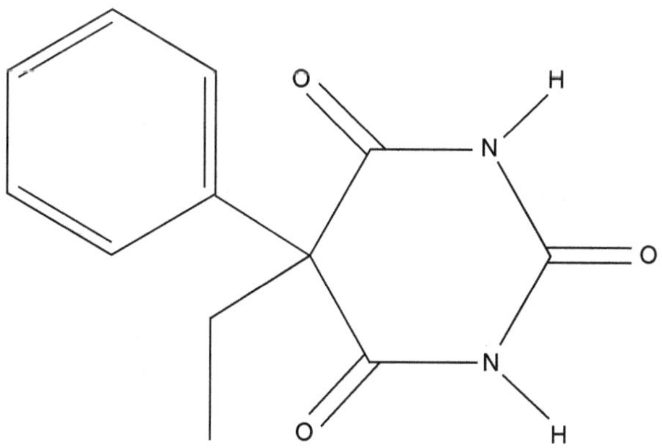

P. N. Patsalos, *Antiseizure Medication Interactions*, https://doi.org/10.1007/978-3-030-82790-8_21

glucuronic acid conjugate, and 9-D-glucopyranosylphenobarbital, an *N*-glucoside conjugate. CYP2C9 plays a major role in the metabolism of phenobarbital to *p*-hydroxyphenobarbital with minor metabolism by CYP2C19 and CYP2E1. Phenobarbital is an enzyme inducer. Phenobarbital undergoes autoinduction so that its clearance can increase, and this may require an upward dosage adjustment when prescribed as monotherapy.

Renal Excretion

In adults, 20–25% of an administered dose is excreted as unchanged phenobarbital in urine.

Elimination

Plasma elimination half-life values are 70–140 h in adults, while in newborns, half-life values are 100–200 h. During the neonatal period, phenobarbital elimination accelerates markedly; thereafter, half-life values are very short, with average values of 63 h during the first year of life and 69 h at ages 1–5 years.

Time to new steady-state phenobarbital blood levels consequent to an inhibition of metabolism interaction:

- Adults = 15–29 days later

Effects on Isoenzymes

No in vitro data on the induction or inhibition potential of phenobarbital on human CYP or UGT isoenzymes have been published.

Therapeutic Drug Monitoring

Optimum seizure control in patients on phenobarbital monotherapy is most likely to occur at plasma phenobarbital levels of 10–40 mg/L (43–172 μmol/L). The conversion factor from mg/L to μmol/L for phenobarbital is 4.31 (i.e., 1 mg/L = 4.31 μmol/L).

Propensity to Be Associated with Pharmacokinetic Interactions

- Phenobarbital affects the pharmacokinetics of other drugs—substantial.
- Other drugs affect the pharmacokinetics of phenobarbital—substantial.

Interactions with ASMs

Acetazolamide	Inhibits the metabolism of phenobarbital
Consequence	Plasma phenobarbital levels can be increased [1]
Brivaracetam	Does not affect the pharmacokinetics of phenobarbital [2]
Cannabidiol	Does not affect the pharmacokinetics of phenobarbital [3]
Carbamazepine	Does not affect the pharmacokinetics of phenobarbital [4]
Cenobamate	Inhibits the metabolism of phenobarbital
Consequence	Plasma phenobarbital AUC values can be increased by 37% [5]
Clobazam	Does not affect the pharmacokinetics of phenobarbital [6]
Clonazepam	Does not affect the pharmacokinetics of phenobarbital [7]
Eslicarbazepine acetate	Does not affect the pharmacokinetics of phenobarbital [8]
Ethosuximide	Does not affect the pharmacokinetics of phenobarbital [9]
Everolimus	The interaction has not been investigated. Theoretically, a pharmacokinetic interaction could occur
Felbamate	Inhibits the metabolism of phenobarbital

Consequence	Mean plasma phenobarbital levels can be increased by 24%. The interaction is the consequence of inhibition of CYP2C19 [10]
Fenfluramine	The interaction has not been investigated. Theoretically, a pharmacokinetic interaction could occur
Gabapentin	Does not affect the pharmacokinetics of phenobarbital [11]
Lacosamide	The interaction has not been investigated. Theoretically, a pharmacokinetic interaction would not be anticipated
Lamotrigine	Does not affect the pharmacokinetics of phenobarbital [12]
Levetiracetam	Does not affect the pharmacokinetics of phenobarbital [13]
Methsuximide	Inhibits the metabolism of phenobarbital
Consequence	Plasma phenobarbital levels can be increased by 23–57%. The interaction is considered to be the consequence of inhibition of CYP2C19 [14]
Oxcarbazepine	Inhibits the metabolism of phenobarbital
Consequence	At oxcarbazepine dosages above 1200 mg/day, mean plasma phenobarbital levels can be increased by 15%. The interaction is the consequence of inhibition of CYP2C19 [15]
Perampanel	Does not affect the pharmacokinetics of phenobarbital [16]
	Perampanel in combination with phenobarbital is associated with increased irritability. This effect may be the consequence of a pharmacodynamic interaction [17]
Phenytoin	Inhibits the metabolism of phenobarbital
Consequence	Plasma phenobarbital levels can be increased by 50–70%. The interaction is the consequence of inhibition of CYP2C19 [18]
Piracetam	Does not affect the pharmacokinetics of phenobarbital [19]
Pregabalin	Does not affect the pharmacokinetics of phenobarbital [20]
Primidone	Not commonly co-prescribed
Rufinamide	Inhibits the metabolism of phenobarbital
Consequence	Plasma clearance of phenobarbital is decreased by 7–12% so that plasma phenobarbital levels are increased by 8–13% [21]
Stiripentol	Inhibits the metabolism of phenobarbital
Consequence	Plasma clearance of phenobarbital is decreased by 30–40% so that plasma phenobarbital levels are increased. The interaction is the consequence of inhibition of CYP2C9 and CYP2C19 [22]
Sulthiame	Inhibits the metabolism of phenobarbital
Consequence	Plasma phenobarbital levels can be increased [23]
Tiagabine	The interaction has not been investigated. Theoretically, a pharmacokinetic interaction would not be anticipated
Topiramate	Does not affect the pharmacokinetics of phenobarbital [24]
Valproic acid	Inhibits the metabolism of phenobarbital
Consequence	The extent of this interaction is characterized by considerable interindividual variability with 30–50% increases in mean plasma phenobarbital levels, probably via an action on CYP2C9 and/or CYP2C19. In children, mean plasma phenobarbital levels can be increased by 112% [25]
Vigabatrin	Does not affect the pharmacokinetics of phenobarbital [26]
	During combination therapy for the treatment of infantile spasms, especially in patients with tuberous sclerosis, phenobarbital appears to delay or prevent the onset of seizure control by vigabatrin. This is considered to be the consequence of a pharmacodynamic interaction [27]
Zonisamide	Does not affect the pharmacokinetics of phenobarbital [28]

References

1. Kelly WN, Richardson AP, Mason MF, Rector FC. Acetazolamide in phenobarbital intoxication. Arch Intern Med. 1966;117:64–9.
2. Moseley BD, Otoul C, Staelens L, Stockis A. Pharmacokinetic interaction of brivaracetam on other antiepileptic drugs in adults with focal seizures: pooled analysis of data from randomized clinical trials. Epilepsy Res. 2019;158:106218.
3. Gaston TE, Bekib EM, Cutter GR, Liu Y, Szaflarski JP, UAB CBD Program. Interactions between cannabidiol and commonly used antiepileptic drugs. Epilepsia. 2017;58:1586–92.
4. Eadie MJ, Lander CM, Hooper WD, Tyrer JH. Factors influencing phenobarbitone levels in epileptic patients. Br J Clin Pharmacol. 1977;4:541–7.
5. Bialer M, Johannessen SI, Koepp MJ, Levy RH, Perucca E, Perucca P, Tomson T, White HS. Progress report on new antiepileptic drugs: a summary of the fifteenth Eilat conference on new antiepileptic drugs and devices (EILAT XV). II. Drugs in more advanced clinical development. Epilepsia. 2020;61:2365–85.
6. Vakil SD, Critchley EMR, Cocks A, Hayward HW. The effect of clobazam on blood levels of phenobarbitone, phenytoin and carbamazepine (preliminary report). Royal Society of Medicine International Congress and Symposium Series no. 43. London; 1981. p. 165–167.
7. Nanda RN, Johnson RH, Keogh HJ, Lambie DG, Melville ID. Treatment of epilepsy with clonazepam and its effect on other anti-convulsants. J Neurol Neurosurg Psychiatry. 1977;40:538–43.
8. Falcao A, Fuseau E, Nunes T, Almeida L, Soares-da-Silva P. Pharmacokinetics, drug interactions and exposure-response relationships of eslicarbazepine acetate in adult patients with partial-onset seizures: population pharmacokinetic and pharmacokinetic/pharmacodynamic analysis. CNS Drugs. 2012;26:79–91.
9. Schmidt D. The effect of phenytoin and ethosuximide on primidone metabolism in patients with epilepsy. J Neurol. 1975;209:115–23.
10. Reidenberg P, Glue P, Banfield CR, Colucci RD, Meehan JW, Radwanski E, Mojavarian P, Lin CC, Nezamis J, Guillaume M, Affrime MB. Effects of felbamate on the pharmacokinetics of phenobarbital. Clin Pharmacol Ther. 1995;58:279–87.
11. Hooper WD, Kavanagh MC, Herkes GK, Eadie MJ. Lack of a pharmacokinetic interaction between phenobarbitone and gabapentin. Br J Clin Pharmacol. 1991;31:171–4.
12. Eriksson AS, Hoppu K, Nergardh A, Boreu L. Pharmacokinetic interactions between lamotrigine and other antiepileptic drugs in children with intractable epilepsy. Epilepsia. 1996;37:769–73.
13. Perucca E, Baltes E, Ledent E. Levetiracetam: absence of pharmacokinetic interactions with other antiepileptic drugs (AEDs). Epilepsia. 2000;41(Suppl):150.
14. Rambeck B. Pharmacological interactions of methsuximide with phenobarbital and phenytoin in hospitalized epileptic patients. Epilepsia. 1979;20:147–56.
15. Barcs G, Walker EB, Elger CE, Scaramelli A, Stefan H, Sturm Y, Moore A, Flesch G, Kramer L, D'Souza J. Oxcarbazepine placebo-controlled, dose-ranging trial in refractory partial epilepsy. Epilepsia. 2000;41:1597–607.
16. Patsalos PN. The clinical pharmacology profile of the new antiepileptic drug perampanel: a novel noncompetitive AMPA receptor antagonist. Epilepsia. 2015;56:12–27.
17. Gidal BE, Ferry J, Majid O, Hussein Z. Concentration-effect relationships with perampanel in patients with pharmacoresistant partial-onset seizures. Epilepsia. 2013;54:1490–7.
18. Lambie DG, Johnson RH. The effect of phenytoin on phenobarbitone and primidone metabolism. J Neurol Neurosurg Psychiatry. 1981;44:148–51.
19. Summary of product characteristics: Piracetam (Nootropil). UCB Pharma Ltd. Last update 9 Feb 2017.
20. Bockbrader HN, Burger P, Knapp L. Pregabalin effect on steady-state pharmacokinetics of carbamazepine, lamotrigine, phenobarbital, phenytoin, topiramate, valproate, and tiagabine. Epilepsia. 2011;52:405–9.

21. Perucca E, Cloyd J, Critchley D, Fuseau E. Rufinamide: clinical pharmacokinetics and concentration-response relationships in patients with epilepsy. Epilepsia. 2008;49:1123–41.
22. Levy RH, Loiseau P, Guyot M, Blehaut H, Tor J, Moreland TA. Stiripentol kinetics in epilepsy: nonlinearity and interactions. Clin Pharmacol Ther. 1984;36:661–9.
23. Summary of product characteristics: Sulthiame (Ospolot). Phebra Pty, Ltd. Last update 21 Nov 2013.
24. Doose DR, Walker SA, Pledger G, Lim P, Reife RA. Evaluation of phenobarbital and primidone/phenobarbital (primidone active metabolite) plasma concentrations during administration of add-on topiramate therapy in five multicenter, double-blind, placebo controlled trials in outpatients with partial seizures. Epilepsia. 1995;36(Suppl 3):158.
25. Kapetanovic IM, Kupferberg HJ, Porter RJ, Theodore W, Schulman E, Penry JK. Mechanism of valproate–phenobarbital interaction in epileptic patients. Clin Pharmacol Ther. 1981;29:480–6.
26. Loiseau P, Hardenberg JP, Pestre M, Guyot M, Schechter PJ, Tell GP. Double-blind, placebo-controlled study of vigabatrin (gamma-vinyl GABA) in drug-resistant epilepsy. Epilepsia. 1986;27:115–20.
27. Spence SJ, Nakagawa J, Sankar R, Shields WD. Phenobarbital interferes with the efficacy of vigabatrin in treating infantile spasms in patients with tuberous sclerosis. Epilepsia. 2000;41(Suppl 7):189.
28. Buchanan RA, Page JG, French JA, Leppik IE, Padgett CS. Zonisamide drug interactions. Epilepsia. 1997;38(Suppl 8):107.

21. Perucca E, Cloyd J, Critchley D, Fuseau E. Rufinamide: clinical pharmacokinetics and concentration-response relationships in patients with epilepsy. Epilepsia. 2008;49:1123–41.
22. Levy RH, Loiseau P, Guyot M, Blehaut H, Tor J, Moreland TA. Stiripentol kinetics in epilepsy: nonlinearity and interactions. Clin Pharmacol Ther. 1984;36:661–9.
23. Summary of product characteristics. Sulthiame (Ospolot). Phebra Pty. Ltd. Last updated: Nov 2017.
24. [illegible] felbamate [illegible] plasma concentrations during monotherapy and add-on therapy in a five-center, double-blind, placebo-controlled trial in outpatients with partial seizures. Epilepsia. 1993;34(Suppl 3):[illegible].
25. Kapetanovic IM, Kupferberg HJ, Porter RJ, Theodore W, Schulman E, Penry JK. Mechanism of valproate-phenobarbital interaction in epileptic patients. Clin Pharmacol Ther. 1981;29:480–6.
26. Loiseau P, Hardenberg JP, Pestre M, Guyot M, Schechter PJ, Tell GP. Double-blind, placebo-controlled study of vigabatrin (gamma-vinyl GABA) in drug-resistant epilepsy. Epilepsia. 1986;27:115–20.
27. Spence SJ, Nakagawa J, Sankar R, Shields WD. Phenobarbital interferes with the efficacy of vigabatrin in treating infantile spasms in patients with tuberous sclerosis. Epilepsia. 2000;41(Suppl 7):189.
28. Buchanan R, Page JG, French JA, Leppik IE, Padgett CS. Zonisamide drug interactions. Epilepsia. 1997;38(Suppl 8):107.

Phenytoin

Phenytoin (Fig. 1) corresponds chemically to 5,5-diphenyl-2,4-imidazolidinedione with an empirical formula of $C_{15}H_{12}N_2O_2$ and a molecular weight of 252.26 for the free acid and a molecular weight of 274.25 for the sodium salt which is equivalent to an acid content of 91.98%.

Fig. 1 Phenytoin

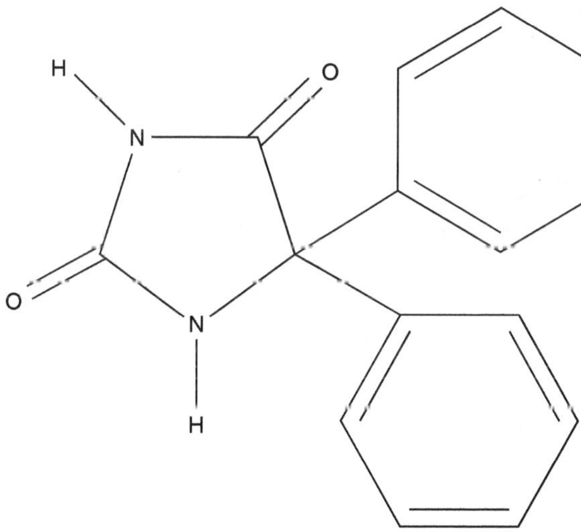

P. N. Patsalos, *Antiseizure Medication Interactions*,
https://doi.org/10.1007/978-3-030-82790-8_22

Pharmacokinetic Characteristics

Absorption and Distribution

After oral ingestion, phenytoin's rate of absorption (T_{max} = 4–12 h) and bioavailability (≥80%) are formulation-dependent. Its volume of distribution is 0.5–0.8 L/kg, and plasma protein binding is 90%.

Biotransformation

Phenytoin undergoes extensive metabolism in the liver by hydroxylation to various metabolites, the principal metabolites being 5-(*p*-hydroxyphenyl)-5-phenylhydantoin (p-HPPH; 67–88%) and a dihydrodiol derivative (7–11%). The isoenzymes responsible for the hydroxylation of phenytoin are CYP2C9 (~80%) and CYP2C19 (~20%). In excess of 60% of p-HPPH is subsequently glucuronidated and excreted in urine. Phenytoin is an enzyme inducer, and additionally, phenytoin undergoes autoinduction, primarily via CYP2C19, so that its clearance can increase and this may require an upward dosage adjustment when prescribed as monotherapy.

Renal Excretion

Approximately 5% of an administered dose is excreted as unchanged phenytoin in urine.

Elimination

In the absence of enzyme-inducing antiseizure medications, plasma elimination half-life values are 30–100 h, while in the presence of enzyme-inducing antiseizure medications, half-life values are 30–100 h.

Phenytoin elimination follows Michaelis–Menten (saturable, zero-order) kinetics so that plasma half-life and clearance are dose-dependent with values decreasing with increasing dose. As a result, phenytoin steady-state plasma levels increase more than proportionately after a dose increment.

Time to new steady-state phenytoin blood levels consequent to an inhibition of metabolism interaction:

- Adults = 6–21 days later

Effects on Isoenzymes

No in vitro data on the induction or inhibition potential of phenytoin on human CYP or UGT isoenzymes have been published.

Therapeutic Drug Monitoring

Optimum seizure control in patients on phenytoin monotherapy is most likely to occur at plasma phenytoin levels of 10–20 mg/L (40–80 μmol/L). The conversion factor from mg/L to μmol/L for phenytoin is 3.96 (i.e., 1 mg/L = 3.96 μmol/L).

Propensity to Be Associated with Pharmacokinetic Interactions

- Phenytoin affects the pharmacokinetics of other drugs—substantial.
- Other drugs affect the pharmacokinetics of phenytoin—substantial.

Interactions with ASMs

Acetazolamide	Inhibits the metabolism of phenytoin
Consequence	Plasma phenytoin levels can increase [1]
Brivaracetam	Inhibits the metabolism of phenytoin
Consequence	Plasma phenytoin Cmax and AUC values can increase by 20% [2]
Cannabidiol	Does not affect the pharmacokinetics of phenytoin [3]
Carbamazepine	Conflicting results are observed
Consequence	Plasma phenytoin levels may decrease, remain the same, or increase after addition of carbamazepine. This is a consequence of intersubject variability in CYP isoenzyme expression of CYP2C19 which carbamazepine inhibits and the fact that carbamazepine may increase the clearance of phenytoin through induction of CYP2C9 and/or CYP2C19 [4]
Cenobamate	Inhibits the metabolism of phenytoin
Consequence	Plasma phenytoin AUC values can increase by 84% [5]
Clobazam	Inhibits the metabolism of phenytoin
Consequence	Plasma phenytoin levels can be increased by 25–74% [6]
Clonazepam	Conflicting results are observed
Consequence	Plasma phenytoin levels may decrease, remain the same, or increase after addition of clonazepam. This may be the consequence of a multi-mechanism interaction, whereby clonazepam induces the metabolism of phenytoin in some patients while in other patients, it acts as an inhibitor of phenytoin metabolism [7, 8]
Eslicarbazepine acetate	Inhibits the metabolism of phenytoin
Consequence	Plasma phenytoin AUC values can increase by 30–35%. The interaction is considered to be the consequence of inhibition of CYP2C19 [9]
Ethosuximide	Does not affect the pharmacokinetics of phenytoin
Everolimus	The interaction has not been investigated. Theoretically, a pharmacokinetic interaction could occur
Felbamate	Inhibits the metabolism of phenytoin
Consequence	Mean plasma phenytoin levels can be increased by 34%, 67%, and 106% at 1200, 1800, and 2400 mg/day felbamate, respectively. The interaction is the consequence of inhibition of phenytoin metabolism through CYP2C19 [10]
Fenfluramine	The interaction has not been investigated. Theoretically, a pharmacokinetic interaction could occur
Gabapentin	Does not affect the pharmacokinetics of phenytoin [11]
Lacosamide	Does not affect the pharmacokinetics of phenytoin [12]
	Neurotoxicity may occur in combination with phenytoin, and other voltage-gated sodium channel blocking antiseizure medications, consequent to a pharmacodynamic interaction [13]
Lamotrigine	Does not affect the pharmacokinetics of phenytoin [14]
	During combination therapy with lamotrigine, a drug-induced chorea can occur. This is considered to be the consequence of a pharmacodynamic interaction [15]
Levetiracetam	Does not affect the pharmacokinetics of phenytoin [16]
Methsuximide	Inhibits the metabolism of phenytoin
Consequence	Plasma phenytoin levels can be increased by 47–102%. The interaction is considered to be the consequence of inhibition of CYP2C19 [17]

Oxcarbazepine	Inhibits the metabolism of phenytoin
Consequence	At oxcarbazepine dosages above 1200 mg/day, mean plasma phenytoin levels can be increased by 40%. The interaction is the consequence of inhibition of CYP2C19 [18]
Perampanel	Does not affect the pharmacokinetics of phenytoin [19] Phenytoin plasma protein binding is not affected by perampanel [20]
Phenobarbital	Conflicting results are observed
Consequence	Plasma phenytoin levels have been reported to increase, decrease, or not change upon the addition of phenobarbital. This variability reflects the fact that phenobarbital is both a CYP enzyme inducer and an inhibitor. In most patients, only small changes in blood levels occur, and no dosage modification is needed. However, because of variability in the magnitude and direction of the interaction, clinical response and plasma phenytoin levels should be monitored [21, 22]
Piracetam	Does not affect the pharmacokinetics of phenytoin [23]
Pregabalin	Does not affect the pharmacokinetics of phenytoin [24]
Primidone	Does not affect the pharmacokinetics of phenytoin [25]
Rufinamide	Inhibits the metabolism of phenytoin
Consequence	Plasma clearance of phenytoin is decreased by 6–17% so that plasma phenytoin levels are increased [26]
Stiripentol	Inhibits the metabolism of phenytoin
Consequence	Plasma clearance of phenytoin is decreased by 78% so that plasma phenytoin levels are increased. The interaction is the consequence of inhibition of CYP2C9 and CYP2C19 [27]
Sulthiame	Inhibits the metabolism of phenytoin
Consequence	Mean plasma phenytoin levels can increase by 74% [28, 29]
Tiagabine	Does not affect the pharmacokinetics of phenytoin [30]
Topiramate	Inhibits the metabolism of phenytoin
Consequence	The magnitude of the interaction is variable with plasma phenytoin levels increasing by up to 25% in some patients. At high phenytoin concentrations, where CYP2C19 contributes to phenytoin metabolism more than at low concentrations, topiramate may inhibit the CYP2C19 minor metabolic pathway [31]
Valproic acid	Conflicting results are observed
Consequence	The effect of valproic acid on plasma phenytoin levels varies among patients and may vary in the same patient during the course of therapy. Thus, a persistent fall, a transient fall, or even a rise can occur in some patients. These effects are the consequence of a displacement of phenytoin from its plasma protein (albumin) binding sites and the concurrent inhibition of CYP2C9 metabolism. The free fraction of phenytoin is increased. Clinically, the need to adjust phenytoin dosage is rare, but if adjustment is necessary, it might best be guided by measurement of free (nonprotein bound) phenytoin levels [32, 33]
Vigabatrin	Plasma phenytoin levels are decreased
Consequence	During comedication with vigabatrin, mean plasma phenytoin levels can decrease by 32%. The mechanism of this interaction is not known but does not involve any absorption, metabolic, or bioavailability processes [34]
Zonisamide	Does not affect the pharmacokinetics of phenytoin [35]

References

1. Norell E, Lilienberg G, Gamstorp I. Systematic determination of the serum phenytoin level as an aid in the management of children with epilepsy. Eur Neurol. 1975;13:232–44.
2. Summary of product characteristics: Brivaracetam (Briviact). UCB Pharma Ltd. Last update 27 Nov 2020.
3. Gaston TE, Bekib EM, Cutter GR, Liu Y, Szaflarski JP, UAB CBD Program. Interactions between cannabidiol and commonly used antiepileptic drugs. Epilepsia. 2017;58:1586–92.
4. Browne TR, Szabo GK, Evans JE, Evans BA, Greenblatt DJ, Mikati MA. Carbamazepine increases phenytoin serum concentration and reduces phenytoin clearance. Neurology. 1988;38:1146–50.
5. Bialer M, Johannessen SI, Koepp MJ, Levy RH, Perucca E, Perucca P, Tomson T, White HS. Progress report on new antiepileptic drugs: a summary of the fifteenth Eilat conference on new antiepileptic drugs and devices (EILAT XV). II. Drugs in more advanced clinical development. Epilepsia. 2020;61:2365–85.
6. Zifkin B, Sherwin A, Alderman F. Phenytoin toxicity due to interaction with clobazam. Neurology. 1991;41:313–4.
7. Nanda RN, Johnson RH, Keogh HJ, Lambie DG, Melville ID. Treatment of epilepsy with clonazepam and its effect on other anticonvulsants. J Neurol Neurosurg Psychiatry. 1977;40:538–43.
8. Saavedra IN, Aguilera LI, Faure E, Galdames DG. Phenytoin/clonazepam interaction. Ther Drug Monit. 1985;7:481–4.
9. Bialer M, Soares-da-Siva P. Pharmacokinetics and drug interactions of eslicarbazepine acetate. Epilepsia. 2012;53:935–46.
10. Glue P, Banfield CR, Perhach JL, Mather GG, Racha JK, Levy RH. Pharmacokinetic interactions with felbamate. In vitro-in vivo correlation. Clin Pharmacokinet. 1997;33:214–24.
11. Anhut H, Leppik I, Schmidt B, Thomann P. Drug interaction study of the new anticonvulsant gabapentin with phenytoin in epileptic patients. Naunyn Schmiedebergs Arch Pharmacol. 1988;337(Suppl):R127.
12. Halasz P, Kalviainen R, Mazurkiewicz-Beldzinska M, Rosenow F, Doty P, Hebert D, Sullivan T. Adjunctive lacosamide for partial-onset seizures: efficacy and safety results from a randomized controlled trial. Epilepsia. 2009;50:443–53.
13. Novy J, Patsalos PN, Sander JW, Sisodiya SM. Lacosamide neurotoxicity associated with concomitant use of sodium-blocking antiepileptic drugs: a pharmacodynamic interaction? Epilepsy Behav. 2011;20:20–3.
14. Grasela TH, Fiedler-Kelly J, Cox E, Womble GP, Risner ME, Chen C. Population pharmacokinetics of lamotrigine adjunctive therapy in adults with epilepsy. J Clin Pharmacol. 1999;39:373–84.
15. Zatreeh M, Tennison M, D'Cruz O, Beach RL. Anticonvulsant-induced chorea: a role for pharmacodynamic drug interaction? Seizure. 2001;10:596–9.
16. Browne TR, Szabo GK, Leppik IE, Josephs E, Paz J, Baltes E, Jensen CM. Absence of pharmacokinetic drug interaction of levetiracetam with phenytoin in patients with epilepsy determined by new technique. J Clin Pharmacol. 2000;40:590–5.
17. Rambeck B. Pharmacological interactions of methsuximide with phenobarbital and phenytoin in hospitalized epileptic patients. Epilepsia. 1979;20:147–56.
18. Barcs G, Walker EB, Elger CE, Scaramelli A, Stefan H, Sturm Y, Moore A, Flesch G, Kramer L, D'Souza J. Oxcarbazepine placebo-controlled, dose-ranging trial in refractory partial epilepsy. Epilepsia. 2000;41:1597–607.
19. Patsalos PN. The clinical pharmacology profile of the new antiepileptic drug perampanel: a novel noncompetitive AMPA receptor antagonist. Epilepsia. 2015;56:12–27.
20. Gidal BE, Ferry J, Laurenza A, Ueno T. Potential protein-binding displacement interactions with perampanel: an in vitro analysis. Epilepsy Res. 2019;149:102–6.

21. Morselli PL, Rizzo M, Garattini S. Interaction between phenobarbital and diphenylhydantoin in animals and in epileptic patients. Ann N Y Acad Sci. 1971;179:88–107.
22. Kutt H. Interactions between anticonvulsants and other commonly prescribed drugs. Epilepsia. 1984;25(Suppl 2):S118–31.
23. Summary of product characteristics: Piracetam (Nootropil). UCB Pharma Ltd. Last update 9 Feb 2017.
24. Brodie MJ, Wilson EA, Wesche DL, Alvey CW, Randinitis EJ, Posvar EL, Hounslow NJ, Bron NJ, Gibson GL, Bockbrader HN. Pregabalin drug interaction studies: lack of effect on the pharmacokinetics of carbamazepine, phenytoin, lamotrigine, and valproate in patients with partial epilepsy. Epilepsia. 2005;46:1407–13.
25. Fincham RW, Schottelius DD, Sahs AL. The influence of diphenylhydantoin on primidone metabolism. Arch Neurol. 1974;30:259–62.
26. Perucca E, Cloyd J, Critchley D, Fuseau E. Rufinamide: clinical pharmacokinetics and concentration-response relationships in patients with epilepsy. Epilepsia. 2008;49:1123–41.
27. Levy RH, Loiseau P, Guyot M, Blehaut H, Tor J, Moreland TA. Stiripentol kinetics in epilepsy: nonlinearity and interactions. Clin Pharmacol Ther. 1984;36:661–9.
28. Hansen JM, Kristensen M, Skovsted L. Sulthiame (Ospolot) an inhibitor of diphenylhydantoin metabolism. Epilepsia. 1968;9:17–22.
29. Houghton GW, Richens A. Phenytoin intoxication induced by sulthiame in epileptic patients. J Neurol Neurosurg Psychiatry. 1974;37:275–81.
30. Gustavson LE, Cato A, Boellner SW, Cao GX, Quian JX, Guenther HJ, Sommerville KW. Lack of pharmacokinetic drug interactions between tiagabine and carbamazepine or phenytoin. Am J Ther. 1998;5:9–16.
31. Sachdeo RC, Sachdeo SK, Levy RH, Streeter AJ, Bishop FE, Kunze KL, Mather GG, Roskos LK, Shen DD, Thummel KE, Trager WF, Curtin CR, Doose DR, Gsclon LG. Topiramate and phenytoin pharmacokinetics during repetitive monotherapy and concomitant therapy in patients with epilepsy. Epilepsia. 2002;3:691–6.
32. Lai ML, Huang JD. Dual effect of valproic acid on the pharmacokinetics of phenytoin. Biopharm Drug Dispos. 1993;14:365–70.
33. Perucca E, Hebdige S, Frigo GM, Gatti G, Lecchini S, Crema A. Interaction between phenytoin and valproic acid: plasma protein binding and metabolic effects. Clin Pharmacol Ther. 1980;28:779–89.
34. Gatti G, Bartoli A, Marchiselli R, Michelucci R, Tassinari CA, Pisani F, Zaccara G, Timmings P, Richens A, Perucca E. Vigabatrin-induced decrease in serum phenytoin concentration does not involve a change in phenytoin bioavailability. Br J Clin Pharmacol. 1993;36:603–6.
35. Levy RH, Ragueneau-Majlessi I, Garnett WR, Schmerler M, Rosenfeld W, Shah J, Pan WJ. Lack of clinically significant effects of zonisamide on phenytoin steady-state pharmacokinetics in patients with epilepsy. J Clin Pharmacol. 2004;44:1230–4.

Piracetam

Piracetam (Fig. 1) corresponds chemically to 2-oxo-1-pyrrolidine acetamide acetamide with an empirical formula of $C_6H_{10}N_2O_2$ and a molecular weight of 142.2.

Fig. 1 Piracetam

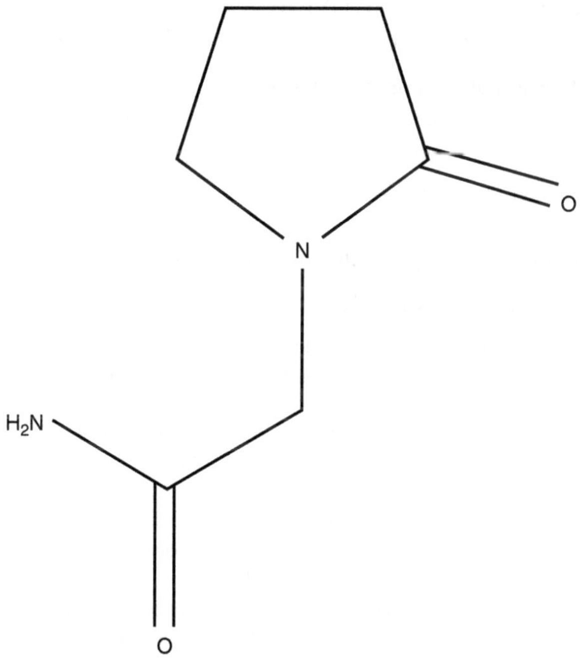

P. N. Patsalos, *Antiseizure Medication Interactions*,
https://doi.org/10.1007/978-3-030-82790-8_23

Pharmacokinetic Characteristics

Absorption and Distribution

After oral ingestion, piracetam is rapidly absorbed (T_{max} = 0.5–1.5 h) with a bioavailability of 100%. Its volume of distribution is 0.6 L/kg and plasma protein binding is 0%.

Biotransformation

Piracetam is not metabolized.

Renal Excretion

Approximately 100% of an administered dose is excreted as unchanged piracetam in urine.

Elimination

Following a single dose, plasma elimination half-life values in young men are 4–6 h.

Effects on Isoenzymes

In vitro piracetam is not an inhibitor of CYP1A2, CYP2B6, CYP2C8, CYP2C9, CYP2C19, CYP2D6, CYP2E1, and CYP4A9/11 at clinically relevant concentrations. Piracetam, in vitro, has a minor inhibitory effect on CYP2A6 and CYP3A4/5.

Therapeutic Drug Monitoring

There are no data relating plasma piracetam levels with that of seizure suppression or adverse effects.

Propensity to Be Associated with Pharmacokinetic Interactions

- Piracetam affects the pharmacokinetics of other drugs—does not interact.
- Other drugs affect the pharmacokinetics of piracetam—does not interact.

Interactions with ASMs

Acetazolamide	The interaction has not been investigated. Theoretically, a pharmacokinetic interaction would not be anticipated
Brivaracetam	The interaction has not been investigated. Theoretically, a pharmacokinetic interaction would not be anticipated
Cannabidiol	The interaction has not been investigated. Theoretically, a pharmacokinetic interaction could occur
Carbamazepine	Does not affect the pharmacokinetics of piracetam [1]
Cenobamate	The interaction has not been investigated. Theoretically, a pharmacokinetic interaction could occur
Clobazam	The interaction has not been investigated. Theoretically, a pharmacokinetic interaction would not be anticipated
Clonazepam	Does not affect the pharmacokinetics of piracetam [2]
Eslicarbazepine acetate	The interaction has not been investigated. Theoretically, a pharmacokinetic interaction would not be anticipated
Ethosuximide	The interaction has not been investigated. Theoretically, a pharmacokinetic interaction would not be anticipated
Everolimus	The interaction has not been investigated. Theoretically, a pharmacokinetic interaction could occur

Felbamate	The interaction has not been investigated. Theoretically, a pharmacokinetic interaction would not be anticipated
Fenfluramine	The interaction has not been investigated. Theoretically, a pharmacokinetic interaction would not be anticipated
Gabapentin	The interaction has not been investigated. Theoretically, a pharmacokinetic interaction would not be anticipated
Lacosamide	The interaction has not been investigated. Theoretically, a pharmacokinetic interaction would not be anticipated
Lamotrigine	The interaction has not been investigated. Theoretically, a pharmacokinetic interaction would not be anticipated
Levetiracetam	The interaction has not been investigated. Theoretically, a pharmacokinetic interaction would not be anticipated
Methsuximide	The interaction has not been investigated. Theoretically, a pharmacokinetic interaction would not be anticipated
Oxcarbazepine	The interaction has not been investigated. Theoretically, a pharmacokinetic interaction would not be anticipated
Perampanel	The interaction has not been investigated. Theoretically, a pharmacokinetic interaction would not be anticipated
Phenobarbital	Does not affect the pharmacokinetics of piracetam [1]
Phenytoin	Does not affect the pharmacokinetics of piracetam [1]
Pregabalin	The interaction has not been investigated. Theoretically, a pharmacokinetic interaction would not be anticipated
Primidone	Does not affect the pharmacokinetics of piracetam [2]
Rufinamide	The interaction has not been investigated. Theoretically, a pharmacokinetic interaction would not be anticipated
Stiripentol	The interaction has not been investigated. Theoretically, a pharmacokinetic interaction would not be anticipated
Sulthiame	The interaction has not been investigated. Theoretically, a pharmacokinetic interaction would not be anticipated
Tiagabine	The interaction has not been investigated. Theoretically, a pharmacokinetic interaction would not be anticipated
Topiramate	The interaction has not been investigated. Theoretically, a pharmacokinetic interaction would not be anticipated
Valproic acid	Does not affect the pharmacokinetics of piracetam [2]
Vigabatrin	The interaction has not been investigated. Theoretically, a pharmacokinetic interaction would not be anticipated
Zonisamide	The interaction has not been investigated. Theoretically, a pharmacokinetic interaction would not be anticipated

References

1. Summary of product characteristics: Piracetam (Nootropil). UCB Pharma Ltd. Last update 9 Feb 2017.
2. Obeso JA, Artieda J, Quinn N, Rothwell JC, Luquin MR, Vaamonde J, Marsden CD. Piracetam in the treatment of different types of myoclonus. Clin Neuropharmacol. 1988;11:529–36.

Pregabalin

Pregabalin (Fig. 1) corresponds chemically to *S*-3-(aminomethyl)-5-methylhexanoic acid with an empirical formula of $C_8H_{17}NO_2$ and a molecular weight of 159.2.

Pharmacokinetic Characteristics

Absorption and Distribution

After oral ingestion, pregabalin is rapidly absorbed (T_{max} = 1–2 h) with a bioavailability of ≥90%. Its volume of distribution is 0.57 L/kg, and plasma protein binding is 0%.

Biotransformation

Pregabalin is not metabolized.

Fig. 1 Pregabalin

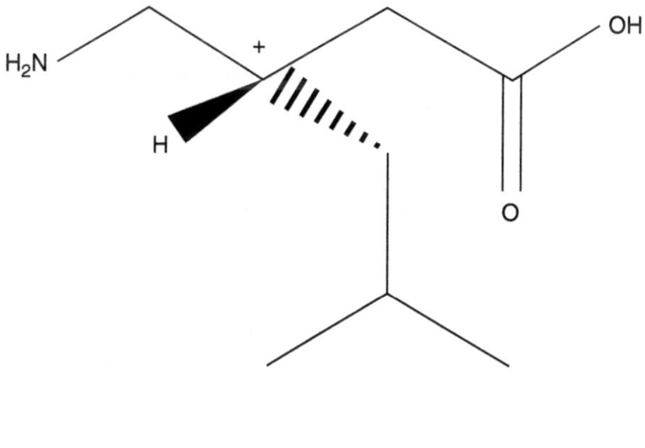

P. N. Patsalos, *Antiseizure Medication Interactions*,
https://doi.org/10.1007/978-3-030-82790-8_24

Renal Excretion

Approximately 98% of an administered dose is excreted as unchanged pregabalin in urine.

Elimination

Following a single dose, plasma elimination half-life values in adults and children (up to 6 years of age) are 5–7 h and 3–4 h, respectively.

Effects on Isoenzymes

No in vitro data on the induction or inhibition potential of pregabalin on human CYP or UGT isoenzymes have been published.

Therapeutic Drug Monitoring

Very little information is available regarding therapeutic plasma concentrations of pregabalin. However, one report states that in samples collected at random times relative to dose from patients maintained on 600 mg/day, serum pregabalin concentrations ranged from 0.9 to 14.2 mg/L (5.6–89.2 μmol/L). The conversion factor from mg/L to μmol/L for pregabalin is 6.28 (1 mg/L = 6.28 /L).

Propensity to Be Associated with Pharmacokinetic Interactions

- Pregabalin affects the pharmacokinetics of other drugs—does not interact.
- Other drugs affect the pharmacokinetics of pregabalin—does not interact.

Interactions with ASMs

Acetazolamide	The interaction has not been investigated. Theoretically, a pharmacokinetic interaction would not be anticipated
Brivaracetam	Does not affect the pharmacokinetics of pregabalin [1]
Cannabidiol	Does not affect the pharmacokinetics of pregabalin [2]
Carbamazepine	Does not affect the pharmacokinetics of pregabalin [3]
Cenobamate	The interaction has not been investigated. Theoretically, a pharmacokinetic interaction would not be anticipated
Clobazam	The interaction has not been investigated. Theoretically, a pharmacokinetic interaction would not be anticipated
Clonazepam	The interaction has not been investigated. Theoretically, a pharmacokinetic interaction would not be anticipated
Eslicarbazepine acetate	The interaction has not been investigated. Theoretically, a pharmacokinetic interaction would not be anticipated
Ethosuximide	The interaction has not been investigated. Theoretically, a pharmacokinetic interaction would not be anticipated
Everolimus	The interaction has not been investigated. Theoretically, a pharmacokinetic interaction would not be anticipated
Felbamate	The interaction has not been investigated. Theoretically, a pharmacokinetic interaction would not be anticipated
Fenfluramine	The interaction has not been investigated. Theoretically, a pharmacokinetic interaction would not be anticipated
Gabapentin	Pregabalin plasma levels are decreased
Consequence	Pregabalin C_{max} values are decreased by 18% [4]

Lacosamide	The interaction has not been investigated. Theoretically, a pharmacokinetic interaction would not be anticipated
Lamotrigine	Does not affect the pharmacokinetics of pregabalin [3]
Levetiracetam	Does not affect the pharmacokinetics of pregabalin [5]
Methsuximide	The interaction has not been investigated. Theoretically, a pharmacokinetic interaction would not be anticipated
Oxcarbazepine	The interaction has not been investigated. Theoretically, a pharmacokinetic interaction would not be anticipated
Perampanel	The interaction has not been investigated. Theoretically, a pharmacokinetic interaction would not be anticipated
Phenobarbital	Does not affect the pharmacokinetics of pregabalin [6]
Phenytoin	Pregabalin plasma levels are decreased
Consequence	Pregabalin mean C_{max} and AUC values are decreased by ~30% and 14%, respectively. However, this is thought to be an effect of food co-ingestion [3]
Piracetam	The interaction has not been investigated. Theoretically, a pharmacokinetic interaction would not be anticipated
Primidone	The interaction has not been investigated. Theoretically, a pharmacokinetic interaction would not be anticipated
Rufinamide	The interaction has not been investigated. Theoretically, a pharmacokinetic interaction would not be anticipated
Stiripentol	The interaction has not been investigated. Theoretically, a pharmacokinetic interaction would not be anticipated
Sulthiame	The interaction has not been investigated. Theoretically, a pharmacokinetic interaction would not be anticipated
Tiagabine	Does not affect the pharmacokinetics of pregabalin [7]
Topiramate	Does not affect the pharmacokinetics of pregabalin [8]
Valproic acid	Does not affect the pharmacokinetics of pregabalin [3]
Vigabatrin	The interaction has not been investigated. Theoretically, a pharmacokinetic interaction would not be anticipated
Zonisamide	The interaction has not been investigated. Theoretically, a pharmacokinetic interaction would not be anticipated

References

1. Moseley BD, Otoul C, Staelens L, Stockis A. Pharmacokinetic interaction of brivaracetam on other antiepileptic drugs in adults with focal seizures: pooled analysis of data from randomized clinical trials. Epilepsy Res. 2019;158:106218.
2. Gaston TE, Bekib EM, Cutter GR, Liu Y, Szaflarski JP, UAB CBD Program. Interactions between cannabidiol and commonly used antiepileptic drugs. Epilepsia. 2017;58:1586–92.
3. Brodie MJ, Wilson EA, Wesche DL, Alvey CW, Randinitis EJ, Posvar EL, Hounslow NJ, Bron NJ, Gibson GL, Bockbrader HN. Pregabalin drug interaction studies: lack of effect on the pharmacokinetics of carbamazepine, phenytoin, lamotrigine, and valproate in patients with partial epilepsy. Epilepsia. 2005;46:1407–13.
4. Ben-Menachem E. Pregabalin pharmacology and its relevance to clinical practice. Epilepsia. 2004;45(Suppl 6):13–8.

5. Patsalos PN. Levetiracetam: pharmacology and therapeutics in the treatment of epilepsy and other neurological conditions. Rev Contemp Pharmacother. 2004;13:1–168.
6. May TW, Rambeck B, Neb R, Jurgens U. Serum concentrations of pregabalin in patients with epilepsy: the influence of dose, age, and comedication. Ther Drug Monit. 2007;29:789–94.
7. Summary of product characteristics: Pregabalin (Lyrica). Upjohn UK Ltd; Last update Nov 2020.
8. Bockbrader HN, Burger PJ, Corrigan BW, Kugler AR, Knapp LE, Garofalo EA, Lalonde RL. Population pharmacokinetic (PK) analysis of commonly prescribed antiepileptic drugs (AEDs) co-administered with pregabalin (PGB) in adult patients with refractory partial seizures. Epilepsia. 2001;42(Suppl 7):84.

Primidone

Primidone (Fig. 1) corresponds chemically to 5-ethyldihydro-5-phenyl-4,6(1-H,5H) pyrimidine-dione with an empirical formula of $C_{12}H_{14}N_2O_2$ and a molecular weight of 218.25.

Pharmacokinetic Characteristics

Absorption and Distribution

After oral ingestion, primidone is rapidly absorbed (T_{max} = 2–4 h, adults; 4–6 h children) with a bioavailability of >90%. Its volume of distribution is 0.5–0.8 L/kg, and plasma protein binding is 10%.

Fig. 1 Primidone

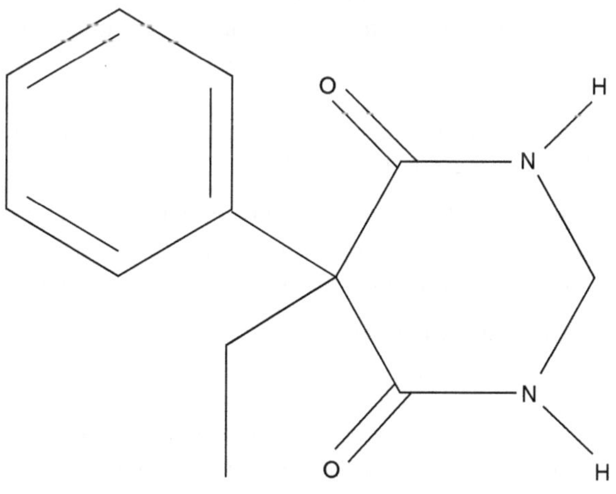

P. N. Patsalos, *Antiseizure Medication Interactions*,
https://doi.org/10.1007/978-3-030-82790-8_25

Biotransformation
Primidone is extensively metabolized in the liver by cleavage of the pyrimidine ring and oxidation of the methylene group to form, respectively, two primary metabolites, namely, phenylethylmalonamide (PEMA) and phenobarbital. Phenobarbital subsequently undergoes metabolism to two metabolites, *p*-hydroxyphenobarbital and 9-d-glucopyranosylphenobarbital. Both phenobarbital and PEMA are pharmacologically active. Primidone, via its metabolite phenobarbital, is an enzyme inducer, and additionally, phenobarbital undergoes autoinduction so that its clearance can increase and this may require an upward dosage adjustment of primidone.

Renal Excretion
Approximately 65% of an administered dose is excreted as unchanged primidone in urine.

Elimination
In the absence of enzyme-inducing antiseizure medications, plasma elimination half-life values in adults are 7–22 h, while in the presence of enzyme-inducing antiseizure medications, half-life values are 3–12 h. In newborns, half-life values are 8–80 h, and in children, they are 5–11 h.

Time to new steady-state blood levels consequent to an inhibition of metabolism interaction:

- Primidone = 2–4 days later
- Phenobarbital (derived) = 15–29 days later

Effects on Isoenzymes
No in vitro data on the induction or inhibition potential of primidone on human CYP or UGT isoenzymes have been published.

Therapeutic Drug Monitoring
Optimum seizure control in patients on primidone monotherapy is most likely to occur at primidone plasma levels of 5–10 mg/L (23–46 μmol/L) and phenobarbital plasma levels of 10–40 mg/L (43–172 μmol/L). The conversion factor from mg/L to μmol/L for primidone is 4.59 (1 mg/L = 4.59 μmol/L), and for phenobarbital, it is 4.31 (i.e., 1 mg/L = 4.31 μmol/L).

Propensity to Be Associated with Pharmacokinetic Interactions
- Primidone affects the pharmacokinetics of other drugs—substantial.
- Other drugs affect the pharmacokinetics of primidone—substantial.

Interactions with ASMs

Acetazolamide	Decreases plasma primidone levels
Consequence	Acetazolamide decreases the absorption of primidone so that plasma primidone levels are low or not detectable [1]
Brivaracetam	Does not affect the pharmacokinetics of primidone [2]
Cannabidiol	The interaction has not been investigated. Theoretically, a pharmacokinetic interaction could occur
Carbamazepine	Enhances the metabolism of primidone

Consequence	Carbamazepine can decrease the mean plasma primidone level to dose ratio by 17% and increase mean plasma phenobarbital to primidone ratio by 59% [3]
Cenobamate	The interaction has not been investigated. Theoretically, a pharmacokinetic interaction could occur
Clobazam	Inhibits the metabolism of primidone
Consequence	Clobazam decreases the plasma clearance of primidone so that plasma primidone levels are increased [4]
Clonazepam	Does not affect the pharmacokinetics of primidone [5]
Eslicarbazepine acetate	The interaction has not been investigated. Theoretically, a pharmacokinetic interaction would not be anticipated
Ethosuximide	Inhibits the metabolism of primidone
Consequence	Ethosuximide can increase the mean plasma primidone level to dose ratio by 7% but does not affect the mean plasma phenobarbital to primidone ratio [3]
Everolimus	The interaction has not been investigated. Theoretically, a pharmacokinetic interaction could occur
Felbamate	The interaction has not been investigated. Theoretically, a pharmacokinetic interaction could occur
Fenfluramine	The interaction has not been investigated. Theoretically, a pharmacokinetic interaction could occur
Gabapentin	The interaction has not been investigated. Theoretically, a pharmacokinetic interaction would not be anticipated
Lacosamide	The interaction has not been investigated. Theoretically, a pharmacokinetic interaction would not be anticipated
Lamotrigine	Does not affect the pharmacokinetics of primidone [6]
Levetiracetam	Does not affect the pharmacokinetics of primidone [7]
Methsuximide	The metabolism of primidone to phenobarbital is unaffected, but the subsequent metabolism of phenobarbital is inhibited
Consequence	Methsuximide may cause a 17% increase in plasma phenobarbital levels. The interaction is considered to be the consequence of inhibition of phenobarbital metabolism through CYP2C9 [8]
Oxcarbazepine	The interaction has not been investigated. Theoretically, a pharmacokinetic interaction could occur
Perampanel	The interaction has not been investigated. Theoretically, a pharmacokinetic interaction would not be anticipated
	Perampanel in combination with primidone is associated with an increased risk of decreased appetite. This effect may be the consequence of a pharmacodynamic interaction [9]
Phenobarbital	Combination not commonly co-prescribed
Phenytoin	Enhances the metabolism of primidone
Consequence	Mean plasma primidone levels can decrease by 33%, and mean plasma phenobarbital levels can increase by 112% [10]
Piracetam	The interaction has not been investigated. Theoretically, a pharmacokinetic interaction would not be anticipated
Pregabalin	The interaction has not been investigated. Theoretically, a pharmacokinetic interaction would not be anticipated
Rufinamide	The interaction has not been investigated. Theoretically, a pharmacokinetic interaction would not be anticipated

Stiripentol	Inhibits the metabolism of primidone. The metabolism of the derived phenobarbital is also inhibited
Consequence	The plasma clearance of phenobarbital is decreased by >48% so that plasma phenobarbital levels are increased. The interaction is the consequence of inhibition of CYP2C9 and CYP2C19 [11]
Sulthiame	The metabolism of primidone to phenobarbital is unaffected, but the subsequent metabolism of phenobarbital is inhibited
Consequence	Sulthiame may increase plasma phenobarbital levels [12]
	During combination therapy, sulthiame adverse effects such as dizziness, uncertain gate, and drowsiness may be enhanced. This is considered to be the consequence of a pharmacodynamic interaction [12]
Tiagabine	The interaction has not been investigated. Theoretically, a pharmacokinetic interaction would not be anticipated
Topiramate	Does not affect the pharmacokinetics of primidone [13]
Valproic acid	The metabolism of primidone to phenobarbital is unaffected, but the subsequent metabolism of phenobarbital is inhibited
Consequence	Mean plasma phenobarbital levels can increase by 51%, probably via an action on CYP2C9 and/or CYP2C19, but plasma primidone levels are unaffected [14]
Vigabatrin	Does not affect the pharmacokinetics of primidone [15]
Zonisamide	Does not affect the pharmacokinetics of primidone [16]

References

1. Syversen GB, Morgan JP, Weintraub M, Myers GJ. Acetazolamide-induced interference with primidone absorption. Case reports and metabolic studies. Arch Neurol. 1977;34:80–4.
2. Moseley BD, Chanteux H, Nicolas JM, Laloyaux C, Gidal B. A review of the drug-drug interactions of the antiepileptic drug brivaracetam. Epilepsy Res. 2020;163:106327.
3. Battino D, Avanzini G, Bossi L, Croci D, Cusi C, Gomeni C, Moise A. Plasma levels of primidone and its metabolite phenobarbital: effect of age and associated therapy. Ther Drug Monit. 1983;5:73–9.
4. Theis JGW, Koren G, Daneman R, Sherwin AL, Menzano E, Cortez M, Hwang P. Interactions of clobazam with conventional antiepileptics in children. J Child Neurol. 1997;12:208–13.
5. Nanda RN, Johnson RH, Keogh HJ, Lambie DG, Melville ID. Treatment of epilepsy with clonazepam and its effect on other anti-convulsants. J Neurol Neurosurg Psychiatry. 1977;40:538–43.
6. Jawad S, Richens A, Goodwin G, Yuen WC. Controlled trial of lamotrigine (lamictal) for refractory partial seizures. Epilepsia. 1989;30:356–63.
7. Perucca E, Baltes E, Ledent E. Levetiracetam: absence of pharmacokinetic interactions with other antiepileptic drugs (AEDs). Epilepsia. 2000;41(Suppl):150.
8. Browne TR, Feldman RG, Buchanan RA, Allen NC, Fawcett-Vickers L, Szabo GK, Mattson GF, Norman SE, Greenblatt DJ. Methsuximide for complex partial seizures: efficacy, toxicity, clinical pharmacology, and drug interactions. Neurology. 1983;33:414–8.
9. Gidal BE, Ferry J, Majid O, Hussein Z. Concentration-effect relationships with perampanel in patients with pharmacoresistant partial-onset seizures. Epilepsia. 2013;54:1490–7.
10. Fincham RW, Schottelius DD, Sahs AL. The influence of diphenylhydantoin on primidone metabolism. Arch Neurol. 1974;30:259–62.

11. Levy RH, Loiseau P, Guyot M, Blehaut H, Tor J, Moreland TA. Stiripentol kinetics in epilepsy: nonlinearity and interactions. Clin Pharmacol Ther. 1984;36:661–9.
12. Summary of product characteristics: Sulthiame (Ospolot). Phebra Pty, Ltd. Last update 21 Nov 2013.
13. Doose DR, Walker SA, Pledger G, Lim P, Reife RA. Evaluation of phenobarbital and primidone/phenobarbital (primidone active metabolite) plasma concentrations during administration of add-on topiramate therapy in five multicenter, double-blind, placebo controlled trials in outpatients with partial seizures. Epilepsia. 1995;36(Suppl 3):158.
14. Kapetanovic IM, Kupferberg HJ, Porter RJ, Theodore W, Schulman E, Penry JK. Mechanism of valproate–phenobarbital interaction in epileptic patients. Clin Pharmacol Ther. 1981;29:480–6.
15. Matilainen R, Pitkanen A, Ruutiainen T, et al. Effect of vigabatrin on epilepsy in mentally retarded patients: a 7-month follow-up study. Neurology. 1988;38:743–7.
16. Schmidt D, Jacob R, Loiseau P, Deisenhammer E, Klinger D, Despland A, Egli M, Basuer G, Stenzel E, Blankenhorn V. Zonisamide for add-on treatment of refractory partial epilepsy: a European double-blind trial. Epilepsy Res. 1993;15:67–73.

11. Levy RH, Loiseau P, Guyot M, Blehaut H, Tor J, Moreland TA. Stiripentol kinetics in epilepsy: nonlinearity and interactions. Clin Pharmacol Ther. 1984;36:661–9.
12. Summary of product characteristics: Sulthiame (Ospolot). Health PG, Ltd. Last update 2? Nov 2017.
13. Doose DR, Walker SA, Pledger G, Lim P, Reife RA. Evaluation of phenobarbital and primidone/phenobarbital (primidone's active metabolite) plasma concentrations during administra [illegible] outpatients with partial seizures. Epilepsia. 1995;36(Suppl 4):158.
14. Kapetanovic IM, Kupferberg HJ, Porter RJ, Theodore W, Schulman E, Penry JK. Mechanism of valproate-phenobarbital interaction in epileptic patients. Clin Pharmacol Ther. 1981;29:480–6.
15. Matilainen R, Pitkänen A, Ruutiainen T, et al. Effect of vigabatrin on epilepsy in mentally retarded patients: a 7-month follow-up study. Neurology. 1988;3[illegible].
16. Schmidt D, Jacob R, Loiseau P, Deisenhammer E, Klinger D, Despland A, Egli M, Bauer G, Stenzel E, Blankenhorn V. Zonisamide for add-on treatment of refractory partial epilepsy: a European double-blind trial. Epilepsy Res. 1993;15:67–73.

Rufinamide

Rufinamide (Fig. 1) corresponds chemically to 1-[(2,6-difluorophenyl) methyl]-1-hydro-1,23-triazole-4 carboxamide with an empirical formula of $C_{10}H_8F_2N_4O$ and a molecular weight of 238.19.

Pharmacokinetic Characteristics

Absorption and Distribution

After oral ingestion, rufinamide is rapidly absorbed (T_{max} = 4–6 h) with a bioavailability of at least 85%. Its volume of distribution is 0.71–1.14 L/kg, and plasma protein binding is 35%.

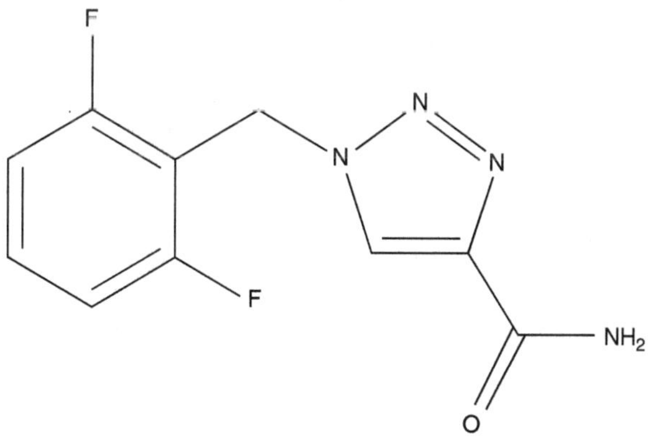

Fig. 1 Rufinamide

P. N. Patsalos, *Antiseizure Medication Interactions*,
https://doi.org/10.1007/978-3-030-82790-8_26

Biotransformation

Rufinamide is extensively metabolized in the liver, primarily by hydrolysis mediated by carboxylesterase 1, to a carboxylic acid derivative CGP 47292. Acyl glucuronide metabolites of CGP 47292 constitute minor components.

Renal Excretion

Approximately 2% of an administered dose is excreted as unchanged rufinamide in urine.

Elimination

Plasma elimination half-life values for rufinamide in adults are 6–10 h.

Time to new steady-state blood levels consequent to an inhibition of metabolism interaction

- Adults = 1–2 days later

Effects on Isoenzymes

At therapeutic concentrations, rufinamide in vitro has no inhibitory effect on the activity of CYP1A2, CYP2A6, CYP2C9, CYP2C19, CYP2D, CYP2E1, CYP3A4/5, and CYP4A9/11. Consequently, pharmacokinetic interactions of metabolic origin with other antiseizure medications and other medicines are not expected.

No in vitro data on the induction potential of rufinamide on human CYP enzymes have been published.

Therapeutic Drug Monitoring

Optimum seizure control in patients on rufinamide monotherapy is most likely to occur at plasma levels of 30–40 mg/L (126–168 μmol/L). The conversion factor from mg/L to μmol/L for rufinamide is 4.20 (i.e., 1 mg/L = 4.20 μmol/L).

Propensity to Be Associated with Pharmacokinetic Interactions

- Rufinamide affects the pharmacokinetics of other drugs—minimal.
- Other drugs affect the pharmacokinetics of rufinamide—minimal.

Interactions with ASMs

Acetazolamide	The interaction has not been investigated. Theoretically, a pharmacokinetic interaction would not be anticipated
Brivaracetam	The interaction has not been investigated. Theoretically, a pharmacokinetic interaction would not be anticipated
Cannabidiol	Inhibits the metabolism of rufinamide
Consequence	Increases mean plasma rufinamide levels by 9% [1]
Carbamazepine	Enhances the metabolism of rufinamide
Consequence	Steady-state plasma rufinamide levels can decrease by 19–26%. This interaction is more substantial in children [2]
Cenobamate	The interaction has not been investigated. Theoretically, a pharmacokinetic interaction would not be anticipated
Clobazam	Does not affect the pharmacokinetics of rufinamide [2]
Clonazepam	The interaction has not been investigated. Theoretically, a pharmacokinetic interaction would not be anticipated
Eslicarbazepine acetate	The interaction has not been investigated. Theoretically, a pharmacokinetic interaction would not be anticipated

Ethosuximide	The interaction has not been investigated. Theoretically, a pharmacokinetic interaction would not be anticipated
Everolimus	The interaction has not been investigated. Theoretically, a pharmacokinetic interaction would not be anticipated
Felbamate	The interaction has not been investigated. Theoretically, a pharmacokinetic interaction could occur
Fenfluramine	The interaction has not been investigated. Theoretically, a pharmacokinetic interaction would not be anticipated
Gabapentin	Does not affect the pharmacokinetics of rufinamide [3]
Lacosamide	The interaction has not been investigated. Theoretically, a pharmacokinetic interaction would not be anticipated
Lamotrigine	Does not affect the pharmacokinetics of rufinamide [2]
Levetiracetam	The interaction has not been investigated. Theoretically, a pharmacokinetic interaction would not be anticipated
Methsuximide	Enhances the metabolism of rufinamide
Consequence	Mean rufinamide plasma levels can decrease by 29% [4]
Oxcarbazepine	Enhances the metabolism of rufinamide
Consequence	Mean rufinamide plasma levels can decrease by 21% [4]
Perampanel	The interaction has not been investigated. Theoretically, a pharmacokinetic interaction would not be anticipated
Phenobarbital	Enhances the metabolism of rufinamide
Consequence	Steady-state plasma rufinamide levels can decrease by 25–46%. This interaction is more substantial in children [2]
Phenytoin	Enhances the metabolism of rufinamide
Consequence	Steady-state plasma rufinamide levels can decrease by 25–46%. This interaction is more substantial in children [2]
Piracetam	The interaction has not been investigated. Theoretically, a pharmacokinetic interaction would not be anticipated
Pregabalin	The interaction has not been investigated. Theoretically, a pharmacokinetic interaction would not be anticipated
Primidone	Enhances the metabolism of rufinamide
Consequence	Steady-state plasma rufinamide levels can decrease by 25–46%. This interaction is more substantial in children [2]
Stiripentol	The interaction has not been investigated. Theoretically, a pharmacokinetic interaction could occur
Sulthiame	The interaction has not been investigated. Theoretically, a pharmacokinetic interaction could occur
Tiagabine	The interaction has not been investigated. Theoretically, a pharmacokinetic interaction would not be anticipated
Topiramate	Does not affect the pharmacokinetics of rufinamide [2]
Valproic acid	Inhibits the metabolism of rufinamide

Consequence	The interaction is more marked in children, and typically, rufinamide plasma levels can increase by 55–70%. Rufinamide plasma levels can increase by ≤26% and <16% in adolescents and adults, respectively. The difference in magnitude of this interaction can be explained by the observation that plasma valproic acid levels were higher in the children rather than effect of age per se. The mechanism for this interaction is unknown but may involve inhibition of the carboxylesterases responsible for the metabolism of rufinamide [2]
Vigabatrin	Enhances the metabolism of rufinamide
Consequence	Steady-state plasma rufinamide levels can decrease by 14–30%. This interaction is more substantial in children [2]
Zonisamide	The interaction has not been investigated. Theoretically, a pharmacokinetic interaction could occur

References

1. Gaston TE, Bekib EM, Cutter GR, Liu Y, Szaflarski JP, UAB CBD Program. Interactions between cannabidiol and commonly used antiepileptic drugs. Epilepsia. 2017;58:1586–92.
2. Perucca E, Cloyd J, Critchley D, Fuseau E. Rufinamide: clinical pharmacokinetics and concentration-response relationships in patients with epilepsy. Epilepsia. 2008;49:1123–41.
3. Brodie MJ, Rosenfeld WE, Vazquez B, et al. Rufinamide for the adjunctive treatment of partial seizures in adults and adolescents a randomized placebo-controlled trial. Epilepsia. 2009;50:1899–909.
4. May TW, Boor R, Rambeck B, Jurgens U, Korn-Merker E, Brandt C. Serum concentrations of rufinamide in children and adults with epilepsy the influence of dose, age, and comedication. Ther Drug Monit. 2011;33:214–21.

Stiripentol

Stiripentol (Fig. 1) corresponds chemically to 4, 4-dimethyl-1[3, 4(methylenedioxy)-phenyl]-1-pentan-3-ol with an empirical formula of $C_{14}H_{18}O_3$ and a molecular weight of 234.

Pharmacokinetic Characteristics

Absorption and Distribution

After oral ingestion, stiripentol is rapidly absorbed (T_{max} = 0.5–2 h) with a bioavailability of ≥70%. Its volume of distribution is not known, and plasma protein binding is 99%.

Biotransformation

Stiripentol is extensively metabolized in the liver, primarily by demethylation and glucuronidation, to 13 different metabolites. The precise identification of the enzymes involved in metabolism is not known, but the principal enzymes are considered to be CYP1A2, CYP2C19, and CYP3A4.

Fig. 1 Stiripentol

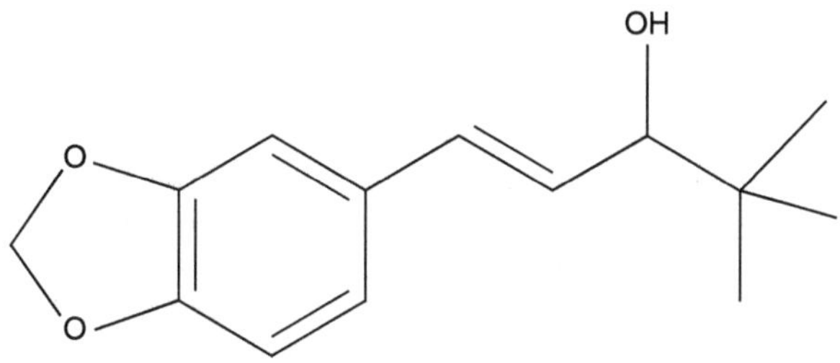

P. N. Patsalos, *Antiseizure Medication Interactions*,
https://doi.org/10.1007/978-3-030-82790-8_27

Renal Excretion
Approximately 3–14% of an administered dose is excreted as unchanged stiripentol in urine.

Elimination
Plasma elimination half-life values in adults are 4.5–13.0 h. Stiripentol elimination follows Michaelis–Menten (saturable, zero-order) kinetics so that plasma half-life and clearance is dose-dependent with values decreasing with increasing dose. As a result, steady-state plasma stiripentol levels increase more than proportionately after a dose increment.

Effects on Isoenzymes
At therapeutic concentrations, stiripentol in vitro substantially inhibits the activity of CYP3A4. CYP1A2, CYP2C19, and CYP2D6.

Therapeutic Drug Monitoring
While the reference range for stiripentol in plasma is not well defined, concentrations of 4–22 mg/L (17–94 μmol/L) correlate with control of absence seizures in children, and in Dravet syndrome, concentrations of 8–12 mg/L (34–51 μmol/L) are reported to be effective. The conversion factor from mg/L to μmol/L for stiripentol is 4.27 (i.e., 1 mg/L = 4.27 μmol/L).

Propensity to Be Associated with Pharmacokinetic Interactions

- Stiripentol affects the pharmacokinetics of other drugs—substantial.
- Other drugs affect the pharmacokinetics of stiripentol—substantial.

Interactions with ASMs

Acetazolamide	The interaction has not been investigated. Theoretically, a pharmacokinetic interaction would not be anticipated
Brivaracetam	The interaction has not been investigated. Theoretically, a pharmacokinetic interaction would not be anticipated
Cannabidiol	Inhibits the metabolism of stiripentol
Consequence	Mean plasma stiripentol AUC values increase by 30–55% [1]
Carbamazepine	Enhances the metabolism of stiripentol
Consequence	Mean plasma clearance of stiripentol is increased by 300% so that stiripentol plasma levels can decrease substantially. The interaction is probably the consequence of induction of CYP3A4 and CYP2C19 [2]
Cenobamate	The interaction has not been investigated. Theoretically, a pharmacokinetic interaction could occur
Clobazam	Inhibits the metabolism of stiripentol
Consequence	Mean plasma stiripentol levels are increased by 25% [3]
Clonazepam	The interaction has not been investigated. Theoretically, a pharmacokinetic interaction would not be anticipated
Eslicarbazepine acetate	The interaction has not been investigated. Theoretically, a pharmacokinetic interaction would not be anticipated
Ethosuximide	The interaction has not been investigated. Theoretically, a pharmacokinetic interaction would not be anticipated

Everolimus	The interaction has not been investigated. Theoretically, a pharmacokinetic interaction could occur
Felbamate	The interaction has not been investigated. Theoretically, a pharmacokinetic interaction could occur
Fenfluramine	Does not affect the pharmacokinetics of stiripentol [4]
Gabapentin	The interaction has not been investigated. Theoretically, a pharmacokinetic interaction would not be anticipated
Lacosamide	The interaction has not been investigated. Theoretically, a pharmacokinetic interaction would not be anticipated
Lamotrigine	The interaction has not been investigated. Theoretically, a pharmacokinetic interaction would not be anticipated
Levetiracetam	The interaction has not been investigated. Theoretically, a pharmacokinetic interaction would not be anticipated
Methsuximide	The interaction has not been investigated. Theoretically, a pharmacokinetic interaction would not be anticipated
Oxcarbazepine	The interaction has not been investigated. Theoretically, a pharmacokinetic interaction could occur
Perampanel	The interaction has not been investigated. Theoretically, a pharmacokinetic interaction would not be anticipated
Phenobarbital	Enhances the metabolism of stiripentol
Consequence	Mean plasma clearance of stiripentol is increased by 300% so that stiripentol plasma levels can decrease substantially. The interaction is probably the consequence of induction of CYP3A4 and CYP2C19 [2]
Phenytoin	Enhances the metabolism of stiripentol
Consequence	Mean plasma clearance of stiripentol is increased by 300% so that stiripentol plasma levels can decrease substantially. The interaction is probably the consequence of induction of CYP3A4 and CYP2C19 [2]
Piracetam	The interaction has not been investigated. Theoretically, a pharmacokinetic interaction would not be anticipated
Pregabalin	The interaction has not been investigated. Theoretically, a pharmacokinetic interaction would not be anticipated
Primidone	Enhances the metabolism of stiripentol
Consequence	Mean plasma clearance of stiripentol is increased by 300% so that stiripentol plasma levels can decrease substantially. The interaction is probably the consequence of induction of CYP3A4 and CYP2C19 [2]
Rufinamide	The interaction has not been investigated. Theoretically, a pharmacokinetic interaction would not be anticipated
Sulthiame	The interaction has not been investigated. Theoretically, a pharmacokinetic interaction could occur
Tiagabine	The interaction has not been investigated. Theoretically, a pharmacokinetic interaction would not be anticipated
Topiramate	The interaction has not been investigated. Theoretically, a pharmacokinetic interaction could occur
Valproic acid	Does not affect the pharmacokinetics of stiripentol [3]
Vigabatrin	The interaction has not been investigated. Theoretically, a pharmacokinetic interaction would not be anticipated
Zonisamide	The interaction has not been investigated. Theoretically, a pharmacokinetic interaction could occur

References

1. Patsalos PN, Szaflarski JP, Gidal B, Van Landingham K, Critchley D, Morrison G. Clinical implications of trials investigating drug-drug interactions between cannabidiol and enzyme inducers or inhibitors or common antiseizure drugs. Epilepsia. 2020;61:1854–68.
2. Levy RH, Loiseau P, Guyot M, Blehaut H, Tor J, Moreland TA. Stiripentol kinetics in epilepsy: nonlinearity and interactions. Clin Pharmacol Ther. 1984;36:661–9.
3. May TW, Boor R, Mayer T, Jurgens U, Rambeck B, Holert N, Korn-Merker E, Brandt C. Concentrations of stiripentol in children and adults with epilepsy: the influence of dose, age and comedication. Ther Drug Monit. 2012;34:390–7.
4. Boyd B, Smith S, Gammaitoni A, Galer BS, Farfel GM. A phase 1, randomized, open-label, single dose, 3 period crossover study to evaluate the drug-drug interaction between ZX008 (fenfluramine HCl oral solution) and a regimen of stiripentol, clobazam, and valproate in healthy subjects. Int J Clin Pharmacol Therapeut. 2019;57:11–9.

Sulthiame

Sulthiame (Fig. 1) corresponds chemically to 4(1, 1-diozothiazinan-2-yl)benzene-sulfonamide with an empirical formula of $C_{10}H_{14}N_2O_4S_2$ and a molecular weight of 290.04.

Fig. 1 Sulthiame

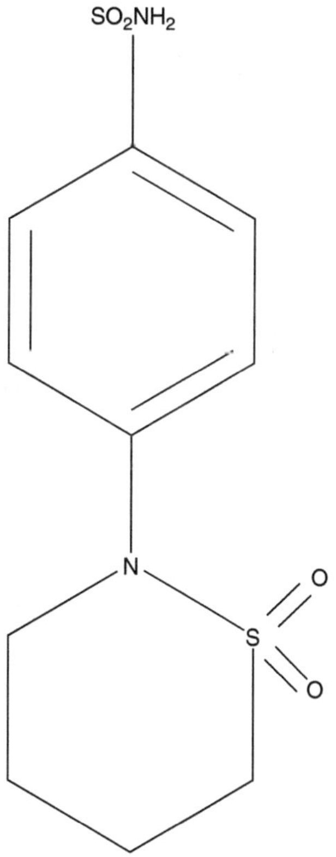

P. N. Patsalos, *Antiseizure Medication Interactions*,
https://doi.org/10.1007/978-3-030-82790-8_28

Pharmacokinetic Characteristics

Absorption and Distribution

After oral ingestion, sulthiame is rapidly absorbed (T_{max} = 1–5 h) with a bioavailability of 100%. Its volume of distribution is not known, and plasma protein binding is 29%.

Biotransformation

Sulthiame undergoes moderate metabolism in the liver via unknown isoenzymes to unknown metabolites.

Renal Excretion

Approximately 32% of an administered dose is excreted unchanged as sulthiame in urine.

Elimination

Plasma elimination half-life values in adults are 8–15 h, and in children, half-life values are 5–7 h.

Effects on Isoenzymes

No in vitro data on the induction or inhibition potential of sulthiame on human CYP or UGT isoenzymes have been published.

Therapeutic Drug Monitoring

Optimum seizure control in adult patients on polytherapy is most likely to occur at plasma sulthiame levels of 2–10 mg/L (7–34 μmol/L), while in children on polytherapy, it is most likely to occur at plasma sulthiame levels of 1–3 mg/L (3–10 μmol/L). The conversion factor from mg/L to μmol/L for sulthiame is 3.45 (i.e., 1 mg/L = 3.45 μmol/L).

Propensity to Be Associated with Pharmacokinetic Interactions

- Sulthiame affects the pharmacokinetics of other drugs—substantial.
- Other drugs affect the pharmacokinetics of sulthiame—minimal.

Interactions with ASMs

Acetazolamide	The interaction has not been investigated. Theoretically, a pharmacokinetic interaction would not be anticipated
	Acetazolamide and sulthiame are both weak inhibitors of carbonic anhydrase and, as a direct result, may independently increase the risk of renal calculi. Consequently, there is a theoretical potential that when they are administered together, an adverse pharmacodynamic interaction will occur [1]
Brivaracetam	The interaction has not been investigated. Theoretically, a pharmacokinetic interaction would not be anticipated
Cannabidiol	The interaction has not been investigated. Theoretically, a pharmacokinetic interaction would not be anticipated
Carbamazepine	Enhances the metabolism of sulthiame
Consequence	Plasma sulthiame levels can decrease [2]

Cenobamate	The interaction has not been investigated. Theoretically, a pharmacokinetic interaction would not be anticipated
Clobazam	The interaction has not been investigated. Theoretically, a pharmacokinetic interaction would not be anticipated
Clonazepam	The interaction has not been investigated. Theoretically, a pharmacokinetic interaction would not be anticipated
Eslicarbazepine acetate	The interaction has not been investigated. Theoretically, a pharmacokinetic interaction would not be anticipated
Ethosuximide	The interaction has not been investigated. Theoretically, a pharmacokinetic interaction would not be anticipated
Everolimus	The interaction has not been investigated. Theoretically, a pharmacokinetic interaction would not be anticipated
Felbamate	The interaction has not been investigated. Theoretically, a pharmacokinetic interaction could occur
Fenfluramine	The interaction has not been investigated. Theoretically, a pharmacokinetic interaction would not be anticipated
Gabapentin	The interaction has not been investigated. Theoretically, a pharmacokinetic interaction would not be anticipated
Lacosamide	The interaction has not been investigated. Theoretically, a pharmacokinetic interaction would not be anticipated
Lamotrigine	The interaction has not been investigated. Theoretically, a pharmacokinetic interaction would not be anticipated
Levetiracetam	The interaction has not been investigated. Theoretically, a pharmacokinetic interaction would not be anticipated
Methsuximide	The interaction has not been investigated. Theoretically, a pharmacokinetic interaction would not be anticipated
Oxcarbazepine	The interaction has not been investigated. Theoretically, a pharmacokinetic interaction would not be anticipated
Perampanel	The interaction has not been investigated. Theoretically, a pharmacokinetic interaction would not be anticipated
Piracetam	The interaction has not been investigated. Theoretically, a pharmacokinetic interaction would not be anticipated
Phenobarbital	The interaction has not been investigated. Theoretically, a pharmacokinetic interaction could occur
Phenytoin	The interaction has not been investigated. Theoretically, a pharmacokinetic interaction could occur
Piracetam	The interaction has not been investigated. Theoretically, a pharmacokinetic interaction would not be anticipated
Pregabalin	The interaction has not been investigated. Theoretically, a pharmacokinetic interaction would not be anticipated
Primidone	Enhances the metabolism of sulthiame
Consequence	Plasma sulthiame levels can decrease
	A pharmacodynamic interaction has also been reported whereby the intensity of the side effects of sulthiame may increase, especially in children (e.g., dizziness, uncertain gait, and drowsiness) [3]
Rufinamide	The interaction has not been investigated. Theoretically, a pharmacokinetic interaction would not be anticipated

Stiripentol	The interaction has not been investigated. Theoretically, a pharmacokinetic interaction could occur
Tiagabine	The interaction has not been investigated. Theoretically, a pharmacokinetic interaction would not be anticipated
Topiramate	The interaction has not been investigated. Theoretically, a pharmacokinetic interaction would not be anticipated
	Topiramate and sulthiame are both weak inhibitors of carbonic anhydrase, and, as a direct result, may independently increase the risk of renal calculi. Consequently, there is a theoretical potential that when they are administered together, an adverse pharmacodynamic interaction will occur [1]
Valproic acid	Does not affect the pharmacokinetics of sulthiame [2]
Vigabatrin	The interaction has not been investigated. Theoretically, a pharmacokinetic interaction would not be anticipated
Zonisamide	The interaction has not been investigated. Theoretically, a pharmacokinetic interaction would not be anticipated
	Zonisamide and sulthiame are both weak inhibitors of carbonic anhydrase and, as a direct result, may independently increase the risk of renal calculi. Consequently, there is a theoretical potential that when they are administered together, an adverse pharmacodynamic interaction will occur [1]

References

1. Patsalos PN, St Louis EK. The epilepsy prescriber's guide to antiepileptic drugs. 3rd ed. Cambridge: Cambridge University Press; 2018.
2. May TW, Korn-Merker E, Rambeck B, Boenigk HE. Pharmacokinetics of sulthiame in epileptic patients. Ther Drug Monit. 1994;16:251–7.
3. Summary of product characteristics: Sulthiame (Ospolot). Phebra Pty, Ltd. Last update 21st Nov 2013.

Tiagabine

Tiagabine (Fig. 1) corresponds chemically to R-*n*-(4, 4-di(3-methyl-thien-2-yl)-but-3-enyl)-nipecotic acid hydrochloride with an empirical formula of $C_{20}H_{25}NO_2S_2$ and a molecular weight of 375.5.

Pharmacokinetic Characteristics

Absorption and Distribution

After oral ingestion, tiagabine is rapidly absorbed (T_{max} = 0.5–2 h) with a bioavailability of ≥90%. Its volume of distribution is 1.0 L/kg, and plasma protein binding is 96%.

Biotransformation

Tiagabine is substantially metabolized (98%) in the liver, primarily by CYP3A4, to two 5-oxo-tiagabine isomers (E5 and Z-5; 60%). The remaining 40% of metabolites have yet to be identified.

Fig. 1 Tiagabine

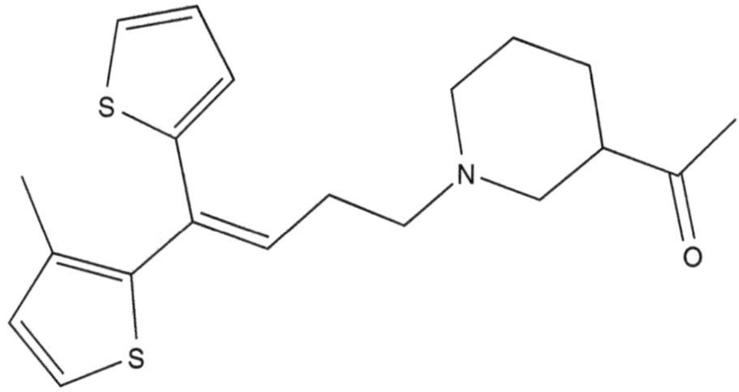

P. N. Patsalos, *Antiseizure Medication Interactions*,
https://doi.org/10.1007/978-3-030-82790-8_29

Renal Excretion

Less than 2% of an administered dose is excreted as unchanged tiagabine in urine.

Elimination

During tiagabine monotherapy, plasma elimination half-life values in adults are 5–9 h, while during polytherapy with enzyme-inducing antiseizure medications, half-life values are 2–4 h.

Effects on Isoenzymes

No in vitro data on the induction or inhibition potential of tiagabine on human CYP or UGT isoenzymes have been published.

Therapeutic Drug Monitoring

Optimum seizure control in patients on tiagabine monotherapy is most likely to occur at plasma tiagabine levels of 20–200 µg/L (53–532 nmol/L). The conversion factor from µg/L to nmol/L for tiagabine is 2.66 (i.e., 1 µg/L = 2.66 nmol/L).

Propensity to Be Associated with Pharmacokinetic Interactions

- Tiagabine affects the pharmacokinetics of other drugs—minimal.
- Other drugs affect the pharmacokinetics of tiagabine—minimal.

Interactions with ASMs

Acetazolamide	The interaction has not been investigated. Theoretically, a pharmacokinetic interaction would not be anticipated
Brivaracetam	The interaction has not been investigated. Theoretically, a pharmacokinetic interaction would not be anticipated
Cannabidiol	The interaction has not been investigated. Theoretically, a pharmacokinetic interaction would not be anticipated
Carbamazepine	Enhances the metabolism of tiagabine
Consequence	Mean tiagabine plasma elimination half-life values in patients taking carbamazepine (plus other enzyme-inducing antiseizure medications) are 3.8–4.9 h compared to 5–8 h in healthy volunteers. Mean plasma tiagabine levels can be expected to be decreased by 40–70%. The interaction is the consequence of induction of CYP3A4 [1]
Cenobamate	The interaction has not been investigated. Theoretically, a pharmacokinetic interaction could occur
Clobazam	The interaction has not been investigated. Theoretically, a pharmacokinetic interaction could occur
Clonazepam	The interaction has not been investigated. Theoretically, a pharmacokinetic interaction could occur
Eslicarbazepine acetate	The interaction has not been investigated. Theoretically, a pharmacokinetic interaction would not be anticipated
Ethosuximide	The interaction has not been investigated. Theoretically, a pharmacokinetic interaction would not be anticipated
Everolimus	The interaction has not been investigated. Theoretically, a pharmacokinetic interaction could occur
Felbamate	The interaction has not been investigated. Theoretically, a pharmacokinetic interaction could occur

Fenfluramine	The interaction has not been investigated. Theoretically, a pharmacokinetic interaction could occur
Gabapentin	The interaction has not been investigated. Theoretically, a pharmacokinetic interaction would not be anticipated
Lacosamide	The interaction has not been investigated. Theoretically, a pharmacokinetic interaction would not be anticipated
Lamotrigine	The interaction has not been investigated. Theoretically, a pharmacokinetic interaction would not be anticipated
Levetiracetam	The interaction has not been investigated. Theoretically, a pharmacokinetic interaction would not be anticipated
Methsuximide	The interaction has not been investigated. Theoretically, a pharmacokinetic interaction could occur
Oxcarbazepine	The interaction has not been investigated. Theoretically, a pharmacokinetic interaction could occur
Perampanel	The interaction has not been investigated. Theoretically, a pharmacokinetic interaction would not be anticipated
Phenobarbital	Enhances the metabolism of tiagabine
Consequence	Mean tiagabine plasma elimination half-life values in patients taking phenobarbital (plus other enzyme-inducing antiseizure medications) are 3.8–4.9 h compared to 5–8 h in healthy volunteers. Mean plasma tiagabine levels can be expected to be decreased by 40–70%. The interaction is the consequence of induction of CYP3A4 [1]
Phenytoin	Enhances the metabolism of tiagabine
Consequence	Mean tiagabine plasma elimination half-life values in patients taking phenytoin (plus other enzyme-inducing antiseizure medications) are 3.8–4.9 h compared to 5–8 h in healthy volunteers. Mean plasma tiagabine levels can be expected to be decreased by 40–70%. The interaction is the consequence of induction of CYP3A4 [1]
Piracetam	The interaction has not been investigated. Theoretically, a pharmacokinetic interaction would not be anticipated
Pregabalin	Enhances the clearance of tiagabine
Consequence	Enhances the clearance of tiagabine by 12% and can decrease plasma tiagabine levels [2]
Primidone	Enhances the metabolism of tiagabine
Consequence	Mean tiagabine plasma elimination half-life values in patients taking primidone (plus other enzyme-inducing antiseizure medications) are 3.8–4.9 h compared to 5–8 h in healthy volunteers. Mean plasma tiagabine levels can be expected to be decreased by 40–70%. The interaction is the consequence of induction of CYP3A4 [1]
Rufinamide	The interaction has not been investigated. Theoretically, a pharmacokinetic interaction would not be anticipated
Stiripentol	The interaction has not been investigated. Theoretically, a pharmacokinetic interaction could occur
Sulthiame	The interaction has not been investigated. Theoretically, a pharmacokinetic interaction could occur
Topiramate	The interaction has not been investigated. Theoretically, a pharmacokinetic interaction could occur
Valproic acid	Does not affect the pharmacokinetics of tiagabine [3]

Vigabatrin	The interaction has not been investigated. Theoretically, a pharmacokinetic interaction would not be anticipated
	Vigabatrin and tiagabine can have a synergistic effect consequent to a pharmacodynamic interaction [4]
Zonisamide	The interaction has not been investigated. Theoretically, a pharmacokinetic interaction would not be anticipated

References

1. So EJ, Wolff D, Graves NM, Leppik IE, Cascino GD, Pixton GC, Gustavson LE. Pharmacokinetics of tiagabine as add-on therapy in patients taking enzyme inducing antiepilepsy drugs. Epilepsy Res. 1995;22:221–6.
2. Bockbrader HN, Burger P, Knapp L. Pregabalin effect on steady-state pharmacokinetics of carbamazepine, lamotrigine, phenobarbital, phenytoin, topiramate, valproate, and tiagabine. Epilepsia. 2011;52:405–9.
3. Wang X, Patsalos PN. The pharmacokinetic profile of tiagabine. Rev Contemp Pharmacother. 2002;12:225–34.
4. Leach JP, Brodie MJ. Synergism with GABAergic drugs in refractory epilepsy. Lancet. 1994;343:1650.

Topiramate

Topiramate (Fig. 1) corresponds chemically to 2, 3:4, 5-bis-*O*-(1-methylethylidene)-β-d-fructopyranose sulfamate with an empirical formula of $C_{12}H_{21}NO_8S$ and a molecular weight of 339.37.

Pharmacokinetic Characteristics

Absorption and Distribution

After oral ingestion, topiramate is rapidly absorbed (T_{max} = 2–4 h) with a bioavailability of ≥80%. Its volume of distribution is 0.6–0.8 L/kg, and plasma protein binding is 15%.

Biotransformation

Topiramate is not extensively metabolized in patients on monotherapy or in patients not prescribed with enzyme-inducing drugs, and typically, 40–50% of a topiramate dose is excreted unchanged via the kidneys. However, in the presence of enzyme-inducing antiseizure medications, this value is doubled. Metabolites thus far

Fig. 1 Topiramate

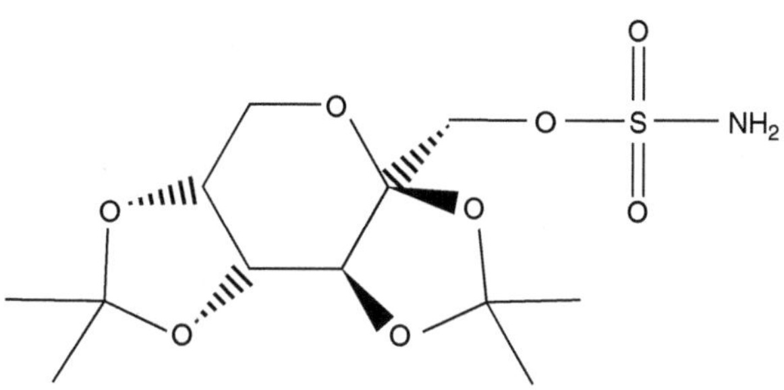

P. N. Patsalos, *Antiseizure Medication Interactions*,
https://doi.org/10.1007/978-3-030-82790-8_30

identified include two hydroxy and two diol metabolites as well as several glucuronide conjugates, none of which constitutes more than 5% of an administered dose. Although the specific CYP isoenzymes for the metabolism of topiramate have not been identified, it is evident that isoenzymes induced by carbamazepine and phenytoin play a major role.

Renal Excretion

Approximately 20–50% of an administered dose is excreted as unchanged topiramate in urine.

Elimination

During monotherapy, plasma elimination half-life values in adults are 20–30 h, while in polytherapy with enzyme-inducing antiseizure medications, half-life values are 10–15 h.

Time to new steady-state blood levels consequent to an inhibition of metabolism interaction:

- Adults = 4–5 days later.

Effects on Isoenzymes

At therapeutic concentrations, topiramate in vitro inhibits the activity of CYP2C19. Consequently, pharmacokinetic interactions of metabolic origin with other antiseizure medications and other medicines can be expected.

Topiramate has no in vitro inhibitory effect on the activity of CYP1A2, CYP2A6, CYP2C9, CYP2D6, CYP2E1, and CYP3A4.

No in vitro data on the induction potential of topiramate on human CYP or UGT isoenzymes have been published.

Therapeutic Drug Monitoring

Optimum seizure control in adult patients on topiramate monotherapy is most likely to occur at plasma topiramate levels of 5–20 mg/L (15–59 μmol/L), while in children aged 6–12 years, it is most likely to occur at plasma topiramate levels of 2–21 mg/L (6–59 μmol/L). The conversion factor from mg/L to μmol/L for topiramate is 2.95 (i.e., 1 mg/L = 2.95 μmol/L).

Propensity to Be Associated with Pharmacokinetic Interactions

- Topiramate affects the pharmacokinetics of other drugs—minimal.
- Other drugs affect the pharmacokinetics of topiramate—moderate.

Interactions with ASMs

Acetazolamide	The interaction has not been investigated. Theoretically, a pharmacokinetic interaction would not be anticipated
	Acetazolamide and topiramate are both weak inhibitors of carbonic anhydrase and, as a direct result, may independently increase the risk of renal calculi. Consequently, there is a theoretical potential that when they are administered together, an adverse pharmacodynamic interaction will occur [1]
Brivaracetam	Does not affect the pharmacokinetics of topiramate [2]
Cannabidiol	Inhibits the metabolism of topiramate

Consequence	Plasma mean topiramate levels can increase by 10% [3]
Carbamazepine	Enhances the metabolism of topiramate
Consequence	Plasma topiramate clearance is increased twofold so that mean plasma topiramate levels can be decreased by 40% [4, 5]
Cenobamate	The interaction has not been investigated. Theoretically, a pharmacokinetic interaction could occur
Clobazam	The interaction has not been investigated. Theoretically, a pharmacokinetic interaction would not be anticipated
Clonazepam	The interaction has not been investigated. Theoretically, a pharmacokinetic interaction would not be anticipated
Eslicarbazepine acetate	Enhances the clearance of topiramate
Consequence	Plasma mean topiramate C_{max} and AUC values are decreased by 8 and 18%, respectively [6]
Ethosuximide	The interaction has not been investigated. Theoretically, a pharmacokinetic interaction would not be anticipated
Everolimus	The interaction has not been investigated. Theoretically, a pharmacokinetic interaction could occur
Felbamate	The interaction has not been investigated. Theoretically a pharmacokinetic interaction could occur
Fenfluramine	The interaction has not been investigated. Theoretically, a pharmacokinetic interaction could occur
Gabapentin	Does not affect the pharmacokinetics of topiramate [7]
Lacosamide	Does not affect the pharmacokinetics of topiramate [8]
Lamotrigine	Does not affect the pharmacokinetics of topiramate [9]
	Lamotrigine and topiramate can have a synergistic antiseizure effect consequent to a pharmacodynamic interaction [10]
Levetiracetam	Does not affect the pharmacokinetics of topiramate [11]
	A pharmacodynamic interaction may occur whereby symptoms of decreased appetite, weight loss, and nervousness present [12]
Methsuximide	Enhances the metabolism of topiramate
Consequence	Plasma topiramate levels can be decreased [7]
Oxcarbazepine	Enhances the metabolism of topiramate
Consequence	Plasma topiramate levels can be decreased [7]
Perampanel	Does not affect the pharmacokinetics of topiramate [13]
Phenobarbital	Enhances the metabolism of topiramate
Consequence	Plasma topiramate clearance is increased twofold so that mean plasma topiramate levels can be decreased by 68% [5, 14]
Phenytoin	Enhances the metabolism of topiramate
Consequence	Plasma topiramate clearance is increased two-fold so that mean plasma topiramate levels can be decreased by 50% [5, 14]
Piracetam	The interaction has not been investigated. Theoretically, a pharmacokinetic interaction would not be anticipated
Pregabalin	Does not affect the pharmacokinetics of topiramate [15]
Primidone	Enhances the metabolism of topiramate
Consequence	Plasma topiramate clearance is increased twofold so that mean plasma topiramate levels can be decreased by 68% [4, 13]

Rufinamide	Does not affect the pharmacokinetics of topiramate [16]
Stiripentol	Does not affect the pharmacokinetics of topiramate [17]
Sulthiame	Does not affect the pharmacokinetics of topiramate [7]
	Sulthiame and topiramate are both weak inhibitors of carbonic anhydrase and, as a direct result, may independently increase the risk of renal calculi. Consequently, there is a theoretical potential that when they are administered together, an adverse pharmacodynamic interaction will occur [1]
Tiagabine	The interaction has not been investigated. Theoretically, a pharmacokinetic interaction would not be anticipated
Valproic acid	Enhances the metabolism of topiramate
Consequence	Mean plasma topiramate AUC values can be decreased by 14% [18]
	A pharmacodynamic interaction has been reported whereby topiramate induces a valproate-induced hyperammonemic encephalopathy in the context of normal liver function [19]
Vigabatrin	The interaction has not been investigated. Theoretically, a pharmacokinetic interaction would not be anticipated
Zonisamide	The interaction has not been investigated. Theoretically, a pharmacokinetic interaction would not be anticipated
	Zonisamide and topiramate are both weak inhibitors of carbonic anhydrase and, as a direct result, may independently increase the risk of renal calculi. Consequently, there is a theoretical potential that when they are administered together, an adverse pharmacodynamic interaction will occur [1]

References

1. Patsalos PN, St Louis EK. The epilepsy prescriber's guide to antiepileptic drugs. 3rd ed. Cambridge: Cambridge University Press; 2018.
2. Moseley BD, Otoul C, Staelens L, Stockis A. Pharmacokinetic interaction of brivaracetam on other antiepileptic drugs in adults with focal seizures: pooled analysis of data from randomized clinical trials. Epilepsy Res. 2019;158:106218.
3. Gaston TE, Bekib EM, Cutter GR, Liu Y, Szaflarski JP, UAB CBD Program. Interactions between cannabidiol and commonly used antiepileptic drugs. Epilepsia. 2017;58:1586–92.
4. Sachdeo RC, Sachdeo SK, Walker SA, Kramer LD, Nayak RK, Doose DR. Steady-state pharmacokinetics of topiramate and carbamazepine in patients with epilepsy during monotherapy and concomitant therapy. Epilepsia. 1996;37:774–80.
5. Bialer M, Doose DR, Murthy B, Curtin C, Wang SS, Twyman RE, Schwabe S. Pharmacokinetic interactions of topiramate. Clin Pharmacokinet. 2004;43:763–80.
6. Nunes T, Sicard E, Almeida L, Falcao A, Rocha JF, Brunet JS, Lefebvre M, Soares-da-Silva P. Pharmacokinetic interaction study between eslicarbazepine acetate and topiramate in healthy subjects. Curr Med Res Opin. 2010;26:1355–62.
7. May TW, Rambeck B, Jurgens U. Serum concentrations of topiramate in patients with epilepsy: influence of dose, age, and comedication. Ther Drug Monit. 2002;24:366–74.
8. Halasz P, Kalviainen R, Mazurkiewicz-Beldzinska M, Rosenow F, Doty P, Hebert D, Sullivan T. Adjunctive lacosamide for partial-onset seizures: efficacy and safety results from a randomized controlled trial. Epilepsia. 2009;50:443–53.
9. Doose DR, Brodie MJ, Wilson EA, Chadwick D, Oxbury J, Berry DJ, Schwabe S, Bialer M. Topiramate and lamotrigine pharmacokinetics during repetitive monotherapy and combination therapy in epileptic patients. Epilepsia. 2003;44:917–22.

10. Stephen LJ, Sills GJ, Brodie MJ. Lamotrigine and topiramate may be a useful combination. Lancet. 1998;351:958–9.
11. Otoul C, De Smedt H, Stockis A. Lack of pharmacokinetic interaction of levetiracetam on carbamazepine, valproic acid, topiramate, and lamotrigine in children with epilepsy. Epilepsia. 2007;48:2111–5.
12. Glauser TA, Pellock JM, Bebin EM, Fountain NB, Ritter FJ, Jensen CM, Shields WD. Efficacy and safety of levetiracetam in children with partial seizures: an open-label trial. Epilepsia. 2002;43:518–24.
13. Patsalos PN. The clinical pharmacology profile of the new antiepileptic drug perampanel: a novel noncompetitive AMPA receptor antagonist. Epilepsia. 2015;56:12–27.
14. Sachdeo RC, Sachdeo SK, Levy RH, Streeter AJ, Bishop FE, Kunze KL, Mather GG, Roskos LK, Shen DD, Thummel KE, Trager WF, Curtin CR, Doose DR, Gsclon LG, Bialer M. Topiramate and phenytoin pharmacokinetics during repetitive monotherapy and concomitant therapy in patients with epilepsy. Epilepsia. 2002;43:691–6.
15. Bockbrader HN, Burger P, Knapp L. Pregabalin effect on steady-state pharmacokinetics of carbamazepine, lamotrigine, phenobarbital, phenytoin, topiramate, valproate, and tiagabine. Epilepsia. 2011;52:405–9.
16. Perucca E, Cloyd J, Critchley D, Fuseau E. Rufinamide: clinical pharmacokinetics and concentration-response relationships in patients with epilepsy. Epilepsia. 2008;49:1123–41.
17. Summary of product characteristics: Stiripentol (Diacomit). Alan Pharmaceuticals. Last update 20th Sept 2018.
18. Rosenfeld WE, Liao S, Kramer LD, Anderson G, Palmer M, Levy RH, Nayak RN. Comparison of the steady-state pharmacokinetics of topiramate and valproate in patients with epilepsy during monotherapy and concomitant therapy. Epilepsia. 1997;38:324–33.
19. Deutsch SI, Burket JA, Rosse RB. Valproate-induced hyperammonemic encephalopathy and normal liver functions; possible synergism with topiramate. Clin Neuropharmacol. 2009;32:350–2.

10. Stephen LJ, Sills GJ, Brodie MJ. Lamotrigine and topiramate may be a useful combination. Lancet. 1998;351:958–9.
11. Dunkel G, De Saeed H, Stockham A. Lack of pharmacokinetic interaction of levetiracetam on carbamazepine, valproic acid, topiramate, and lamotrigine in children with epilepsy. Epilepsia. 2007;48:2111–5.
12. Glauser TA, Pellock JM, Bebin EM, Fountain NB, Ritter FJ, Jensen CM, Shields WD. Efficacy [illegible] 2002;43:518–24.
13. Patsalos PN. The clinical pharmacology profile of the new antiepileptic drug perampanel: a novel noncompetitive AMPA receptor antagonist. Epilepsia. 2015;56:12–27.
14. Sachdeo RC, Sachdeo SK, Levy RH, Streeter AJ, Bishop FE, Kunze KL, Mather GG, Roskos LK, Shen DD, Thummel KE, Trager WF, Curtin CR, Doose DR, Gisclon LG, Bialer M. Topiramate and phenytoin pharmacokinetics during repetitive monotherapy and combination therapy in patients with epilepsy. Epilepsia. 2002;43:691–6.
15. Brodie HN, Burger P, Knapp L. Pregabalin effect on steady-state pharmacokinetics of carbamazepine, lamotrigine, phenobarbital, phenytoin, topiramate, valproate, and tiagabine. Epilepsia. 2011;52:405–9.
16. Perucca E, Cloyd J, Critchley D, Fuseau E. Rufinamide: clinical pharmacokinetics and concentration-response relationships in patients with epilepsy. Epilepsia. 2008;49:1123–41.
17. Summary of product characteristics: Stiripentol (Diacomit). Alan Pharmaceuticals. last update 20th Sept 2018.
18. Rosenfeld WE, Liao S, Kramer LD, Anderson G, Palmer M, Levy RH, Nayak RK. Comparison of the steady-state pharmacokinetics of topiramate and valproate in patients with epilepsy during monotherapy and concomitant therapy. Epilepsia. 1997;38:324–33.
19. Deutsch SI, Burket JA, Rosse RB. Valproate-induced hyperammonemic encephalopathy and normal liver functions: possible synergism with topiramate. Clin Neuropharmacol. 2009;32:350–2.

Valproic Acid

Valproic acid (Fig. 1) corresponds chemically to *N*-dipropylacetic acid with an empirical formula of $C_8H_{16}O_2$ and a molecular weight of 144.21.

Pharmacokinetic Characteristics

Absorption and Distribution

After oral ingestion, valproic acid is rapidly absorbed (T_{max} is formulation-dependent) with a bioavailability of >90%. Its volume of distribution in adults is 0.13–0.19 L/kg, while in children, it is 0.20–0.30 L/kg, and plasma protein binding is 90%. Valproic acid exhibits saturable plasma protein binding and, as a result, valproic acid steady-state plasma levels increase less than proportionately after a dose increment.

Biotransformation

Valproic acid is extensively metabolized in the liver and involves multiple metabolic pathways including *O*-glucuronidation, β-oxidation, ω-oxidation hydroxylation, ketone formation, and desaturation. To date, in excess of 25 metabolites have been identified with valproic acid glucuronide and 3-oxo-valproic acid being by far the most abundant metabolites (~40 and 33% of an administered dose, respectively).

Fig. 1 Valproic acid

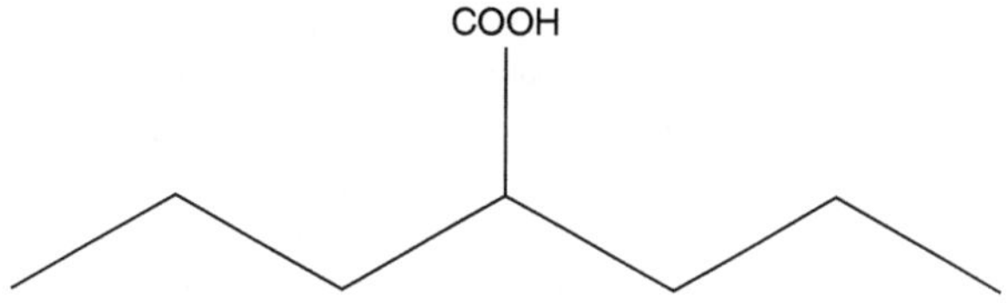

P. N. Patsalos, *Antiseizure Medication Interactions*,
https://doi.org/10.1007/978-3-030-82790-8_31

Hydroxylation to form 4-ene-valproic acid and other metabolites is via the action of CYP2A6, CYP2C9, CYP2C19, and CYP2B6 isoenzymes while *O*-glucuronidation is mediated by UGT1A3 and UGT2B7 isoenzymes.

Renal Excretion

Approximately 1–3% of an administered dose is excreted as unchanged valproic acid in urine.

Elimination

In the absence of enzyme-inducing antiseizure medications, plasma elimination half-life values for adults are 12–16 h, while in children, they are 8.6–12.3 h, and in infants, they are 8.4–12.5 h. In the presence of enzyme-inducing antiseizure medications, valproic acid half-life values for adults are 5–9 h, while in children, half-life values are 7–9.4 h, and in infants, they are 4–8 h. Newborns eliminate valproic acid slowly with half-life values of 20–40 h.

Time to new steady-state blood levels consequent to an inhibition of metabolism interaction:

- Adults = 2–4 days later.

Effects on Isoenzymes

No in vitro data on the induction or inhibition potential of valproic acid on human CYP or UGT isoenzymes have been published.

Therapeutic Drug Monitoring

Optimum seizure control in patients on valproic acid monotherapy is most likely to occur at plasma valproic acid levels of 50–100 mg/L (350–700 μmol/L). The conversion factor from mg/L to μmol/L for valproic acid is 6.93 (i.e., 1 mg/L = 6.93 μmol/L).

Propensity to Be Associated with Pharmacokinetic Interactions

- Valproic acid affects the pharmacokinetics of other drugs—substantial.
- Other drugs affect the pharmacokinetics of valproic acid—substantial.

Interactions with ASMs

Acetazolamide	The interaction has not been investigated. Theoretically, a pharmacokinetic interaction would not be anticipated
Brivaracetam	Does not affect the pharmacokinetics of valproic acid [1]
Cannabidiol	Enhances the metabolism of valproic acid
Consequence	Mean plasma valproic acid AUC values decrease by 17%, while mean AUC values of the metabolite 3-ene-valproic acid are decreased by 30% [2] A synergistic increase in aspartate aminotransferase can occur consequent to a pharmacodynamic interaction [3]
Carbamazepine	Enhances the metabolism of valproic acid
Consequence	Mean plasma valproic acid levels can be decreased by 39% [4]
	Co-administration with carbamazepine, and other enzyme-inducing antiseizure medications, does not only increase the clearance of valproic acid but may also change metabolic pathways. That patients treated with polytherapy have a greater incidence of valproic acid hepatotoxicity may be due to an increase in plasma levels of the 4-en and 2–4-en hepatotoxic metabolites [5]
	During combination therapy, carbamazepine may synergistically enhance the antiseizure efficacy (partial seizures) of valproic acid. This effect may probably be the consequence of a pharmacodynamic interaction [6]

Cenobamate	Does not affect the pharmacokinetics of valproic acid [7]
Clobazam	Inhibits the metabolism of valproic acid
Consequence	Decreases the plasma clearance of valproic acid so that plasma valproic acid levels are increased [8]
Clonazepam	Does not affect the pharmacokinetics of valproic acid [9]
Eslicarbazepine acetate	Enhance the metabolism of valproic acid
Consequence	Median plasma valproic acid levels are decreased by 12% [10, 11]
Ethosuximide	Enhance the metabolism of valproic acid
Consequence	Mean plasma valproic acid levels can be decreased by 28% [12]
	During combination therapy, ethosuximide synergistically enhances the antiseizure efficacy (absence seizures) and toxicity of valproic acid. These effects are probably the consequence of a pharmacodynamic interaction [13]
Everolimus	The interaction has not been investigated. Theoretically, a pharmacokinetic interaction could occur
Felbamate	Inhibits the metabolism of valproic acid
Consequence	Mean plasma valproic acid levels can be increased by 28–54%. The interaction is the consequence of inhibition of β-oxidation [14]
Fenfluramine	Does not affect the pharmacokinetics of valproic acid [15]
Gabapentin	Does not affect the pharmacokinetics of valproic acid [16]
Lacosamide	Enhances the metabolism of valproic acid
Consequence	Plasma valproic acid levels are decreased [17]
	Hyperammonemic encephalopathy may occur in combination with valproic acid consequent to a pharmacodynamic interaction [18]
Lamotrigine	Enhance the metabolism of valproic acid
Consequence	Mean plasma valproic acid levels can be decreased by 25%. The interaction is considered to be the consequence of induction of glucuronidation and β-oxidation [19]
	Concurrent valproic acid therapy is a risk factor for the development of skin rash with lamotrigine. The introduction of lamotrigine to patients already taking valproic acid should be undertaken with caution, using a low starting dose and a slow-dose escalation rate. However, there is no risk of rash if valproic acid is introduced to patients already stabilized on lamotrigine [20]
	During combination therapy, valproic acid synergistically enhances the antiseizure efficacy (partial and generalized seizures) and toxicity of lamotrigine. This is considered to be the consequence of a pharmacodynamic interaction [21–23]
Levetiracetam	Does not affect the pharmacokinetics of valproic acid [24]
Methsuximide	Enhance the metabolism of valproic acid
Consequence	Plasma valproic acid levels can be decreased by 7–60% [25]
Oxcarbazepine	Does not affect the pharmacokinetics of valproic acid [26]
Perampanel	Enhances the metabolism of valproic acid
Consequence	Mean plasma valproic acid clearance is increased by 5.0% [27] Perampanel does not affect the plasma protein binding of valproic acid [28]
Phenobarbital	Enhances the metabolism of valproic acid

Consequence	Mean plasma valproic acid levels can decrease by 37%, and the mean plasma level to dose ratio for valproic acid can be decreased by 45% [29]
	Co-administration with phenobarbital, and other enzyme-inducing antiseizure medication, does not only increase the clearance of valproic acid but may also change metabolic pathways. That patients treated with polytherapy have a greater incidence of valproic acid hepatotoxicity may be due to an increase in plasma levels of the 4-en and 2–4-en hepatotoxic metabolites [6]
Phenytoin	Enhances the metabolism of valproic acid
Consequence	Mean plasma valproic acid levels can decrease by 37%, and the mean plasma level to dose ratio for valproic acid can be decreased by 59% [29]
	Co-administration with phenytoin, and other enzyme-inducing antiseizure medications, does not only increase the clearance of valproic acid but may also change metabolic pathways. That patients treated with polytherapy have a greater incidence of valproic acid hepatotoxicity may be due to an increase in plasma levels of the 4-en and 2–4-en hepatotoxic metabolites [6, 29]
Piracetam	Does not affect the pharmacokinetics of valproic acid [30]
Pregabalin	Does not affect the pharmacokinetics of valproic acid [31]
Primidone	Enhances the metabolism of valproic acid
Consequence	Mean plasma valproic acid levels can be decreased by 50% [29]
	Co-administration with primidone, and other enzyme-inducing antiseizure medications, does not only increase the clearance of valproic acid but may also change metabolic pathways. That patients treated with polytherapy have a greater incidence of valproic acid hepatotoxicity may be due to an increase in plasma levels of the 4-en and 2–4-en hepatotoxic metabolites [6]
Rufinamide	Does not affect the pharmacokinetics of valproic acid [32]
Stiripentol	Inhibits the metabolism of valproic acid
Consequence	Plasma valproic acid levels are increased. The interaction is considered to be the consequence of inhibition of CYP2C9 and CYP2C19 [6]
Sulthiame	The interaction has not been investigated. Theoretically, a pharmacokinetic interaction could occur
Tiagabine	Enhances the clearance of valproic acid
Consequence	Mean plasma valproic acid Cmax and and AUC values are decreased by 10% and 12%, respectively via an unknown mechanism [33]
Topiramate	Enhances the metabolism of valproic acid
Consequence	Mean plasma valproic acid AUC values can be decreased by 13%. This is a consequence of the induction of β-oxidation (42%) and ω-oxidation (36%) and inhibition of the glucuronide conjugation pathway (35%). The changes in metabolite production are noteworthy, particularly since the 4-ene metabolite has been implicated as a potential hepatotoxin [34]
	A pharmacodynamic interaction has been reported whereby topiramate induces a valproate-induced encephalopathy [35]
Vigabatrin	Does not affect the pharmacokinetics of valproic acid [36]
Zonisamide	Does not affect the pharmacokinetics of valproic acid [37]

References

1. Moseley BD, Otoul C, Staelens L, Stockis A. Pharmacokinetic interaction of brivaracetam on other antiepileptic drugs in adults with focal seizures: pooled analysis of data from randomized clinical trials. Epilepsy Res. 2019;158:106218.
2. Ben-Menachem E, Gunning B, Cabrera CMA, Van Landingham K, Crockett J, Critchley D, Wray L, Tayo B, Morrison G, Toledo M. A phase II randomized trial to explore the potential for pharmacokinetic drug-drug interactions with stiripentol or valproate when combined with cannabidiol in patients with epilepsy. CNS Drugs. 2020;34:661–72.
3. Patsalos PN, Szaflarski JP, Gidal B, Van Landingham K, Critchley D, Morrison G. Clinical implications of trials investigating drug-drug interactions between cannabidiol and enzyme inducers or inhibitors or common antiseizure drugs. Epilepsia. 2020;61:1854–68.
4. Panesar SK, Orr JM, Farrell K, Burton RW, Kassahun K, Abbott FS. The effect of carbamazepine on valproic acid disposition. Br J Clin Pharmacol. 1989;27:323–8.
5. Levy R, Rettenmeier AW, Anderson GD, Wilensky AJ, Friel PN, Bailie TA, Acheampong A, Tor J, Guyot M, Loiseau P. Effects of polytherapy with phenytoin, carbamazepine, and stiripentol on formation of 4-ene-valproate, a hepatotoxic metabolite of valproic acid. Clin Pharmacol Ther. 1990;48:225–35.
6. Brodie MJ, Mumford JP. Double-blind substitution of vigabatrin and valproate in carbamazepine-resistant partial epilepsy. 012 study group. Epilepsy Res. 1999;34:199–205.
7. Bialer M, Johannessen SI, Koepp MJ, Levy RH, Perucca E, Perucca P, Tomson T, White HS. Progress report on new antiepiletis drugs: a summary of the fifteenth Eilat conference on new antiepileptic drugs and devices (EILAT XV). II. Drugs in more advanced clinical development. Epilepsia. 2020;61:2365–85.
8. Theis JGW, Koren G, Daneman R, Sherwin AL, Menzano E, Cortez M, Hwang P. Interactions of clobazam with conventional antiepileptics in children. J Child Neurol. 1997;12:208–13.
9. Wang L, Wang XD. Pharmacokinetic and pharmacodynamic effects of clonazepam in children with epilepsy treated with valproate: a preliminary study. Ther Drug Monit. 2002;24:632–6.
10. Elger C, Halasz P, Maia J, Almeidas L, Soares-da-Silva P, BIA-2093-301 Investigators Study Group. Efficacy and safety of eslicarbazepine acetate as adjunctive treatment in adults with refractory partial seizures: a randomized, double-blind, placebo-controlled, parallel-group phase III study. Epilepsia. 2009;50:454–63.
11. Falcao A, Fuseau E, Nunes T, Almeida L, Soares-da-Silva P. Pharmacokinetics, drug interactions and exposure-response relationships of eslicarbazepine acetate in adult patients with partial-onset seizures: population pharmacokinetic and pharmacokinetic/pharmacodynamic analysis. CNS Drugs. 2012;26:79–91.
12. Salke-Kellermann RA, May T, Boenigk HE. Influence of ethosuximide on valproic acid serum concentrations. Epilepsy Res. 1997;26:345–9.
13. Rowan AJ, Meijer JW, de Beer-Pawlikowski N, van der Geest P, Meinardi H. Valproate-ethosuximide combination therapy for refractory seizures. Arch Neurol. 1983;40:797–802.
14. Wagner ML, Graves NM, Leppik IE, Remmel RP, Shmaker RC, Ward D, Perhach JL. The effect of felbamate on valproic acid disposition. Clin Pharmacol Ther. 1994;56:494–502.
15. Boyd B, Smith S, Gammaitoni A, Galer BS, Farfel GM. A phase 1, randomized, open-label, single dose, 3 period crossover study to evaluate the drug-drug interaction between ZX008 (fenfluramine HCl oral solution) and a regimen of stiripentol, clobazam, and valproate in healthy subjects. Int J Clin Pharmaol Therapeut. 2019;57:11–9.
16. Radulovic LL, Wilder BJ, Leppik IE, Bockbrader HN, Chang T, Posvar EL, Sedman AJ, Uthman BM, Erdman GR. Lack of interaction of gabapentin with carbamazepine and valproate. Epilepsia. 1994;35:155–61.
17. Toutopoulou M, Weshke B, Kaindl AM. Lacsamide lowers valproate and levetiracetam levels. Neuropediatrics. 2017;48:188–9.
18. Jones GL, Popli GS, Silvia MT. Lacosamide-induced valproic acid toxicity. Pediatr Neurol. 2013;48:308–10.

19. Anderson GD, Yau MK, Gidal BE, Harris SJ, Levy RH, Lai AA, Wolf KB, Wargin WA, Dren AT. Bidirectional interaction of valproate and lamotrigine in healthy subjects. Clin Pharmacol Ther. 1996;60:145–56.
20. Kanner AM. When thinking of lamotrigine and valproic acid, think "pharmacokinetically". Epilepsy Curr. 2004;4:206–7.
21. Brodie MJ, Yuen AW. Lamotrigine substitution study: evidence for synergism with sodium valproate? 105 Study Group. Epilepsy Res. 1997;26:423–33.
22. Pisani F, Oteri G, Russo MF, Di Perri R, Perucca E, Richens A. The efficacy of valproate-lamotrigine comedication in refractory complex partial seizures: evidence for a pharmacodynamic interaction. Epilepsia. 1999;40:1141–6.
23. Reutens DC, Duncan JS, Patsalos PN. Disabling tremor after lamotrigine with sodium valproate. Lancet. 1993;342:185–6.
24. Coupez R, Nicolas JM, Browne TR. Levetiracetam, a new antiepileptic agent: lack of in vitro and in vivo pharmacokinetic interaction with valproic acid. Epilepsia. 2003;44:171–8.
25. Besag FM, Berry DJ, Vasey M. Methsuximide reduces valproic acid serum levels. Ther Drug Monit. 2001;23:694–7.
26. McKee PJW, Blacklaw J, Forrest G, Gillham RA, Walker SM, Connelly D, Brodie MJ. A double-blind, placebo-controlled interaction study between oxcarbazepine and carbamazepine, sodium valproate and phenytoin in epileptic patients. Br J Clin Pharmacol. 1994;37:27.32.
27. Majid O, Laurenza A, Ferry J, Hussein Z. Impact of perampanel on pharmacokinetics of concomitant antiepileptics in patients with partial-onset seizures: pooled analysis of clinical trials. Br J Clin Pharmacol. 2016;82:422–30.
28. Gidal BE, Ferry J, Laurenza A, Ueno T. Potential protein-binding displacement interactions with perampanel: an in vitro analysis. Epilepsy Res. 2019;149:102–6.
29. Sackellares JC, Sato S, Dreifuss FE, Penry JK. Reduction of steady-state valproate levels by other antiepileptic drugs. Epilepsia. 1981;22:437–41.
30. Summary of product characteristics: Piracetam (Nootropil). UCB Pharma Ltd. Last update 9th Feb 2017.
31. Brodie MJ, Wilson EA, Wesche DL, Alvey CW, Randinitis EJ, Posvar EL, Hounslow NJ, Bron NJ, Gibson GL, Bockbrader HN. Pregabalin drug interaction studies: lack of effect on the pharmacokinetics of carbamazepine, phenytoin, lamotrigine, and valproate in patients with partial epilepsy. Epilepsia. 2005;46:1407–13.
32. Perucca E, Cloyd J, Critchley D, Fuseau E. Rufinamide: clinical pharmacokinetics and concentration-response relationships in patients with epilepsy. Epilepsia. 2008;49:1123–41.
33. Gustavson LE, Sommerville KW, Boellner SW, Witt GF, Guenther HJ, Granneman GR. Lack of a clinically significant pharmacokinetic interaction between tiagabine and valproate. Am J Ther. 1998;5:73–9.
34. Rosenfeld WE, Liao S, Kramer LD, Anderson G, Palmer M, Levy RH, Nayak RN. Comparison of the steady-state pharmacokinetics of topiramate and valproate in patients with epilepsy during monotherapy and concomitant therapy. Epilepsia. 1997;38:324–33.
35. Noh Y, Kim DW, Chu K, Lee ST, Jung KH, Moon HJ, Lee SK. Topiramate increases the risk of valproic acid-induced encephalopathy. Epilepsia. 2013;54:e1–4.
36. Armijo JA, Arteaga R, Valdizan EM, Herranz JL. Coadministration of vigabatrin and valproate in children with refractory epilepsy. Clin Neuropharmacol. 1992;15:459–69.
37. Ragueneau-Majlessi I, Levy RH, Brodie MJ, Smith D, Shah J, Grundy JS. Lack of pharmacokinetic interactions between steady-state zonisamide and valproic acid in patients with epilepsy. Clin Pharmacokinet. 2005;44:517–23.

Vigabatrin

Vigabatrin (Fig. 1) corresponds chemically to (±)-amino-hex-5-enoic acid with an empirical formula of $C_6H_{11}NO_2$ and a molecular weight of 129.2.

Pharmacokinetic Characteristics

Absorption and Distribution

After oral ingestion, vigabatrin is rapidly absorbed (T_{max} = 1 2 days) with a bioavailability of 60–80%. Its volume of distribution in adults is 0.8 L/kg, and plasma protein binding is 0%.

Biotransformation

Vigabatrin is not metabolized.

Renal Excretion

Approximately 100% of an administered dose is excreted as unchanged vigabatrin in urine.

Elimination

Following a single dose, plasma elimination half-life values in adults are 5–8 h.

Fig. 1 Vigabatrin

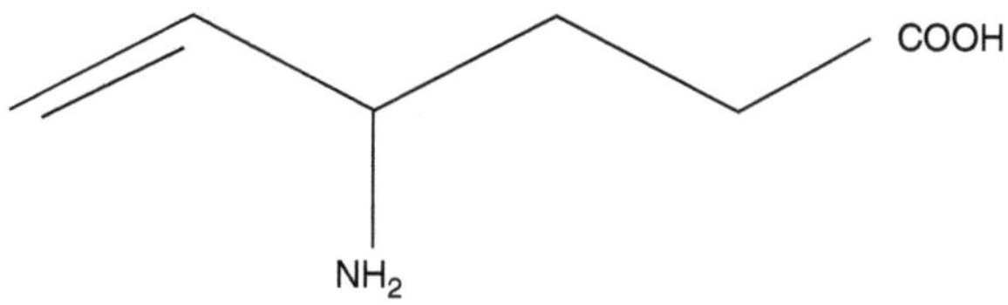

P. N. Patsalos, *Antiseizure Medication Interactions*,
https://doi.org/10.1007/978-3-030-82790-8_32

Effects on Isoenzymes

No in vitro data on the induction or inhibition potential of vigabatrin on human CYP or UGT isoenzymes have been published.

Therapeutic Drug Monitoring

At doses between 1000 and 3000 mg/day, the expected trough plasma vigabatrin levels are in the range of 0.8–36 mg/L (6–279 μmol/L). The conversion factor from mg/L to μmol/L for vigabatrin is 7.74 (i.e., 1 mg/L = 7.74 μmol/L).

Propensity to Be Associated with Pharmacokinetic Interactions

- Vigabatrin affects the pharmacokinetics of other drugs—does not interact.
- Other drugs affect the pharmacokinetics of vigabatrin—does not interact.

Interactions with ASMs

Acetazolamide	The interaction has not been investigated. Theoretically, a pharmacokinetic interaction would not be anticipated
Brivaracetam	The interaction has not been investigated. Theoretically, a pharmacokinetic interaction would not be anticipated
Cannabidiol	Does not affect the pharmacokinetics of vigabatrin [1]
Carbamazepine	Does not affect the pharmacokinetics of vigabatrin [2]
	During combination therapy, carbamazepine may synergistically enhance the antiseizure efficacy (partial seizures) of vigabatrin. This effect may probably be the consequence of a pharmacodynamic interaction [3]
Cenobamate	The interaction has not been investigated. Theoretically, a pharmacokinetic interaction would not be anticipated
Clobazam	The interaction has not been investigated. Theoretically, a pharmacokinetic interaction would not be anticipated
Clonazepam	The interaction has not been investigated. Theoretically, a pharmacokinetic interaction would not be anticipated
Eslicarbazepine acetate	The interaction has not been investigated. Theoretically, a pharmacokinetic interaction would not be anticipated
Ethosuximide	The interaction has not been investigated. Theoretically, a pharmacokinetic interaction would not be anticipated
Everolimus	The interaction has not been investigated. Theoretically, a pharmacokinetic interaction would not be anticipated
Felbamate	Increases the excretion of vigabatrin
Consequence	Mean plasma AUC values of the pharmacologically active S(+)-enantiomer is increased by 13%, and urinary excretion is increased by a mean of 8% [4]
Fenfluramine	The interaction has not been investigated. Theoretically, a pharmacokinetic interaction would not be anticipated
Gabapentin	The interaction has not been investigated. Theoretically, a pharmacokinetic interaction would not be anticipated
Lacosamide	The interaction has not been investigated. Theoretically, a pharmacokinetic interaction would not be anticipated
Lamotrigine	The interaction has not been investigated. Theoretically, a pharmacokinetic interaction would not be anticipated
	Lamotrigine and vigabatrin in combination may be associated with substantial efficacy in patients with partial and secondary generalized tonic-clonic seizures consequent to a pharmacodynamic interaction [5]
Levetiracetam	Does not affect the pharmacokinetics of vigabatrin [6]

Methsuximide	The interaction has not been investigated. Theoretically, a pharmacokinetic interaction would not be anticipated
Oxcarbazepine	The interaction has not been investigated. Theoretically, a pharmacokinetic interaction would not be anticipated
Perampanel	The interaction has not been investigated. Theoretically, a pharmacokinetic interaction would not be anticipated
Phenobarbital	Does not affect the pharmacokinetics of vigabatrin [2]
	During combination therapy for the treatment of infantile spasms, especially in patients with tuberous sclerosis, phenobarbital appears to delay or prevent the onset of seizure control by vigabatrin. This is considered to be the consequence of a pharmacodynamic interaction [7]
Phenytoin	Does not affect the pharmacokinetics of vigabatrin [2]
Piracetam	The interaction has not been investigated. Theoretically, a pharmacokinetic interaction would not be anticipated
Pregabalin	The interaction has not been investigated. Theoretically, a pharmacokinetic interaction would not be anticipated
Primidone	Does not affect the pharmacokinetics of vigabatrin [2]
Rufinamide	The interaction has not been investigated. Theoretically, a pharmacokinetic interaction would not be anticipated
Stiripentol	The interaction has not been investigated. Theoretically, a pharmacokinetic interaction would not be anticipated
Sulthiame	The interaction has not been investigated. Theoretically, a pharmacokinetic interaction would not be anticipated
Tiagabine	The interaction has not been investigated. Theoretically, a pharmacokinetic interaction would not be anticipated
	Tiagabine and vigabatrin can have a synergistic anticonvulsant effect consequent to a pharmacodynamic interaction [8]
Topiramate	The interaction has not been investigated. Theoretically, a pharmacokinetic interaction would not be anticipated
Valproic acid	Does not affect the pharmacokinetics of vigabatrin [9]
Zonisamide	The interaction has not been investigated. Theoretically, a pharmacokinetic interaction would not be anticipated

References

1. Gaston TE, Bekib EM, Cutter GR, Liu Y, Szaflarski JP, UAB CBD Program. Interactions between cannabidiol and commonly used antiepileptic drugs. Epilepsia. 2017;58:1586–92.
2. Armijo JA, Cuadrado A, Bravo J, Arteaga R. Vigabatrin serum concentration to dosage ratio: influence of age and associated antiepileptic drugs. Ther Drug Monit. 1997;19:491–8.
3. Brodie MJ, Mumford JP. Double-blind substitution of vigabatrin and valproate in carbamazepine-resistant partial epilepsy. 012 Study group. Epilepsy Res. 1999;34:199–205.
4. Reidenberg P, Glue P, Banfield C, Colucci R, Meehan J, Rey E, Radwanski E, Nomeir A, Lim J, Lin C, Guillaume M, Affrime MB. Pharmacokinetic interaction studies between felbamate and vigabatrin. Br J Clin Pharmacol. 1995;40:157–60.
5. Stolarek I, Blacklaw J, Forrest G, Brodie MJ. Vigabatrin and lamotrigine in refractory epilepsy. J Neurol Neurosurg Psychiatry. 1994;57:921–4.
6. Perucca E, Baltes E, Ledent E. Levetiracetam: absence of pharmacokinetic interactions with other antiepileptic drugs (AEDs). Epilepsia. 2000;41(Suppl 6):150.

7. Spence SJ, Nakagawa J, Sankar R, Shields WD. Phenobarbital interferes with the efficacy of vigabatrin in treating infantile spasms in patients with tuberous sclerosis. Epilepsia. 2000;41(Suppl 7):189.
8. Leach JP, Brodie MJ. Synergism with GABAergic drugs in refractory epilepsy. Lancet. 1994;343:1650.
9. Armijo JA, Arteaga R, Valdizan EM, Herranz JL. Coadministration of vigabatrin and valproate in children with refractory epilepsy. Clin Neuropharmacol. 1992;15:459–69.

Zonisamide

Zonisamide (Fig. 1) corresponds chemically to 1, 2-benzisoxazole-3-methanesulfonamide with an empirical formula of $C_8H_8N_2O_3S$ and a molecular weight of 212.23.

Pharmacokinetic Characteristics

Absorption and Distribution

After oral ingestion, zonisamide is rapidly absorbed (T_{max} = 2–5 days) with a bioavailability of >90%. Its volume of distribution in adults is 1.0–1.9 L/kg, and plasma protein binding is 40%.

Biotransformation

Zonisamide undergoes moderate metabolism in the liver, primarily acetylation to form *N*-acetyl zonisamide (20%) and reduction to form 2-sulfamoylacetylphenol (50%), the latter being subsequently glucuronidated. The reduction of zonisamide to 2-sulfamoylacetylphenol is mediated by the CYP3A4 isoenzyme.

Fig. 1 Zonisamide

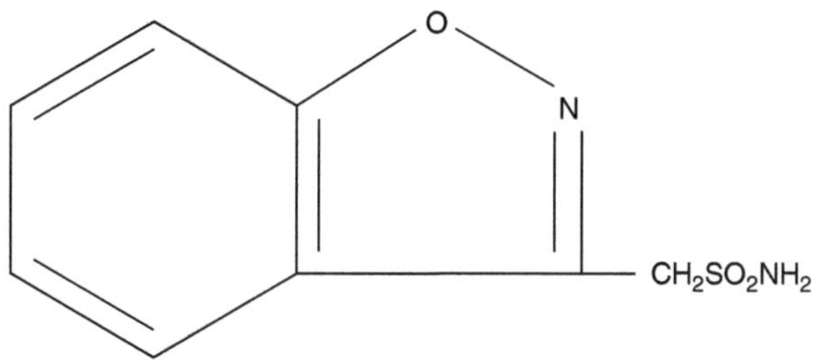

P. N. Patsalos, *Antiseizure Medication Interactions*,
https://doi.org/10.1007/978-3-030-82790-8_33

Renal Excretion
Approximately 30% of an administered dose is excreted as unchanged zonisamide in urine.

Elimination
In the absence of enzyme-inducing antiseizure medications, plasma elimination half-life values in adults are 50–70 h, while in the presence of enzyme-inducing antiseizure medications, half-life values are 25–35 h.

Effects on Isoenzymes
At therapeutic concentrations, zonisamide in vitro inhibits the activity of CYP2C19, CYP2C9, CYP2A6, and CYP2E1. Consequently, pharmacokinetic interactions of metabolic origin with other antiseizure medications and other medicines can be expected.

Zonisamide has no in vitro inhibitory effect on the activity of CYP1A2, CYP2D6, and CYP3A4.

No in vitro data on the induction potential of zonisamide on human CYP or UGT isoenzymes have been published.

Therapeutic Drug Monitoring
Optimum seizure control in patients on zonisamide monotherapy is most likely to occur at plasma zonisamide levels of 10–40 mg/L (47–188 μmol/L). The conversion factor from mg/L to μmol/L for zonisamide is 4.71 (i.e., 1 mg/L = 4.71 μmol/L).

Propensity to Be Associated with Pharmacokinetic Interactions

- Zonisamide affects the pharmacokinetics of other drugs—minimal.
- Other drugs affect the pharmacokinetics of zonisamide—minimal.

Interactions with ASMs

Acetazolamide	The interaction has not been investigated. Theoretically, a pharmacokinetic interaction would not be anticipated
	Acetazolamide and zonisamide are both weak inhibitors of carbonic anhydrase and, as a direct result, may independently increase the risk of renal calculi. Consequently, there is a theoretical potential that when they are administered together, an adverse pharmacodynamic interaction will occur [1]
Brivaracetam	Does not affect the pharmacokinetics of zonisamide [2]
Cannabidiol	Inhibits the metabolism of zonisamide
Consequence	Increases mean plasma zonisamide levels by 9% [3]
Carbamazepine	Enhances the metabolism of zonisamide
Consequence	Plasma zonisamide half-life values can be decreased to ~36 h compared to 60 h observed in untreated volunteers. Concurrent oral clearance values are increased to 0.98 L/h from 0.7 L/h. The interaction is the consequence of induction of zonisamide metabolism through CYP3A4 [4]
Cenobamate	The interaction has not been investigated. Theoretically, a pharmacokinetic interaction could occur
Clobazam	The interaction has not been investigated. Theoretically, a pharmacokinetic interaction would not be anticipated

Clonazepam	Does not affect the pharmacokinetics of zonisamide [5]
Eslicarbazepine acetate	The interaction has not been investigated. Theoretically, a pharmacokinetic interaction would not be anticipated
Ethosuximide	The interaction has not been investigated. Theoretically, a pharmacokinetic interaction would not be anticipated
Everolimus	The interaction has not been investigated. Theoretically, a pharmacokinetic interaction could occur
Felbamate	The interaction has not been investigated. Theoretically, a pharmacokinetic interaction could occur
Fenfluramine	The interaction has not been investigated. Theoretically, a pharmacokinetic interaction could occur
Gabapentin	The interaction has not been investigated. Theoretically, a pharmacokinetic interaction would not be anticipated
Lacosamide	Does not affect the pharmacokinetics of zonisamide [6]
Lamotrigine	Does not affect the pharmacokinetics of zonisamide [7]
Levetiracetam	The interaction has not been investigated. Theoretically, a pharmacokinetic interaction would not be anticipated
Methsuximide	The interaction has not been investigated. Theoretically, a pharmacokinetic interaction would not be anticipated
Oxcarbazepine	The interaction has not been investigated. Theoretically, a pharmacokinetic interaction would not be anticipated
Perampanel	Does not affect the pharmacokinetics of zonisamide [8]
Phenobarbital	Enhances the metabolism of zonisamide
Consequence	Plasma zonisamide half-life values can be decreased to ~38 h compared to 60 h observed in untreated volunteers. Concurrent clearance values are increased by 27%. The interaction is the consequence of induction of zonisamide metabolism through CYP3A4 [9]
Phenytoin	Enhances the metabolism of zonisamide
Consequence	Plasma zonisamide half-life values can be decreased to ~28 h compared to 60 h observed in untreated volunteers. Concurrent oral clearance values are increased to 1.29 L/h from 0.7 L/h. The interaction is the consequence of induction of zonisamide metabolism through CYP3A4 [10]
Piracetam	The interaction has not been investigated. Theoretically, a pharmacokinetic interaction would not be anticipated
Pregabalin	The interaction has not been investigated. Theoretically, a pharmacokinetic interaction would not be anticipated
Primidone	The interaction has not been investigated. Theoretically, a pharmacokinetic interaction could occur
Consequence	As primidone is metabolized to phenobarbital, the same interaction as that described for phenobarbital can be expected
Rufinamide	The interaction has not been investigated. Theoretically, a pharmacokinetic interaction would not be anticipated
Stiripentol	The interaction has not been investigated. Theoretically, a pharmacokinetic interaction could occur
Sulthiame	The interaction has not been investigated. Theoretically, a pharmacokinetic interaction could occur
	Sulthiame and zonisamide are both weak inhibitors of carbonic anhydrase and, as a direct result, may independently increase the risk of renal calculi. Consequently, there is a theoretical potential that when they are administered together, an adverse pharmacodynamic interaction will occur [1]

Tiagabine	The interaction has not been investigated. Theoretically, a pharmacokinetic interaction would not be anticipated
Topiramate	The interaction has not been investigated. Theoretically, a pharmacokinetic interaction would not be anticipated
	Topiramate and zonisamide are both weak inhibitors of carbonic anhydrase and, as a direct result, may independently increase the risk of renal calculi. Consequently, there is a theoretical potential that when they are administered together, an adverse pharmacodynamic interaction will occur [1]
Valproic acid	Does not affect the pharmacokinetics of zonisamide [11]
Vigabatrin	The interaction has not been investigated. Theoretically, a pharmacokinetic interaction would not be anticipated

References

1. Patsalos PN, St Louis EK. The epilepsy prescriber's guide to antiepileptic drugs. 3rd ed. Cambridge: Cambridge University Press; 2018.
2. Moseley BD, Chanteux H, Nicolas JM, Laloyaux C, Gidal B. A review of the drug-drug interactions of the antiepileptic drug brivaracetam. Epilepsy Res. 2020;163:106327.
3. Gaston TE, Bekib EM, Cutter GR, Liu Y, Szaflarski JP, UAB CBD Program. Interactions between cannabidiol and commonly used antiepileptic drugs. Epilepsia. 2017;58:1586–92.
4. Ragueneau-Majlessi I, Levy RH, Bergen D, Garnet W, Rosenfeld W, Mather G, Shah J, Grundy JS. Carbamazepine pharmacokinetics are not affected by zonisamide: in vitro mechanistic study and in vivo clinical study in epileptic patients. Epilepsy Res. 2004;62:1–11.
5. Shinoda M, Akita M, Hasegawa M, Hasegawa T, Nabeshima T. The necessity of adjusting the dosage of zonisamide when coadministered with other anti-epileptic drugs. Biol Pharm Bull. 1996;19:1090–2.
6. Sachdeo R. Lacosamide. In: Shorvon SD, Perucca E, Engel J, editors. The treatment of epilepsy. 3rd ed. Oxford: Blackwell Publishing; 2009. p. 527–34.
7. Levy RH, Ragueneau-Majlessi I, Brodie MJ, Smith DF, Shah J, Pan WJ. Lack of clinically significant pharmacokinetic interactions between zonisamide and lamotrigine at steady state in patients with epilepsy. Ther Drug Monit. 2005;27:193–8.
8. Patsalos PN. The clinical pharmacology profile of the new antiepileptic drug perampanel: a novel noncompetitive AMPA receptor antagonist. Epilepsia. 2015;56:12–27.
9. Buchanan RA, Page JG, French JA, Leppik IE, Padgett CS. Zonisamide drug interactions. Epilepsia. 1997;38(Suppl 8):107.
10. Levy RH, Ragueneau-Majlessi I, Garnett WR, Schmerler M, Rosenfeld W, Shah J, Pan WJ. Lack of clinically significant effects of zonisamide on phenytoin steady-state pharmacokinetics in patients with epilepsy. J Clin Pharmacol. 2004;44:1230–4.
11. Ragueneau-Majlessi I, Levy RH, Brodie MJ, Smith D, Shah J, Grundy JS. Lack of pharmacokinetic interactions between steady-state zonisamide and valproic acid in patients with epilepsy. Clin Pharmacokinet. 2005;44:517–23.

Part II
Drug Interactions Between ASMs and Non-ASMs: Interactions Affecting ASMs

Acetazolamide

There have been no reports of the effect of non-ASM drugs on the pharmacokinetics or pharmacodynamics of acetazolamide.

P. N. Patsalos, *Antiseizure Medication Interactions*,
https://doi.org/10.1007/978-3-030-82790-8_34

Brivaracetam

Alcohol	Alcohol does not affect the pharmacokinetics of brivaracetam [1]
	Brivaracetam approximately doubled the effect of alcohol on psychomotor function, attention and memory consequent to a pharmacodynamic interaction [1]
Gemfibrozil	Gemfibrozil does not affect the pharmacokinetics of brivaracetam [2]
Oral contraceptives	Oral contraceptives do not affect the pharmacokinetics of brivaracetam [3]
Rifampicin	Rifampicin enhances the metabolism of brivaracetam, via an action on CYP2C19, and decreases mean plasma brivaracetam AUC values by 45% [4]

References

1. Kruithof AC, Watanabe S, Peeters PA, de Kam ML, Zuiker RG, Stevens J, van Gerven JM, Stockis A. Pharmacological interactions between brivaracetam and healthy males. J Psychopharmacol. 2017;31:915–26.
2. Nicolas JM, Chanteux H, Rosa M, Watanabe S, Stockis A. Effect of gemfibrozil on the metabolism of brivaracetam in vitro and in human subjects. Drugs Metab Dispos. 2012;40:1466–72.
3. Stockis A, Watanabe S, Fauchoux N. Interaction between brivaracetam (100 mg/kg) and a combination oral contraceptive: a randomized, double-blind, placebo-controlled study. Epilepsia. 2014;55:e27–31.
4. Stockis A, Watanabe S, Scheen AJ, Tytgat D, Gerin B, Rosa M, Chanteux H, Nicolas JM. Effect of rifampin on the disposition of brivaracetam in human subjects: further insights into brivaracetam hydrolysis. Drug Metab Dispos. 2016;44:792–9.

P. N. Patsalos, *Antiseizure Medication Interactions*, https://doi.org/10.1007/978-3-030-82790-8_35

Cannabidiol

Rifampicin	Rifampicin enhances the metabolism of cannabidiol and decreases mean plasma cannabidiol and 7-hydroxy-cannabidiol, the pharmacologically active metabolite of cannabidiol, by 30% and 60%, respectively [1]

Reference

1. Summary of product characteristics: Cannabidiol (Epidyolex). GW Pharma Ltd. Last update 27th July 2020.

P. N. Patsalos, *Antiseizure Medication Interactions*,
https://doi.org/10.1007/978-3-030-82790-8_36

Carbamazepine

Analgesics

Aspirin	Salicylic acid does not affect the pharmacokinetics of carbamazepine [1]
Propoxyphene (dextropropoxyphene)	Propoxyphene inhibits the metabolism of carbamazepine, probably via an action on CYP3A4. Typically, mean plasma carbamazepine levels can increase by 24–64%, but occasionally larger increases can occur (800%). Concurrent mean plasma carbamazepine-10, 11-epoxide levels can be decreased by 42% [2–4]
Paracetamol	Paracetamol does not affect the pharmacokinetics of carbamazepine [1]
Phenylbutazone	Phenylbutazone does not affect the pharmacokinetics of carbamazepine [1]
Tolfenamic acid	Tolfenamic acid does not affect the pharmacokinetics of carbamazepine [1]

Antibacterials

Azithromycin	Azithromycin does not affect the pharmacokinetics of carbamazepine [5]
Ciprofloxacin	Ciprofloxacin can increase plasma carbamazepine levels [6]
Clarithromycin	Clarithromycin inhibits the metabolism of carbamazepine, probably via an action on CYP3A4, and can increase mean plasma carbamazepine levels by 100%. Plasma carbamazepine-10, 11-epoxide levels have been reported either to be unaffected or to decrease [7, 8]
Dirithromycin	Dirithromycin does not affect the pharmacokinetics of carbamazepine [9]
Erythromycin	Erythromycin inhibits the metabolism of carbamazepine, probably via an action on CYP3A4, and can increase plasma carbamazepine levels two–threefold. Plasma carbamazepine-10, 11-epoxide levels can be concurrently decreased by 41% [10]
Flurithromycin	Flurithromycin inhibits the metabolism of carbamazepine, probably via an action on CYP3A4, and can increase mean plasma carbamazepine AUC values by 18%. Mean plasma carbamazepine-10, 11-epoxide levels can be concurrently decreased by 23% [11]

P. N. Patsalos, *Antiseizure Medication Interactions*,
https://doi.org/10.1007/978-3-030-82790-8_37

Isotretinoin	Isotretinoin can increase plasma carbamazepine AUC values by 11–24% and can decrease plasma carbamazepine-10, 11-epoxide AUC values by 21–24% [12]
Josamycin	Josamycin inhibits the metabolism of carbamazepine, probably via an action on CYP3A4, and can increase mean plasma carbamazepine AUC values by 18%. Plasma carbamazepine-10, 11-epoxide levels are unaffected [13]
Metronidazole	Metronidazole can increase plasma carbamazepine levels by ~60%. The mechanism of this interaction is not known [14]
Ponsinomycin (miocamycin)	Ponsinomycin inhibits the metabolism of carbamazepine, probably via an action on CYP3A4, and can increase mean plasma carbamazepine AUC values by 13% and decrease mean plasma carbamazepine-10, 11-epoxide levels by 26% [15]
Roxithromycin	Roxithromycin does not affect the pharmacokinetics of carbamazepine [16]
Troleandomycin	Troleandomycin inhibits the metabolism of carbamazepine, probably via an action on CYP3A4, and can increase plasma carbamazepine levels twofold–threefold [17]

Antifungal Agents

Fluconazole	Fluconazole inhibits the metabolism of carbamazepine, probably by inhibiting CYP3A4, and can increase plasma carbamazepine levels by 147% [18]
Ketoconazole	Ketoconazole inhibits the metabolism of carbamazepine and can increase mean plasma carbamazepine levels by 29%. Plasma carbamazepine-10, 11-epoxide levels are not affected. The mechanism is considered to be via an action on CYP3A4 [19]
Miconazole	Miconazole inhibits the metabolism of carbamazepine and can increase plasma carbamazepine levels [20]

Antineoplastic Agents

Cisplatin	Cisplatin may decrease plasma carbamazepine levels by decreasing cisplatin absorption [21]
Tamoxifen	Tamoxifen does not affect the pharmacokinetics of carbamazepine [22]

Antituberculous Agents

Isoniazid	Isoniazid inhibits the metabolism of carbamazepine and can result in a 45% decrease in clearance and an increase in plasma carbamazepine levels of up to 85% [23, 24]
Rifampicin	Rifampicin enhances the metabolism of carbamazepine and can decrease plasma carbamazepine levels [25]

Antiulcer Drugs

Histamine H_2-Receptor Antagonists

Cimetidine	Cimetidine inhibits the metabolism of carbamazepine via an action on CYP3A4 and can increase plasma carbamazepine levels by 17%. In many patients, this interaction does not occur or is transient [26, 27]
Ranitidine	Ranitidine does not affect the pharmacokinetics of carbamazepine [28]

Proton Pump Inhibitors

Omeprazole	Conflicting effects have been reported
	A single-dose carbamazepine study of patients found an increase in mean plasma carbamazepine AUC values of 75%, a decrease in mean plasma carbamazepine clearance values of 40%, and an increase in mean plasma carbamazepine half-life values of 118%
	However, another patient study whereby carbamazepine treatment was long-term found a small nonsignificant decrease in carbamazepine plasma levels [29, 30]
Pantoprazole	Pantoprazole does not affect the pharmacokinetics of carbamazepine [31]

Antiviral Agents

Efavirenz	Efavirenz enhances the metabolism of carbamazepine via an action on CYP3A4 and can decrease mean plasma carbamazepine Cmax values by 29% and mean plasma carbamazepine AUC values by 27%. Plasma carbamazepine-10, 11-epoxide levels are not affected [32]
Lopinavir/ritonavir	Lopinavir combined with ritonavir can inhibit the metabolism of carbamazepine via an action on CYP3A4 and can increase plasma carbamazepine levels by 46% [33]
Nelfinavir	Nelfinavir inhibits the metabolism of carbamazepine via an action on CYP3A4 and can increase plasma carbamazepine levels by 53% [33]
Ritonavir	Ritonavir inhibits the metabolism of carbamazepine via an action on CYP3A4 and can increase plasma carbamazepine levels by 180% [34]

Cardiovascular Drugs

Antiarrhythmics

Amiodarone	Amiodarone does not affect the pharmacokinetics of carbamazepine [36]

Antihypertensive Agents

Diltiazem	Diltiazem inhibits the metabolism of carbamazepine and can increase plasma carbamazepine levels by 55–100% [37]
Nifedipine	Nifedipine does not affect the pharmacokinetics of carbamazepine [38]
Verapamil	Verapamil inhibits the metabolism of carbamazepine and can increase mean plasma carbamazepine levels by 46%. Plasma carbamazepine-10, 11-epoxide levels are unaffected [39]

Antiplatelet Drugs

Ticlopidine	Ticlopidine inhibits the metabolism of carbamazepine, perhaps via an action on CYP3A4, and can increase plasma carbamazepine levels by up to 74% [40]

Lipid-Lowering Drugs

Cholestyramine	Cholestyramine does not affect the pharmacokinetics of carbamazepine [41]
Colestipol	Colestipol can reduce the absorption of carbamazepine by 10% [41]
Gemfibrozil	Gemfibrozil can increase plasma carbamazepine levels by 30–65%. The suggested mechanism is that the clearance of carbamazepine is increased in those patients with elevated cholesterol and total lipids; thus when the condition is treated with gemfibrozil, clearance becomes more normal resulting in an increase in plasma carbamazepine levels [42]

Oral Anticoagulants

Pentoxifylline	Pentoxifylline does not affect the pharmacokinetics of carbamazepine [43]

Herbal Remedies

Coca–Cola	Coca-Cola can enhance the rate and extent of carbamazepine absorption and increase plasma carbamazepine levels [44]
Free and Easy Wanderer Plus	Free and Easy Wanderer Plus can decrease mean plasma carbamazepine levels by 57% [45]
Grapefruit juice (furanocoumarins)	Grapefruit juice inhibits the metabolism of carbamazepine via an action on CYP3A4 and can increase mean plasma carbamazepine levels by 39% [46]
Honey	Honey does not affect the pharmacokinetics of carbamazepine [47]
Kinnow juice	Kinnow juice, probably via an inhibition of CYP3A4, can increase plasma carbamazepine levels [48]
Piperine	Piperine can increase mean plasma carbamazepine AUC values, probably via inhibition of CYP3A, by 48% [49]
Resveratrol	Resveratrol inhibits the metabolism of carbamazepine via an action on CYP3A4 and can increase mean Cmax and AUC values by 46% and 37%, respectively [50]
St John's Wort (Hypericum perforatum)	St John's Wort enhances the metabolism of carbamazepine by inducing CYP3A4 and possibly by affecting the activity of drug transporters in the gastrointestinal tract. Indeed, St John's Wort has been shown to decrease plasma carbamazepine levels after a single dose of carbamazepine, although no interaction was identified at a steady state [51]

Psychotropic Drugs

Antidepressants

Amoxapine	Amoxapine does not affect plasma carbamazepine levels. However, plasma carbamazepine-10, 11-epoxide levels can be increased [52]
Citalopram	Citalopram does not affect the pharmacokinetics of carbamazepine [53]
Fluoxetine	Fluoxetine inhibits the metabolism of carbamazepine
	Mean plasma carbamazepine AUC values are increased by 27%, while mean plasma AUC values of its pharmacologically active metabolite, carbamazepine-10, 11-epoxide, are increased by 31%. However, the interaction appears to be variable, with some studies reporting no effect [54, 55]
Fluvoxamine	Conflicting effects have been reported
	The interaction appears to be variable with plasma levels of carbamazepine and its metabolite, carbamazepine-10, 11-epoxide, ranging from no effect to a 71% increase in levels [55, 56]
Nefazodone	Nefazodone inhibits the metabolism of carbamazepine. Plasma carbamazepine levels are increased by up to threefold [57–59]
Paroxetine	Paroxetine does not affect the pharmacokinetics of carbamazepine [60]
Sertraline	Sertraline does not affect the pharmacokinetics of carbamazepine [61]
Trazodone	Trazodone inhibits the metabolism of carbamazepine and can increase plasma carbamazepine levels by 26% [62]
Venlafaxine	Venlafaxine does not affect the pharmacokinetics of carbamazepine [63]
Viloxazine	Viloxazine inhibits the metabolism of carbamazepine and can increase mean plasma carbamazepine levels by 55% and mean plasma carbamazepine-10, 11-epoxide levels by 16% [64]

Antipsychotics

Haloperidol	Haloperidol inhibits the metabolism of carbamazepine and can increase plasma carbamazepine levels by 40% [65]
Loxapine	Loxapine does not affect plasma carbamazepine levels. However, plasma carbamazepine-10, 11-epoxide levels can be increased [51]
Quetiapine	Quetiapine increases plasma carbamazepine-10, 11-epoxide levels so that the plasma carbamazepine-10, 11-epoxide/carbamazepine ratio is increased by three to fourfold [66]
Risperidone	Risperidone inhibits the metabolism of carbamazepine and can increase mean plasma carbamazepine levels, probably via inhibition of CYP3A4, by 19% [67]
Thioridazine	Thioridazine does not affect the pharmacokinetics of carbamazepine [68]

Steroids

Danazol	Danazol inhibits the metabolism of carbamazepine and can increase plasma carbamazepine levels by 38–123% [69]

Miscellanea

Armodafinil	Armodafinil enhances the metabolism of carbamazepine via an action on CYP3A4 and can decrease mean plasma carbamazepine AUC values by 25% and can increase mean carbamazepine-epoxide AUC values by 40% [70]
Atkins diet (modified)	The modified Atkins diet can decrease mean carbamazepine plasma levels by 23% [35]
Disulfiram	Disulfiram does not affect the pharmacokintics of carbamazepine [71]
Influenza vaccination	Influenza vaccination can increases plasma carbamazepine levels [72]
Iron supplementation (ferrous sulfate)	Iron supplementation can decrease mean carbamazepine levels, possibly by the formation of insoluble chelate complexes, by 33% [73]
Ketogenic diet	The ketogenic diet can decrease plasma carbamazepine levels [74]
Nicotinamide	Nicotinamide inhibits the metabolism of carbamazepine and can decrease carbamazepine clearance by 58–81% and increases plasma carbamazepine levels [75]
Orlistat	Orlistat does not affect the pharmacokinetics of carbamazepine [76]
Oxiracetam	Oxiracetam does not affect the pharmacokinetics of carbamazepine [77]
Probenecid	Probenecid enhances the metabolism of carbamazepine via an action on CYP3A4 and CYP2C8 and can decrease mean carbamazepine AUC values by 19% and can increase mean carbamazepine-epoxide AUC values by 33% [78]
Terfenadine	Terfenadine displaces carbamazepine from its plasma protein binding sites and can increase free carbamazepine plasma levels resulting in carbamazepine toxicity [79]
Theophylline	Theophylline enhances the metabolism of carbamazepine and can decrease mean plasma carbamazepine AUC values by 29% [80]

References

1. Neuvonen PJ, Lehtovaara R, Bardy A, Elomaa E. Antipyretic analgesics in patients on antiepileptic drug therapy. Eur J Clin Pharmacol. 1979;15:263–8.
2. Hansen SB, Dam M, Brandt J, Hvidberg EF, Angelo H, Christensen JM, Lous P. Influence of dextropropoxyphene on steady state serum levels and protein binding of three anti-epileptic drugs in man. Acta Neurol Scand. 1980;61:357–67.
3. Bergendal L, Friberg A, Schaffrath AM, Holmdahl M, Landahl S. The clinical relevance of the interaction between carbamazepine and dextropropoxyphene in elderly patients in Gothenburg, Sweden. Eur J Clin Pharmacol. 1997;53:203–6.
4. Yu YL, Huang CY, Chin D, Woo E, Chang CM. Interaction between carbamazepine and dextropropoxyphene. Postgrad Med J. 1986;62:231–3.
5. Garey KW, Amsden GW. Intravenous azithromycin. Ann Pharmacother. 1999;33:218–28.
6. Shahzadi A, Javed I, Aslam B, Muhammad F, Asi MR, Ashraf MY. Zia-ur-Rahman. Therapeutic effects of ciprofloxacin on the pharmacokinetics of carbamazepine in healthy adult male volunteers. Pak J Pharm Sci. 2011;24:63–8.
7. Albani F, Riva R, Baruzzi A. Clarithromycin-carbamazepine interaction: a case report. Epilepsia. 1993;34:161–2.
8. Yasui N, Otani K, Kaneko S, Shimoyama R, Ohkubo T, Sugawara K. Carbamazepine toxicity induced by clarithromycin coadministration in psychiatric patients. Int Clin Psychopharmacol. 1997;12:225–9.

9. Watkins VS, Polk RE, Stotka JL. Drug interactions of macrolides: emphasis on dirithromycin. Ann Pharmacother. 1997;31:349–56.
10. Barzaghi N, Gatti G, Crema F, Monteleone M, Amione C, Leone L, Perucca E. Inhibition by erythromycin of the conversion of carbamazepine to its active 10, 11-epoxide metabolite. Br J Clin Pharmacol. 1987;24:836–8.
11. Barzaghi N, Gatti G, Crema F, Faja A, Monteleone M, Amione C, Leone L, Perucca E. Effect of flurithromycin, a new macrolide antibiotic, on carbamazepine disposition in normal subjects. Int J Clin Pharmacol Res. 1988;8:101–5.
12. Marsden JR. Effect of isotretinoin on carbamazepine pharmacokinetics. Br J Dermatol. 1988;119:403–4.
13. Vincon G, Albin H, Demotes-Mainard F, Guyot M, Bistue C, Loiseau P. Effects of josamycin on carbamazepine kinetics. Eur J Clin Pharmacol. 1987;32:321–3.
14. Patterson BD. Possible interaction between metronidazole and carbamazepine. Ann Pharmacother. 1994;28:1303–4.
15. Couet W, Istin B, Ingrand I, Girault J, Fourtillan JB. Effect of ponsinomycin on single-dose kinetics and metabolism of carbamazepine. Ther Drug Monit. 1990;12:144–9.
16. Saint-Salvi B, Tremblay D, Surjus A, Lefebve MA. A study of the interaction of roxithromycin with theophylline and carbamazepine. J Antimicrob Chemother. 1987;20(Suppl B):121–9.
17. Mesdjian E, Dravet C, Cenraud B, Roger J. Carbamazepine intoxication due to triacetyloleandomycin administration in epileptic patients. Epilepsia. 1980;21:489–96.
18. Ulivelli M, Rubegni P, Nuti D, Bartalini S, Giannini S, Rossi S. Clinical evidence of fluconazole-induced carbamazepine toxicity. J Neurol. 2004;251:622–3.
19. Spina E, Arena S, Scordo MG, Fazio A, Pisan F, Perucca E. Elevation of plasma carbamazepine concentrations by ketoconazole in patients with epilepsy. Ther Drug Monit. 1997;19:535–8.
20. Loupi E, Descotes J, Lery N, Evreux JC. Interactions medicamenteuses et miconazole. A propos de 10 observations. Therapie. 1982;37:437–41.
21. Neef C, de Voogd-van der Straaten I. An interaction between cytostatic and anticonvulsant drugs. Clin Pharmacol Ther. 1988;43:372–5.
22. Rabinowicz AL, Hinton DR, Dyck P, Couldwell WT. High-dose tamoxifen in treatment of brain tumors: interaction with antiepileptic drugs. Epilepsia. 1995;36:513–5.
23. Valsalan VC, Cooper GL. Carbamazepine intoxication caused by interaction with isoniazid. Br Med J. 1982;285:261–2.
24. Block SH. Carbamazepine-isoniazid interaction. Pediatrics. 1982;69:494–5.
25. Desai J. Perspectives on interactions between antiepileptic drugs (AEDs) and antimicrobials. Epilepsia. 2008;49(Suppl 6):47–9.
26. Sonne J, Luhdorf K, Larsen NE, Andreasen PB. Lack of interaction between cimetidine and carbamazepine. Acta Neurol Scand. 1983;68:253–6.
27. Dalton MJ, Powell R, Messenheimer JA, Clark J. Cimetidine and carbamazepine: a complex drug interaction. Epilepsia. 1986;27:553–8.
28. Webster LK, Mihaly GW, Jones DB, Smallwood RA, Philips JA, Vajda FJ. Effect of cimetidine and ranitidine on carbamazepine and sodium valproate pharmacokinetics. Eur J Clin Pharmacol. 1984;27:341–3.
29. Bottiger Y, Bertilsson L. No effect on plasma carbamazepine concentration with concomitant omeprazole. Drug Investig. 1995;9:180–1.
30. Naidu MUR, Shoba J, Dixit VK, Kumar TR, Sekhar EC. Effect of multiple dose omeprazole on the pharmacokinetics of carbamazepine. Drug Investig. 1994;7:8–12.
31. Huber R, Bliesath H, Hartmann M, Steinijans VW, Koch H, Mascher H, Wurst W. Pantoprazole does not interact with the pharmacokinetics of carbamazepine. Int J Clin Pharmacol Ther. 1998;36:521–4.
32. Ji P, Damle B, Xie J, Unger SE, Grasela DM, Kaul S. Pharmacokinetic interaction between efavirenz and carbamazepine after multiple-dose administration in healthy subjects. J Clin Pharmacol. 2008;48:948–56.
33. Bates DE, Herman RJ. Carbamazepine toxicity induced by lopinavir/ritonavir and nelfinavir. Ann Pharmacother. 2006;40:1190–5.

34. Garcia AB, Ibarra AL, Etessam JP, Salio AM, Martinez DAP, Diaz RS, Hera MT. Protease inhibitor-induced carbamazepine toxicity. Clin Neuropharmacol. 2000;23:216–8.
35. Kvemeland M, Taubull E, Molteberg E, Veierod MB, Selmer KK, Nakken KO, Iversen PO. Pharmacokinetic interaction between modified Atkins diet and antiepileptc drugs in adults with drug-resistant epilepsy. Epilepsia. 2019;60:2235–440.
36. Leite SAO, Leite PJM, Rocha GA, Routledge PA, Bittencourt PRM. Carbamazepine kinetics in cardiac patients before and during amiodarone. Arq Neuropsiquiatr. 1994;52:210–5.
37. Shaughnessy AF, Mosley MR. Elevated carbamazepine levels associated with diltiazem use. Neurology. 1992;42:937–8.
38. Brodie MJ, Macphee GJA. Carbamazepine neurotoxicity precipitated by diltiazem. Br Med J. 1986;292:1170–1.
39. Macphee GA, McInnes GT, Thompson GG, Brodie MJ. Verapamil potentiates carbamazepine neurotoxicity: a clinically important inhibitory interaction. Lancet. 1986;1:700–3.
40. Brown RIG, Cooper TG. Ticlopidine-carbamazepine interaction in a coronary stent patient. Can J Cardiol. 1997;13:853–4.
41. Neuvonen PJ, Kivisto K, Hirvisalo EL. Effects of resins and activated charcoal on the absorption of digoxin, carbamazepine and frusemide. Br J Clin Pharmacol. 1988;25:229–33.
42. Denio L, Drake ME, Pakalnis A. Gemfibrozil-carbamazepine interaction in epileptic patients. Epilepsia. 1988;29:654.
43. Poondru S, Devaraj R, Boinpally RR, Yamsani MR. Time-dependent influence of pentoxifylline on the pharmacokinetics of orally administered carbamazepine in human subjects. Pharmacol Res. 2001;43:301–5.
44. Malhotra S, Dixit RK, Garg SK. Effect of an acidic beverage (Coca-Cola) on the pharmacokinetics of carbamazepine in healthy volunteers. Methods Find Exp Clin Pharmacol. 2002;24:31–3.
45. Zhang ZJ, Kang WH, Li Q, Tan QR. The beneficial effects of the herbal medicine free and easy wanderer plus for mood disorders: double-blind, placebo-controlled studies. J Psychiatr Res. 2007;41:828–36.
46. Garg SK, Kumar N, Bhargava VK, Prabhakar SK. Effect of grapefruit juice on carbamazepine bioavailability in patients with epilepsy. Clin Pharmacol Ther. 1998;64:286–8.
47. Malhotra S, Garg SK, Dixit RK. Effect of concomitantly administered honey on the pharmacokinetics of carbamazepine in healthy volunteers. Methods Find Exp Clin Pharmacol. 2003;25:537–40.
48. Garg SK, Bhargava VK, James H, KuJan-Mar N, Prabhakar S, Naresh KM. Influence of kinnow juice on the bioavailability of carbamazepine in healthy male volunteers. Neurol India. 1998;46:229–31.
49. Badada SK, Appani R, Boga PK. Effect of piperine on the metabolism and pharmacokinetics of carbamazepine in healthy volunteers. Drug Res (Stuttg). 2017;67:46–51.
50. Bedada SK, Nearati P. Effect of resveratrol on the pharmacokinetics of carbamazepine in healthy human volunteers. Phytother Res. 2015;29:701–6.
51. Burstein AH, Horton RL, Dunn T, Alfaro RM, Piscitelli SC, Theodore W. Lack of effect of St. John's Wort on carbamazepine pharmacokinetics in healthy volunteers. Clin Pharmacol Ther. 2000;68:605–12.
52. Pitterle ME, Collins DM. Carbamazepine-10, 11-epoxide evaluation associated with coadministration of loxitane and amoxapine. Epilepsia. 1998;29:654.
53. Moller SE, Larsen F, Khant AZ, Rolan PE. Lack of effect of citalopram on the steady-state pharmacokinetics of carbamazepine in healthy male subjects. J Clin Psychopharmacol. 2001;21:493–9.
54. Grimsley SR, Jann MW, Carter JG, D'Mello AP, D'Souza MJ. Increased carbamazepine plasma concentrations after fluoxetine coadministration. Clin Pharmacol Ther. 1991;50:10–5.
55. Spina E, Avenoso A, Pollicino AM, Caputi AP, Fazio A, Pisani F. Carbamazepine coadministration with fluoxetine and fluvoxamine. Ther Drug Monit. 1993;15:247–50.
56. Fritze J, Unsorg B, Lanczik M. Interaction between carbamazepine and fluvoxamine. Acta Psychiatr Scand. 1991;84:583–4.
57. Ashton AK, Wolin RE. Nefazodone-induced carbamazepine toxicity. Am J Psychiatry. 2001;153:733.

58. Roth L, Bertschy G. Nefazodone may inhibit the metabolism of carbamazepine: three case reports. Eur Psychiatry. 2001;16:320–1.
59. Laroudie C, Salazar DE, Cosson JP, Cheuvart B, Istin B, Girault J, Ingrand I, Decourt JP. Carbamazepine-nefazodone interaction in healthy subjects. J Clin Psychopharmacol. 2000;20:46–53.
60. Andersen BB, Mikkelsen M, Vesterager A, Dam M, Kristensen HB, Pedersen B, Lund J, Mengel H. No influence of the antidepressant paroxetine on carbamazepine, valproate and phenytoin. Epilepsy Res. 1991;10:201–4.
61. Rapeport WG, Williams SA, Muirhead DC, Dewland PM, Tanner T, Wesnes K. Absence of a sertraline-mediated effect on the pharmacokinetics and pharmacodynamics of carbamazepine. J Clin Psychiatry. 1996;57(Suppl):20–3.
62. Romero AS, Delgado RG, Pena MF. Interaction between trazodone and carbamazepine. Ann Pharmacother. 1999;33:1370.
63. Wiklander B, Danjou P, Rolan P, Tamin SK, Toon S. Evaluation of the potential pharmacokinetic interaction of venlafaxine and carbamazepine. Eur Neuropsychopharmacol. 1995;6:310–1.
64. Pisani F, Fazio A, Oteri G, Perucca E, Russo M, Trio R, Pisani B, Di Perri R. Carbamazepine-viloxazine interaction in patients with epilepsy. J Neurol Neurosurg Psychiatry. 1986;49:1142–5.
65. Iwahashi K, Miyatake R, Suwaki H, Hosokawa K, Ichikawa Y. The drug-drug interaction effects of haloperidol on plasma carbamazepine levels. Clin Neuropharmacol. 1995;18:233–6.
66. Fitzgerald BJ, Okos AJ. Elevation of carbamazepine-10, 11-epoxide by quetiapine. Pharmacotherapy. 2002;22:1500–3.
67. Mula M, Monaco F. Carbamazepine-risperidone interactions in patients with epilepsy. Clin Neuropharmacol. 2002;25:97–100.
68. Spina E, Amendola D'Agostino AM, Ioculano MP, Oteri G, Fazio A, Pisani F. No effect of thioridazine on plasma concentrations of carbamazepine and its active metabolite carbamazepine-10, 11-epoxide. Ther Drug Monit. 1990;12:511–3.
69. Zielinski JJ, Lichten EM, Haidukewych D. Clinically significant danazol-carbamazepine interaction. Ther Drug Monit. 1987;9:24–7.
70. Darwish M, Bond M, Yang R, Hellriegel ET, Robertson P. Evaluation of the potential for pharmacokinetic drug-drug interaction between armodafinil and carbamazepine in healthy adults. Clin Ther. 2015;37:325–37.
71. Krag B, Dam M, Angelo H, Christensen JM. Influence of disulfiram on the serum concentration of carbamazepine in patients with epilepsy. Acta Neurol Scand. 1981;63:395–8.
72. Robertson WC. Carbamazepine toxicity after influenza vaccination. Pediatr Neurol. 2003;26:61–3.
73. Ahn JE, Bathena SPR, Brundage RC, Conway JM, Leppik IE, Birnbaum AK. Iron supplementation in nursing home patients associated with reduced carbamazepine absorption. Epilepsy Res. 2018;147:115–8.
74. Heo C, Kim SH, Chang MJ. Effect of ketogenic diet and other dietary therapies on anti-epileptic drug comedication in patients with epilepsy. J Clin Pharm Ther. 2007;42:758–64.
75. Bourgeois BFD, Dodson WE, Ferrendelli JA. Interactions between primidone, carbamazepine, and nicotinamide. Neurology. 1982;32:1122–6.
76. Hilgar E, Quiner S, Ginzel I, Walter H, Saria L, Barnas C. The effect of orlistat on plasma levels of psychotropic drugs in patients with long-term psychopharmacology. J Clin Psychopharmacol. 2002;22:68–70.
77. van Wieringen A, Meijer JWA, van Emde BW, Vermeij TAC. Pilot study to determine the interaction of oxiracetam with antiepileptics. Clin Pharmacokinet. 1990;18:332–8.
78. Kim KA, Oh SO, Park PW, Park JY. Effect of probenecid on the pharmacokinetics of carbamazepine in healthy subjects. Eur J Clin Pharmacol. 2005;61:275–80.
79. Hirschfeld S, Jarosinska P. Drug interaction of terfenadine and carbamazepine. Ann Intern Med. 1993;118:907–8.
80. Kulkarni C, Vaz J, David J, Joseph T. Aminophylline alters pharmacokinetics of carbamazepine but not that of sodium valproate – a single dose pharmacokinetic study in human volunteers. Indian J Physiol Pharmacol. 1995;39:122–6.

Cenobamate

Alcohol	Alcohol does not affect the pharmacokinetics of cenobamate [1]

Reference

1. Summary of product characteristics: Cenobamate (XCopri). SK Life Science Inc. Last update Aug 2020.

P. N. Patsalos, *Antiseizure Medication Interactions*,
https://doi.org/10.1007/978-3-030-82790-8_38

Clobazam

Atkins diet (*modified*)	The modified Atkins diet can decrease mean clobazam plasma levels 34% [1]
Cimetidine	The effect of cimetidine on the pharmacokinetics of clobazam is conflicting
	Cimetidine can increase mean plasma clobazam AUC values by 17% and increase mean half-life values by 11% without affecting the pharmacokinetics of N-desmethylclobazam (the pharmacologically active metabolite of clobazam). Also, cimetidine has been reported to increase mean plasma clobazam AUC values by 59%, and increase mean plasma half-life values by 40%, along with a concurrent increase in mean N-desmethylclobazam AUC and half-life values of 57% and 90%, respectively [2, 3]
Esmoprazole	Esmaprozole increases mean plasma clobazam levels sevenfold [4]
Etravirine	Etravirine inhibits the metabolism of clobazam and can increase plasma clobazam and plasma N-desmethylclobazam levels [5]
Ketoconazole	Ketoconazole inhibits the metabolism of clobazam and can increase mean plasma clobazam and N-desmethylclobazam AUC values by 54% and 18%, respectively [6]
Miconazole	Miconazole inhibits the metabolism of clobazam and its pharmacologically active metabolite N-desmethylclobazam and can increase plasma clobazam levels by 85% and plasma N-desmethylclobazam levels by 6.5-fold [7]
Omeprazole	Omeprazole inhibits the metabolism of clobazam and can increase mean plasma clobazam and N-desmethylclobazam AUC values by 30% and 36%, respectively [5]
Oxiracetam	Oxiracetam does not affect the pharmacokinetics of clobazam [8]
Pantoprazole	Pantoprazole increases mean plasma clobazam levels tenfold [4]

P. N. Patsalos, *Antiseizure Medication Interactions*,
https://doi.org/10.1007/978-3-030-82790-8_39

References

1. Kvemeland M, Taubull E, Molteberg E, Veierod MB, Selmer KK, Nakken KO, Iversen PO. Pharmacokinetic interaction between modified Atkins diet and antiepileptc drugs in adults with drug-resistant epilepsy. Epilepsia. 2019;60:2235–440.
2. Grigoleit HG, Hajdu P, Hundt HKL, Koeppen D, Malerczyk V, Meyer BH, Muller FO, Witte PU. Pharmacokinetic aspects of the interaction between clobazam and cimetidine. Eur J Clin Pharmacol. 1983;25:139–42.
3. Pullar T, Edwards D, Haigh JR, Peaker S, Feely MP. The effect of cimetidine on the single dose pharmacokinetics of oral clobazam and N-desmethylclobazam. Br J Clin Pharmacol. 1987;23:317–21.
4. Pasupuleti B, Gone V, Baddam R, Venisetty RK, Prasad OP. Clinical impact of co-medications of levetiracetam and clobazam with proton pump inhibitors: a drug interaction study. Curr Drug Metab. 2020;21:126–31.
5. Naccarato M, Yoong D, Kovacs C, Gough K. A case of potential drug interaction between clobazam and etravirine-based antiviral therapy. Antivir Ther. 2012;17:589–92.
6. Walzer M, Bekersky I, Blum RA, Tolbert D. Pharmacokinetic drug interactions between clobazam and drugs metabolized by cytochrome P450 isoenzymes. Pharmacotherapy. 2012;32:340–53.
7. Goldsmith J, McKnight C, Dickson S, Heenan M, Berezowski R. Miconazole and clobazam; a useful interaction in Dravet's syndrome? Arch Dis Child. 2004;89:89.
8. van Wieringen A, Meijer JWA, van Emde BW, Vermeij TAC. Pilot study to determine the interaction of oxiracetam with antiepileptics. Clin Pharmacokinet. 1990;18:332–8.

Clonazepam

Amiodarone	Clonazepam toxicity was observed in a patient co-prescribed amiodarone, which resolved upon clonazepam withdrawal [1]
Fluoxetine	Fluoxetine does not affect the pharmacokinetics of clonazepam [2]
Ketogenic diet	The ketogenic diet does not affect the pharmacokinetics of phenobarbital [3]
Sertraline	Sertraline does not affect the pharmacokinetics of clonazepam [4]

References

1. Witt DM, Ellsworth AJ, Leversee JH. Amiodarone-clonazepam interaction. Ann Pharmacother. 1993;27:1463–4.
2. Greenblatt DJ, Preskorn SH, Cotreau MM, Horst WD, Harmatz JS. Fluoxetine impairs clearance of alprazolam but not clonazepam. Clin Pharmacol Ther. 1992;52:479–86.
3. Dahlin MG, Beck OM, Amrk PE. Plasma levels of antiepileptic drugs in children on the ketogenic diet. Pediatr Neurol. 2006;35:6–10.
4. Bonate PL, Kroboth PD, Smith RB, Suarez E, Oo C. Clonazepam and sertraline: absence of drug interaction in a multiple-dose study. J Clin Psychopharmacol. 2000;20:19–27.

P. N. Patsalos, *Antiseizure Medication Interactions*,
https://doi.org/10.1007/978-3-030-82790-8_40

Eslicarbazepine Acetate

Rosuvastatin	Rosuvastatin does not affect the pharmacokinetics of eslicarbazepine [1]

Reference

1. Gidal BE, Mintzer S, Schwab M, Schutz R, Kharidia J, Blum D, Grinnell T, Sunkaraneni S. Evidence for a pharmacokinetic interaction between eslicarbazepine and rosuvastatin: potential effects on xenobiotic trasporters. Epileepsy Res. 2017;135:64–70.

P. N. Patsalos, *Antiseizure Medication Interactions*, https://doi.org/10.1007/978-3-030-82790-8_41

Ethosuximide

Isoniazid	Isoniazid inhibits the metabolism of ethosuximide and can increase plasma ethosuximide levels by 42% [1]
Rifampicin	Rifampicin enhances the metabolism of ethosuximide and can decrease plasma ethosuximide levels [2]

References

1. van Wieringen A, Vrijlandt CM. Ethosuximide intoxication caused by interaction with isoniazid. Neurology. 1983;33:1227–8.
2. Desai J. Perspectives on interactions between antiepileptic drugs (AEDs) and antimicrobials. Epilepsia. 2008;49(Suppl 6):47–9.

P. N. Patsalos, *Antiseizure Medication Interactions*,
https://doi.org/10.1007/978-3-030-82790-8_42

Everolimus

Ciclosporin	Ciclosporin inhibits the metabolism of everolimus, probably via an action on CYP3A4, and can increase mean plasma everolimus AUC values by 2.7-fold [1]
Erythromycin	Erythromycin inhibits the metabolism of everolimus, probably via an action on CYP3A4, and can increase mean plasma everolimus AUC values by 15.4-fold [1]
Imatinib	Imatinib inhibits the metabolism of everolimus, probably via an action on CYP3A4, and can increase mean plasma everolimus AUC values by 3.7-fold [1]
Ketoconazole	Ketoconazole inhibits the metabolism of everolimus, probably via an action on CYP3A4, and can increase mean plasma everolimus AUC values by 15.3-fold [1]
Rifampicin	Rifampicin enhances the metabolism of everolimus, probably via an action on CYP3A4, and can decrease mean plasma everolimus AUC values by 63% [1]
Verapamil	Verapamil inhibits the metabolism of everolimus, probably via an action on CYP3A4, and can increase mean plasma everolimus AUC values by 3.5-fold [1]

Reference

1. Summary of product characteristics: Everolimus. Accord Healthcare Ltd. Last update 9th Nov 2020.

P. N. Patsalos, *Antiseizure Medication Interactions*,
https://doi.org/10.1007/978-3-030-82790-8_43

Felbamate

Antacids	Concurrent administration of antacids (Maalox Plus; aluminum/magnesium hydroxides) does not affect the rate or extent of felbamate absorption [1]
Erythromycin	Erythromycin does not affect the pharmacokinetics of felbamate [2]

References

1. Sachdeo RC, Narang-Sachdeo SK, Howard JR, Dix RK, Shumaker RC, Perhach JL, Rosenberg A. Effect of antacid on absorption of felbamate in subjects with epilepsy. Epilepsia. 1993;34(Suppl 6):79–80.
2. Sachdeo RJ, Narang-Sachdeo SK, Montgomery PA, Shumaker RC, Perhach JL, Lyness WH, Rosenberg A. Evaluation of the potential interaction between felbamate and erythromycin in patients with epilepsy. J Clin Pharmacol. 1998;38:184–90.

P. N. Patsalos, *Antiseizure Medication Interactions*,
https://doi.org/10.1007/978-3-030-82790-8_44

Fenfluramine

There have been no reports of the effect of non-ASM drugs on the pharmacokinetics or pharmacodynamics of fenfluramine.

P. N. Patsalos, *Antiseizure Medication Interactions*,
https://doi.org/10.1007/978-3-030-82790-8_45

Gabapentin

Antacids	Antacids (Maalox aluminum hydroxide/magnesium hydroxide) can reduce the oral bioavailability of gabapentin by 20%. To avoid problems, administration of gabapentin and antacids should be separated by at least 2 h [1]
Cetirizine	Cetirizine can decrease mean plasma gabapentin levels, probably via interaction with renal drug transporters [2]
Cimetidine	Cimetidine can increase mean plasma gabapentin AUC values by 24% [3]
Hydrocodone	Hydrocodone can increase gabapentin absorption and increase plasma gabapentin levels [4]
Morphine	Morphine can increase gabapentin absorption and increase plasma gabapentin levels [3]
Naproxen	Naproxen can increase gabapentin absorption and increase mean plasma gabapentin AUC values by 13% [4]
Probenecid	Probenecid does not affect the pharmacokinetics of gabapentin [5]
Shiitake mushroom	Shiitake mushroom can increase mean renal clearance of gabapentin by 18% and decrease mean plasma gabapentin Cmax values by 14% [6]

References

1. Busch JA, Radulovic LL, Bockbrader HN, Underwood BA, Sedman AJ, Chang T. Effect of maalox TC on single-dose pharmacokinetics of gabapentin capsules in healthy subjects. Pharm Res. 1992;9(Suppl 2):S315.
2. Costa ACC, Yamemoto PA, Lauretti GR, de Lima Benzi JT, Zanelli CF, Barz V, Ciarimboli G, de Moraes NV. Cetirizine reduces gabapentin plasma concentrations and effect: role of renal drug transporters for organic cations. J Clin Pharmacol. 2022;60:1076–86.
3. Lal R, Sukbuntherng J, Luo W, Vicente V, Blumenthal R, Ho J, Cundy KC. Clinical pharmacokinetic drug interaction studies of gabapentin enacarbil, a novel transporter prodrug of gabapentin, with naproxen and cimetidine. Br J Clin Pharmacol. 2010;69:498–507.
4. Sternieri E, Coccio CPR, Pinetti D, Guerzoni S, Ferrari A. Pharmacokinetics and interactions of headache medications, part II: prophylactic treatments. Expert Opin Drug Metab Toxicol. 2006;2:981–1007.

P. N. Patsalos, *Antiseizure Medication Interactions*,
https://doi.org/10.1007/978-3-030-82790-8_46

5. Busch JA, Bockbrader HN, Randinitis EJ, Chang T, Welling PG, Reece PA, Underwood B, Sedman AJ, Vollmer KO, Turck D. Lack of clinically significant drug interactions with Neurontin (Gabapentin). In: 20th international epilepsy congress, Oslo. 1993; Abstract 013958.
6. Toh DSL, Limenta LMG, Yee JY, Wang LZ, Goh BC, Murray M, Lee EJD. Effect of mushroom diet on pharmacokinetics of gabapentin in healthy Chinese subjects. Br J Clin Pharmacol. 2013;78:129–34.

Lacosamide

Digoxin	Digoxin does not affect the pharmacokinetics of lacosamide [1]
Metformin	Metformin does not affect the pharmacokinetics of lacosamide [2]
Modified Atkins diet	Modified Atkins diet can decrease mean lacosamide plasma levels by 15% [3]
Omeprazole	Omeprazole does not affect the pharmacokinetics of lacosamide [4]
Oral contraceptives	Oral contraceptives do not affect the pharmacokinetics of lacosamide [5]

References

1. Cawello W, Mueller-Voessing C, Andreas JO. Effect of lacosamide on steady-state pharmacokinetics of digoxin: results from a phase I, multiple-dose, double-blind, randomised, placebo-controlled, crossover trial. Clin Drug Investig. 2014;34:327–34.
2. Thomas D, Scharfenecker U, Schiltmeyer B, Koch B, Rudd D, Cawello W, Horstmann R. Lacosamide has a low potential for drug-drug interactions. Epilepsia. 2007;48(Suppl 5):562.
3. Kvemeland M, Taubull E, Molteberg E, Veierod MB, Selmer KK, Nakken KO, Iversen PO. Pharmacokinetic interaction between modified Atkins diet and antiepileptc drugs in adults with drug-resistant epilepsy. Epilepsia. 2019;60:2235–440.
4. Cawello W, Mueller-Voessing C, Fichtner A. Pharmacokinetics of omeprazole coadministration in healthy volunteers: results from a phase I randomized, crossover trial. Clin Drug Investig. 2014;34:317–25.
5. Cawello W, Rosenkranz B, Schmid B, Wierich W. Pharmacodynamic and pharmacokinetic evaluation of lacosamide and an oral contraceptive (levonorgestrel plus ethinylestradiol) in healthy female volunteers. Epilepsia. 2013;54:530–6.

P. N. Patsalos, *Antiseizure Medication Interactions*,
https://doi.org/10.1007/978-3-030-82790-8_47

Lamotrigine

Analgesics

Acetaminophen	Acetaminophen can decrease mean plasma lamotrigine AUC values by 20% and mean plasma lamotrigine levels by 25% [1]

Antimicrobials

Antituberculous Agents

Ethambutol	Ethambutol enhances the metabolism of lamotrigine and can increase plasma lamotrigine clearance threefold [2]
Isoniazid	Isoniazid inhibits the metabolism of lamotrigine and can decrease plasma lamotrigine clearance by 15% [2]
Rifampicin	Rifampicin enhances the metabolism of lamotrigine via an action on glucuronidation and can decrease mean plasma lamotrigine AUC values by 73% [3]

Antifungal Agents

Fluconazole	Fluconazole does not affect the pharmacokinetics of lamotrigine [4]

Antiviral Agents

Atazanavir	Atazanavir can enhance the metabolism of lamotrigine via an action on UGT1A4 and can decrease mean plasma lamotrigine AUC values by 12% and mean plasma lamotrigine half-life values by 9% [5]
Atazanavir/ritonavir	Atazanavir in combination with ritonavir can enhance the metabolism of lamotrigine via an action on UGT1A4 and can decrease mean plasma lamotrigine AUC values by 32% and mean plasma lamotrigine half-life values by 27% [5]

P. N. Patsalos, *Antiseizure Medication Interactions*,
https://doi.org/10.1007/978-3-030-82790-8_48

Lopinavir/ritonavir	Lopinavir combined with low dose ritonavir can enhance the metabolism of lamotrigine via an action on UGT1A4 and can decrease mean plasma lamotrigine levels by 55% [6]
Raltegravir	Raltegravir does not affect the pharmacokinetics of lamotrigine [7]
Ritonavir	Ritonavir can enhance the metabolism of lamotrigine via induction of UDP-glucuronyltransferases and can decrease plasma lamotrigine levels [5]

Antiulcer Drugs

Histamine H_2-Receptor Antagonists

Cimetidine	Cimetidine does not affect the pharmacokinetics of lamotrigine [3]

Psychotropic Drugs

Antidepressants

Paroxetine	Paroxetine does not affect the pharmacokinetics of lamotrigine [8]
Sertraline	Sertraline can increase plasma lamotrigine levels twofold. Inhibition of lamotrigine glucuronidation by sertraline has been proposed to explain this interaction [9]

Antipsychotics

Aripiprazole	Aripiprazole can decrease mean plasma lamotrigine Cmax and AUC values by 12% and 9%, respectively [10]
Clozapine	Clozapine does not affect the pharmacokinetics of lamotrigine [11]
Olanzapine	Olanzapine can decrease mean plasma lamotrigine Cmax and AUC values by 20% and 24%, respectively. Induction of lamotrigine glucuronidation by olanzapine has been proposed to explain this interaction [12]
Risperidone	Risperidone does not affect the pharmacokinetics of lamotrigine [11]

Steroids

Hormone replacement therapy	Hormone replacement therapy enhances the metabolism of lamotrigine and can decrease mean plasma lamotrigine levels [13]
Oral contraceptives	Oral contraceptives enhance the metabolism of lamotrigine and can decrease plasma lamotrigine levels by 40–65% [14]

Miscellanea

Atkins diet (modified)	The modified Atkins diet can decrease mean plasma lamotrigine levels by 12% [15]
Bupropion	Bupropion does not affect the pharmacokinetics of lamotrigine [16]

Cigarette use	Cigarette use does not affect the pharmacokinetics of lamotrigine [17]
Coffee	Coffee can decrease mean plasma AUC values either by inducing lamotrigine metabolism or decreasing absorption [17]
Ketogenic diet	The ketogenic diet can decrease plasma lamotrigine levels [18]
Orlistat	Orlistat can decrease plasma lamotrigine levels by reducing lamotrigine gastrointestinal absorption [19]
Transdermal patch contraception	Mean plasma lamotrigine levels are decreased [20]
Vaginal ring contraception	Mean plasma lamotrigine levels are decreased [20]

References

1. Gastrup S, Stage TB, Fruekilde PBN, Damker P. Paracetamol decreases steady-state lamotrigine by induction of glucuronidation in healthy subjects. Br J Clin Pharmacol. 2015;81:735–41.
2. Haan GJD, Edelbroek P, Bartels C. Changes in lamotrigine pharmacokinetics induced by anti-tubercular drugs. Epilepsia. 2010;51(Suppl 4):26.
3. Wimpelman J, Hovnik H, Riedel B, Slordal L. The interaction between rifampicin and lamotrigine: a case report. Br J Clin Pharmacol. 2019;85:1859–60.
4. Ulivelli M, Rubegni P, Nuti D, Bartalini S, Giannini S, Rossi S. Clinical evidence of fluconazole-induced carbamazepine toxicity. J Neurol. 2004;251:622–3.
5. Burger DM, Huisman A, van Ewijk N, Neisingh H, van Uden P, Rongen GA, Koopmans P, Bertz RJ. The effect of atazanavir and atazanavir/ritonavir on UDP-glucuronosyltransferase using lamotrigine as a phenotypic probe. Clin Pharmacol Ther. 2008;84:698–703.
6. Van der Lee MJ, Dawood L, ter Hofstede HJM, de Graaff-Teulen MJA, van Ewijk-Beneken-Kolmer EWJ, Caliskan-Yassen N, Koopmans PP, Burger DM. Lopinavir/ritonavir reduces lamotrigine plasma concentrations in healthy volunteers. Clin Pharmacol Ther. 2006;80:159–68.
7. van Luin M, Colbers A, Verwey-van Wissen CP, van Ewijk-Beneken-Kolmer EWJ, van der Kolk M, Hoitsam A, Gomesda Silva H, da Gomes SH, Burger DM. The effect of raltegravir on the glucuronidation of lamotrigine. J Clin Pharmacol. 2009;49:1220–7.
8. Normann C, Hummel B, Scharer LO, Horn M, Grunze H, Walden J. Lamotrigine as adjunctive to paroxetine in acute depression: a placebo-controlled, double-blind study. J Clin Psychiatry. 2002;63:337–44.
9. Kaufman KR, Gerner R. Lamotrigine toxicity secondary to sertraline. Seizure. 1998;7:163–5.
10. Schieber FC, Boulton DW, Balch AH, Croop R, Mallikaarjun S, Benson J, Carlson BX. A non-randomized study to investigate the effects of the atypical antipsychotic aripiprazole on the steady-state pharmacokinetics of lamotrigine in patients with bipolar I disorder. Hum Psychopharmacol. 2009;24:145–52.
11. Reimers A, Skogvoll E, Sund JK, Spiget O. Drug interaction between lamotrigine and psychoactive drugs: evidence from a therapeutic drug monitoring service. J Clin Psychopharmacol. 2005;25:342–8.
12. Sidhu J, Job S, Bullman J, Francis E, Abbott R, Asher J, Theis JGW. Pharmacokinetics and tolerability of lamotrigine and olanzapine coadministered to healthy subjects. Br J Clin Pharmacol. 2006;61:420–6.
13. Reimers A. Hormone replacement therapy with estrogen may reduce lamotrigine serum concentrations: a matched case-controlled study. Epilepsia. 2017;58:e6–9.

14. Sabers A, Ohman I, Christensen J, Tomson T. Oral contraceptives reduce lamotrigine plasma levels. Neurology. 2003;61:570–1.
15. Kvemeland M, Taubull E, Molteberg E, Veierod MB, Selmer KK, Nakken KO, Iversen PO. Pharmacokinetic interaction between modified Atkins diet and antiepileptc drugs in adults with drug-resistant epilepsy. Epilepsia. 2019;60:2235–440.
16. Odishaw J, Chen C. Effects of steady-state bupropion on the pharmacokinetics of lamotrigine in healthy subjects. Pharmacotherapy. 2000;20:1448–53.
17. Welty TE, Gidal BE, Privitera DJ, Berg M, Krebill R, Szaflarski J, Diaz FS. Coffee and cigarette smoking interaction with lamotrigine. Epilepsy Behav. 2021:116. In Press
18. Heo C, Kim SH, Chang MJ. Effect of the ketogenic diet and other dietary therapies on anti-epileptic drug comedication in patients with epilepsy. J Clin Pharm Ther. 2007;42:758–64.
19. Bigham S, McGuigan C, MacDonald BK. Reduced absorption of lipophilic anti-epileptic medications when used concomitantly with the anti-obesity drug orlistat. Epilepsia. 2006;47:2207.
20. King A, Bachman E, Macken M, Lee J, Gerard EE. Contraceptive vaginal ring reduces lamotrigine levels. Epilepsy Behav. 2020:111. In Press

Levetiracetam

Antacids	The antacids calcium carbonate and aluminum hydroxide do not affect the pharmacokinetics of levetiracetam [1]
Atkins diet (modified)	The modified Atkins diet does not affect plasma levetiracetam levels [2]
Digoxin	Digoxin does not affect the pharmacokinetics of levetiracetam [3]
Esmoprazole	Esmoprazole does not affect the pharmacokinetics of levetiracetam [4]
Ketogenic diet	The ketogenic diet can decrease plasma levetiracetam levels [5]
Meropenem	Meropenem does not affect the pharmacokinetics of levetiracetam [6]
Pantoprazole	Pantoprazole does not affect the pharmacokinetics of levetiracetam [4]
Probenecid	Probenecid does not affect the pharmacokinetics of levetiracetam. However, the plasma level of its primary non pharmacologically active metabolite, ucbLO59, increases 2.5-fold consequent to a 61% decrease in tubular excretion [7]
Oral contraceptives	Oral contraceptives do not affect the pharmacokinetics of levetiracetam [8]
Warfarin	Warfarin does not affect the pharmacokinetics of levetiracetam [9]

References

1. Patsalos PN. Clinical pharmacokinetics of levetiracetam. Clin Pharmacokinet. 2004;43:707–24.
2. Kvemeland M, Taubull E, Molteberg E, Veierod MB, Selmer KK, Nakken KO, Iversen PO. Pharmacokinetic interaction between modified Atkins diet and antiepileptc drugs in adults with drug-resistant epilepsy. Epilepsia. 2019;60:2235–440.
3. Levy RH, Ragueneau-Majlessi I, Baltes E. Repeated administration of the novel antiepileptic agent levetiracetam does not alter digoxin pharmacokinetics and pharmacodynamics in healthy volunteers. Epilepsy Res. 2001;46:93–9.
4. Pasupuleti B, Gone V, Baddam R, Venisetty RK, Prasad OP. Clinical impact of co-medications of levetiracetam and clobazam with proton pump inhibitors: a drug interaction study. Curr Drug Metab. 2020;21:126–31.

P. N. Patsalos, *Antiseizure Medication Interactions*,
https://doi.org/10.1007/978-3-030-82790-8_49

5. Heo C, Kim SH, Chang MJ. Effect of ketogenic diet and other dietery tharapies on anti-epileptic drug comedication in patients with epilepsy. J Clin Pharm Ther. 2017;42:758–64.
6. Mink S, Muroi C, Bjeljac M, Keller E. Levetiracetam compared to valproic acid: plasma concentration levels, adverse effects and interactions in aneurismal subarachnoid haemorrhage. Clin Neurol Neurosurg. 2011;113:644–8.
7. Patsalos PN. Pharmacokinetic profile of levetiracetam: toward ideal characteristics. Pharmacol Ther. 2000;85:77–85.
8. Sabers A, Christensen J. No effect of oral contraceptives on the metabolism of levetiracetam. Epilepsy Res. 2011;95:277–9.
9. Ragueneau-Majlessi I, Levy RH, Meyerhoff C. Lack of effect of repeated administration of levetiracetam on the pharmacodynamic and pharmacokinetic profiles of warfarin. Epilepsy Res. 2001;47:55–63.

Methsuximide

There have been no reports of the effect of non-ASM drugs on the pharmacokinetics or pharmacodynamics of methsuximide.

P. N. Patsalos, *Antiseizure Medication Interactions*,
https://doi.org/10.1007/978-3-030-82790-8_50

Oxcarbazepine

Atkins diet (modified)	The modified Atkins diet can decrease plasma 10-hydroxycarbazepine levels [1]
Cimetidine	Cimetidine does not affect the pharmacokinetics of oxcarbazepine [2]
Erythromycin	Erythromycin does not affect the pharmacokinetics of oxcarbazepine [3]
Propoxyphene (dextropropoxyphene)	Propoxyphene does not affect the pharmacokinetics of oxcarbazepine [4]
Rifampicin	Rifampicin can decrease plasma 10-hydroxycarbazepine levels by 19% [5]
Temozolomide	Temozolomide does not affect the pharmacokinetics of oxcarbazepine [6]
Verapamil	Verapamil can decrease mean plasma 10-hydroxycarbazepine AUC values by 20% [7]
Viloxazine	Viloxazine can increase mean plasma 10-hydroxycarbazepine levels by 11% [8]

References

1. Kvemeland M, Taubull E, Molteberg E, Veierod MB, Selmer KK, Nakken KO, Iversen PO. Pharmacokinetic interaction between modified Atkins diet and antiepileptc drugs in adults with drug-resistant epilepsy. Epilepsia. 2019;60:2235–440.
2. Keranen T, Jolkkonen J, Klosterskov-Jense P, Menge GP. Oxcarbazepine does not interact with cimetidine in healthy volunteers. Acta Neurol Scand. 1992;85:239–42.
3. Keranen T, Jolkkonen J, Jensen PK, Menge GP, Andersson P. Absence of interaction between oxcarbazepine and erythromycin. Acta Neurol Scand. 1992;86:120–3.
4. Mogensen PH, Jorgensen L, Boas J, Dam M, Vesterager A, Flesch G, Jensen PK. Effects of dextropropoxyphene on the steady-state kinetics of oxcarbazepine and its metabolites. Acta Neurol Scand. 1992;85:14–7.

P. N. Patsalos, *Antiseizure Medication Interactions*,
https://doi.org/10.1007/978-3-030-82790-8_51

5. Sigaroudi A, Kullak-Ublik GA, Weiler S. Concomitant administration of rifampicin and oxcarbazepine results in a significant decrease of the active MHD metabolite of oxcarbazepine. Eur J Pharmacol. 2016;72:377–8.
6. Maschio M, Albani F, Jandolo B, Zarabla A, Contin M, Dinapoli L, Fabi A, Pace A, Baruzzi A. Temozolomide treatment does not affect topiramate and oxcarbazepine plasma concentrations in chronically treated patients with brain tumor-related epilepsy. J Neuro-Oncol. 2008;90:217–21.
7. de Jesus AN, Wichert-Ana L, Coelho EB, Pasqua OD, Junior VA, Takayanagui OM, Tozatto E, Marques MP, Lanchote VL. Influence of verapamil on the pharmacokinetics of oxcarbazepine and of enantiomer of its 10-hydroxy metabolite in healthy volunteers. Eur J Clin Pharmcol. 2016;72:195–201.
8. Pisani F, Fazio A, Oteri G, Artesi C, Xiao B, Perucca E, Di Perri R. Effects of the antidepressant drug viloxazine on oxcarbazepine and its hydroxylated metabolites in patients with epilepsy. Acta Neurol Scand. 1994;90:130–2.

Perampanel

Ketoconazole	Ketoconazole can increase mean plasma perampanel AUC values [1]
Oral contraceptives (ethinylestradiol / levonorgestrel)	Oral contraceptives do not affect the pharmacokinetics of perampanel [2]
Warfarin	Warfarin does not affect the plasma protein binding of perampanel [3]

References

1. Gidal BE, Maganti R, Laurenza A, Yag H, Verbel DA, Schuck E, Ferry J. Effect of enzyme inhibition on perampanel pharmacokinetics: why study design matters. Epilepsy Res. 2017;134:41–8.
2. Patsalos PN. The clinical pharmacology profile of the new antiepileptic drug perampanel: a novel noncompetitive AMPA receptor antagonist. Epilepsia. 2015;56:12–27.
3. Gidal BE, Ferry J, Laurenza A, Ueno T. Potential protein-binding displacement interactions with perampanel: an in vitro analysis. Epilepsy Res. 2019;149:102–6.

P. N. Patsalos, *Antiseizure Medication Interactions*,
https://doi.org/10.1007/978-3-030-82790-8_52

Phenobarbital

BCNU (13-bis (2-chloroethyl)- 1 - nitrosourea)	BCNU does not affect the pharmacokinetics of phenobarbital [1]
Bleomycin	Bleomycin does not affect the pharmacokinetics of phenobarbital [2]
Chloramphenicol	Chloramphenicol inhibits the metabolism of phenobarbital and can increase plasma phenobarbital levels [3]
Cisplatin	Cisplatin does not affect the pharmacokinetics of phenobarbital [1]
Dicoumarol	Dicoumarol can decrease plasma phenobarbital levels [4]
Disulfiram	Disulfiram does not affect the pharmacokinetics of phenobarbital [5]
Ketogenic diet	The ketogenic diet can increase plasma phenobarbital levels [6]
Pindolol	Pindolol does not affect the pharmacokinetics of phenobarbital [7]
Propoxyphene (dextropropoxyphene)	Propoxyphene can increase plasma phenobarbital levels by 20% [8]
Teniposide	Teniposide does not affect the pharmacokinetics of phenobarbital [9]
Thioridazine	Thioridazine can decrease plasma phenobarbital levels [10]
Tipranavir/ritonavir	Tipranavir combined with ritonavir can enhance the metabolism of phenobarbital and can decrease plasma phenobarbital levels by 50% [11]
Troleandomycin	Troleandomycin can decrease plasma phenobarbital levels by 23% [12]
Vinblastine	Vinblastine does not affect the pharmacokinetics of phenobarbital [13]

P. N. Patsalos, *Antiseizure Medication Interactions*,
https://doi.org/10.1007/978-3-030-82790-8_53

References

1. Grossman SA, Sheidler VR, Gilbert MR. Decreased phenytoin levels in patients receiving chemotherapy. Am J Med. 1989;87:505–10.
2. Fincham RW, Schottelius DD. Decreased phenytoin levels in antineoplastic therapy. Ther Drug Monit. 1979;1:277–83.
3. Koup JR. Interaction of chloramphenicol with phenytoin and phenobarbital. A case report. Clin Pharmacol Ther. 1978;24:393–402.
4. Cucinell SA, Conney AH, Sansur MS, Burns JJ. Drug interactions in man. I. Lowering effect of phenobarbital on plasma levels of bishydroxycoumarin (Dicoumarol®) and diphenylhydantoin (Dilantin®). Clin Pharmacol Ther. 1965;6:420–9.
5. Olesen OV. The influence of disulfiram and calcium carbimide on the serum diphenylhydantoin. Excretion of HPPH in the urine. Arch Neurol. 1967;16:642–4.
6. Heo C, Kim SH, Chang MJ. Effect of ketogenic diet and other dietery tharapies on anti-epileptic drug comedication in patients with epilepsy. J Clin Pharm Ther. 207(42):758–64.
7. Greendyke RM, Gulya A. Effect of pindolol administration on serum levels of thioridazine, haloperidol, phenytoin, and phenobarbital. J Clin Psychiatry. 1988;49:105–7.
8. Hansen SB, Dam M, Brandt J, Hvidberg EF, Angelo H, Christensen MJ, Lous P. Influence of dextropropoxyphene on steady state serum levels and protein binding of three anti-epileptic drugs in man. Acta Neurol Scand. 1980;61:357–67.
9. Baker DK, Relling MV, Pui CH, Christensen ML, Evans WE, Rodman JH. Increased teniposide clearance with concomitant anticonvulsant therapy. J Clin Oncol. 1992;10:311–5.
10. Gay PE, Madsen JA. Interaction between phenobarbital and thioridazine. Neurology. 1983;33:1631–2.
11. Bonaro S, Calgagno A, Fontana S, D'Avolio A, Siccardi M, Gobbi F, Di Perri G. Clinically significant interaction between tipranavir ritonavir and phenobarbital in an HIV-infected patient. Clin Infect Dis. 2007;45:1654–5.
12. Dravet C, Mesdjian E, Cenraud B, Roger J. Interaction between carbamazepine and triacetyloleandomycin. Lancet. 1997;1:810–1.
13. Bollini P, Riva R, Albani F, Ida N, Cacciari L, Bollini C, Baruzzi A. Decreased phenytoin level during antineoplastic therapy: a case report. Epilepsia. 1983;24:75–8.

Phenytoin

Analgesics

Aspirin	Salicylic acid does not affect the pharmacokinetics of phenytoin [1]
Propoxyphene (dextropropoxyphene)	Propoxyphene can increase plasma phenytoin levels. This interaction is consistent with in vitro and clinical reports of inhibition of other CYP2C9 substrates by propoxyphene [2]
Fenyramidol	Fenyramidol inhibits the metabolism of phenytoin and can increase plasma phenytoin levels [3]
Ibuprofen	Ibuprofen does not affect the pharmacokinetics of phenytoin [4]
Paracetamol	Paracetamol does not affect the pharmacokinetics of phenytoin [1]
Phenylbutazone	The interaction between phenylbutazone and phenytoin is complex in that initially, plasma phenytoin levels can decrease (~20%), and then they increase. The mechanism of this interaction involves a concurrent plasma protein binding displacement interaction and an inhibition of phenytoin metabolism by phenylbutazone [1]
Tolfenamic acid	Tolfenamic acid does not affect the pharmacokinetics of phenytoin [1]

Antibacterials

Amoxicillin	Amoxicillin does not affect the pharmacokinetics of phenytoin [5]
Chloramphenicol	Chloramphenicol inhibits the metabolism of phenytoin and can increase plasma phenytoin levels by 177% [6]
Ciprofloxacin	Ciprofloxacin can decrease plasma phenytoin levels by 80% [7]
	There have been conflicting data on a possible interaction of ciprofloxacin with phenytoin, with no change, a decrease or an increase in plasma phenytoin level having all been reported [8]
Clarithromycin	Clarithromycin can increase mean plasma phenytoin levels by 82% [9]
Clinafloxacin	Clinafloxacin can decrease mean clearance values by 15% and increase mean plasma phenytoin AUC values by 20% [10]

P. N. Patsalos, *Antiseizure Medication Interactions*,
https://doi.org/10.1007/978-3-030-82790-8_54

Co-trimoxazole	Co-trimoxazole (a mixture of sulfamethoxazole and trimethoprim) inhibits the metabolism of phenytoin and can increase plasma phenytoin levels [5]
Erythromycin	Erythromycin does not affect the pharmacokinetics of phenytoin [11]
Isotretinoin	Isotretinoin does not affect the pharmacokinetics of phenytoin [12]
Metronidazole	There have been conflicting data on a possible interaction of metronidazole with phenytoin, with no change or an inhibition of phenytoin metabolism and a decrease in phenytoin clearance by 15% resulting in an increase in plasma phenytoin levels [13, 14]
Sulfadiazine	Sulfadiazine inhibits the metabolism of phenytoin and can decrease mean plasma phenytoin clearance values by 45% and increase mean plasma phenytoin half-life values by 80% [15]
Sulfadimethoxine	Sulfadimethoxine does not affect the pharmacokinetics of phenytoin [15]
Sulfamethizole	Sulfamethizole inhibits the metabolism of phenytoin and can decrease mean plasma phenytoin clearance values by 36% and increase mean plasma phenytoin half-life values by 66% [15]
Sulfaphenazole	Sulfaphenazole inhibits the metabolism of phenytoin and can decrease mean plasma phenytoin clearance values by 67% and increase mean plasma phenytoin half-life values by 237% [15]
Sulfamethoxazole	Sulfamethoxazole inhibits the metabolism of phenytoin and can increase mean plasma phenytoin half-life values but does not affect mean plasma phenytoin clearance values [15]
Sulfamethoxazole/trimethoprim	Sulfamethoxazole/trimethoprim in combination inhibits the metabolism of phenytoin and can decrease mean plasma phenytoin clearance values by 27% and increase mean plasma phenytoin half-life values by 39% [15]
Sulfamethoxydiazine	Sulfamethoxydiazine does not affect the pharmacokinetics of phenytoin [15]
Sulfamethoxypyridazine	Sulfamethoxypyridazine does not affect the pharmacokinetics of phenytoin [15]
Trimethoprim	Trimethoprim inhibits the metabolism of phenytoin and can increase mean phenytoin half-life values by 51% and decrease mean clearance values by 30% [15]
	Some of these sulfonamides concurrently displace phenytoin from plasma protein binding sites (primarily albumin), and therefore a measurement of total phenytoin level may underestimate the increase in the level of the free, pharmacologically active drug. In this setting, patient management may benefit from monitoring free phenytoin plasma levels [15]

Antifungal Agents

Fluconazole	Fluconazole inhibits phenytoin metabolism, via an action on CYP2C9 and CYP2C19, and can increase mean plasma phenytoin levels by 128% [16]
Itraconazole	Itraconazole can increase mean plasma phenytoin AUC values by 10% [17]
Ketoconazole	Ketoconazole does not affect the pharmacokinetics of phenytoin [18]
Miconazole	Miconazole can increase plasma phenytoin levels by 50–181% [19]

Posaconazole	Posaconazole inhibits phenytoin metabolism and can increase mean plasma phenytoin AUC values by 25% [20]
Voriconazole	Voriconazole inhibits the metabolism of phenytoin, via an action on CYP2C9 and CYP2C19, and can increase mean plasma phenytoin AUC values by 80% and mean plasma phenytoin levels by 70% [21]

Antineoplastic Agents

BCNU (13-bis (2-chloroethyl)-1-nitrosourea)	BCNU does not affect the pharmacokinetics of phenytoin [22]
Bleomycin	Bleomycin can significantly decrease plasma phenytoin levels, but this may be a consequence of antineoplastic damage to the intestinal mucosa and impaired phenytoin absorption. Only a mean 32% of a phenytoin dose is absorbed during combination therapy with cisplatin, vinblastine, and bleomycin [23]
Capecitabine	Capecitabine can increase plasma phenytoin levels [24, 25]
Carboplatin	Carboplatin can decrease plasma phenytoin levels by 50%. This interaction may be the consequence of enhanced hepatic metabolism or a displacement of phenytoin from its plasma protein binding sites [26]
Cisplatin	Cisplatin can decrease plasma phenytoin levels by up to 78%. Cisplatin possibly enhances the metabolism of phenytoin, although a change in volume of distribution could also be responsible for this interaction [22]
Doxifluridine	Doxifluridine inhibits the metabolism of phenytoin, probably via an action on CYP2C9, and can increase plasma phenytoin levels fourfold [27]
Erlotinib	Erlotinib can increase plasma phenytoin levels threefold [28]
5-Fluorouracil	5-Fluorouracil inhibits the metabolism of phenytoin, via an action on CYP2C9, and can increase plasma phenytoin levels [29]
Methotrexate	Methotrexate can decrease plasma phenytoin levels, but this may be a consequence of antineoplastic damage to the intestinal mucosa and impaired phenytoin absorption [30]
POMP-24	POMP-24 (a mixture of prednisone, vincristine, methotrexate, and 6-mercaptopurine) enhances the metabolism of phenytoin and can decrease plasma phenytoin levels by 72% [31]
Tamoxifen	Tamoxifen inhibits the metabolism of phenytoin, via an action on CYP2C9, and can increase plasma phenytoin levels by 44% [32]
Teniposide	Teniposide does not affect the pharmacokinetics of phenytoin [33]
UFT	UFT (a mixture of uracil and the 5-fluorouracil prodrug tegafur) inhibits the metabolism of phenytoin and can increase plasma phenytoin levels [34]
Vinblastine	Vinblastine can decrease plasma phenytoin levels by 39%. This interaction may be a consequence of antineoplastic damage to the intestinal mucosa and impaired phenytoin absorption [30]. During combination treatment with cisplatin, vinblastine, and bleomycin, as little as a mean 32% of a phenytoin dose is absorbed [23]

Antituberculous Agents

Isoniazid	Isoniazid inhibits the metabolism of phenytoin resulting in a threefold increase in plasma phenytoin levels. However, this interaction is only relevant in those patients that are "slow metabolizers (acetylators)" of isoniazid (which is genetically determined) and attain sufficiently high plasma isoniazid levels so as to inhibit the metabolism of phenytoin [35, 36]
Rifampicin	Rifampicin enhances the metabolism of phenytoin and can increase mean phenytoin clearance by up to 109% [37]
	When rifampicin and isoniazid are administered in combination, rifampicin counteracts the inhibiting effect of isoniazid on phenytoin metabolism [38]

Antiulcer Drugs

Antacids and Surface-Acting Drugs

Antacids	A significant reduction in phenytoin absorption can occur when phenytoin is co-ingested with calcium-containing and aluminum hydroxide-magnesium salt antacids. However, this has not been a consistent finding in all studies. Factors affecting the extent of interaction include antacid dose, administration times, motility of the gastrointestinal tract, and plasma phenytoin levels. To avoid this interaction, the administration of phenytoin and antacids should be separated by at least 2 h [38]
Sucralfate	Phenytoin bioavailability can be decreased by 20% by sucralfate, but the interaction is avoided when phenytoin is ingested at least 2 h before sucralfate ingestion [39]

Histamine H_2-Receptor Antagonists

Cimetidine	Cimetidine inhibits the metabolism of phenytoin, via an action on CYP2C19, and can increase mean plasma phenytoin AUC values by 20% [40]
Famotidine	Famotidine does not affect the pharmacokinetics of phenytoin [41]
Nizatidine	Nizatidine does not affect the pharmacokinetics of phenytoin [42]
Ranitidine	With the exception of an isolated case report where phenytoin plasma levels were increased by 50%, ranitidine has not been found to affect the pharmacokinetics of phenytoin [43, 44]

Proton Pump Inhibitors

Lansoprazole	Lansoprazole does not affect the pharmacokinetics of phenytoin [45]
Omeprazole	Omeprazole inhibits the metabolism of phenytoin, via an action on CYP2C19, and can increase mean plasma phenytoin AUC values by 25% [46]
Pantoprazole	Pantoprazole does not affect the pharmacokinetics of phenytoin [47]

Antiviral Agents

Acyclovir	Acyclovir can decrease plasma phenytoin levels by 71%. The exact mechanism of this interaction is not known but is considered to be an effect on gastrointestinal absorption [48]
Efavirenz	Efavirenz inhibits the metabolism of phenytoin, via an action on CYP2C9 and CYP2C19, and can increase plasma phenytoin levels [49]
Lopinavir/ritonavir	Lopinavir combined with ritonavir enhances the metabolism of phenytoin and can decrease mean plasma phenytoin AUC values by 31% [50]
Nelfinavir	Nelfinavir can decrease plasma phenytoin levels [51]
Nevirapine	Nevirapine enhances the metabolism of phenytoin and can decrease plasma phenytoin levels [52]
Ritonavir	Ritonavir inhibits the metabolism of phenytoin and can increase plasma phenytoin levels [53]
Zidovudine	Zidovudine does not affect the pharmacokinetics of phenytoin [9]

Cardiovascular Drugs

Antiarrhythmics

Amiodarone	Amiodarone inhibits the metabolism of phenytoin and can increase plasma phenytoin levels threefold [54, 55]

Antihypertensive Agents

Diazoxide	Diazoxide enhances the metabolism of phenytoin and can decrease plasma phenytoin levels to undetectable levels [56]
Diltiazem	Diltiazem can increase phenytoin plasma levels by 90% [57]
Losartan	Losartan does not affect the pharmacokinetics of phenytoin [58]
Nifedipine	Nifedipine can increase plasma phenytoin levels [59]
Pindolol	Pindolol does not affect the pharmacokinetics of phenytoin [60]
Verapamil	Verapamil can increase plasma phenytoin levels by 20% [61]

Antiplatelet Drugs

Ticlopidine	Ticlopidine inhibits the metabolism of phenytoin, probably via an action on CYP2C19, and can increase plasma phenytoin levels by 450% [62]

Digoxin

Digoxin	Digoxin does not affect the pharmacokinetics of phenytoin [62]

Lipid-Lowering Drugs

Cholestyramine	Cholestyramine does not affect the pharmacokinetics of phenytoin [63, 64]
Colestipol	Colestipol does not affect the pharmacokinetics of phenytoin [65]
Colesevelam	Colesevelam does not affect the pharmacokinetics of phenytoin [63]

Oral Anticoagulants

Dicoumarol	Dicoumarol can increase plasma phenytoin levels by up to 126% [66]
Phenindione	Phenindione does not affect the pharmacokinetics of phenytoin [67]
Warfarin	Warfarin does not affect the pharmacokinetics of phenytoin [67]

Herbal Remedies

Grapefruit juice (furanocoumarins)	Grapefruit juice does not affect the pharmacokinetics of phenytoin [68]
Noni juice	Noni juice can decrease plasma phenytoin levels, sometimes to undetectable concentrations [69]
Piperine	Piperine can inhibit the metabolism of phenytoin, probably via an action on CYP2C9 and/or CYP2C19, and increase mean plasma phenytoin levels by 22% and mean phenytoin AUC values by 17% [70]
Shankhapushpi (ayurvedic preparation)	Shankhapushpi can enhance the metabolism of phenytoin, probably via an action on CYP2C9 and/or CYP2C19, and decreases plasma phenytoin levels. Shankhapushpi also appears to lower seizure threshold [71]

Psychotropic Drugs

Antidepressants

Fluoxetine	Fluoxetine inhibits the metabolism of phenytoin, via an action on CYP2C9, and can increase plasma phenytoin levels by up to 309% [72]
Fluvoxamine	Fluvoxamine can increase plasma phenytoin levels by up to 200% [73]
Imipramine	Imipramine can increase plasma phenytoin levels by 68–100% [74]
Mirtazapine	Mirtazapine does not affect the pharmacokinetics of phenytoin [75]
Nefazodone	Nefazodone does not affect the pharmacokinetics of phenytoin [76]
Nortriptyline	Nortriptyline can increase plasma phenytoin levels [77]
Paroxetine	Paroxetine does not affect the pharmacokinetics of phenytoin [78]
Sertraline	Conflicting results have been reported. In one report, sertraline had no effect on the pharmacokinetics of phenytoin, while in another, sertraline was observed to inhibit the metabolism of phenytoin, via an action on CYP2C9, and to increase plasma phenytoin levels by 187% [79, 80]

Trazodone	Trazodone can increase plasma phenytoin levels by 158% [81]
Viloxazine	Viloxazine can increase mean plasma phenytoin levels by 37% [82]

Antipsychotics

Chlorpromazine	There have been conflicting data on a possible interaction of chlorpromazine with phenytoin, with no change, a decrease, or an increase in plasma phenytoin level having all been reported [77, 83, 84]
Loxapine	Loxapine can decrease plasma phenytoin levels [85]
Risperidone	Risperidone inhibits the metabolism of phenytoin, probably via an action on CYP2C9, and can increase plasma phenytoin levels [86]
Thioridazine	A variable effect is seen with an increase in plasma phenytoin levels and neurotoxicity in some patients, a decrease in plasma phenytoin levels in others, and with most patients experiencing no change in plasma phenytoin levels after the addition of thioridazine [87, 88]

Steroids

Dexamethasone	The effects of dexamethasone on the pharmacokinetics of phenytoin are conflicting, with both a decrease in plasma phenytoin levels (30–50%) and an increase in plasma phenytoin levels (38%) observed [89–91]
Danazol	The effects of danazol on the pharmacokinetics of phenytoin are conflicting with both an increase and a decrease in plasma phenytoin levels observed [92]

Miscellanea

Allopurinol	Allopurinol inhibits the metabolism of phenytoin and can increase mean plasma phenytoin AUC values by 50–120%, and mean plasma phenytoin levels can increase by 26–37% [93]
Atovaquone	Atovaquone does not affect t0macokinetics of phenytoin [94]
Azapropazone	Azapropazone inhibits the metabolism of phenytoin and can decrease phenytoin clearance by 35–59%, and can increase plasma phenytoin levels at least twfold [95]
Chlorphenamine (Chlorpheniramine)	Chlorphenamine inhibits phenytoin metabolism and can increase plasma phenytoin levels [96, 97]
Cola	Cola containing drinks can increase plasma phenytoin levels [98]
Diazepam	Data are conflicting with case reports and controlled studies reporting both increases and decreases in plasma phenytoin levels [83, 99]
Disulfiram	Disulfiram inhibits the metabolism of phenytoin and can increase mean plasma phenytoin half-life values by 73%, decrease mean plasma phenytoin clearance values by 66%, and increase plasma phenytoin levels by 100–400% [100, 101]
Flunarizine	Flunarizine does not affect the pharmacokinetics of phenytoin [102]
Methaqualone (Mandrax)	Methaqualone can increase plasma phenytoin levels [103]

Methylphenidate	The effects of methylphenidate on the pharmacokinetics of phenytoin are conflicting, with both an increase in plasma phenytoin levels and no effect observed [104–106]
Orlistat	Orlistat does not affect the pharmacokinetics of phenytoin [107]
Sulfinpyrazone	Sulfinpyrazone inhibits the metabolism of phenytoin and can increase plasma phenytoin levels by 100% [108]
Tacrolimus	Tacrolimus can increase plasma phenytoin levels by 97% [109]
Theophylline	Theophylline can decrease phenytoin plasma levels by 21%. The interaction may be attributable to diminished oral absorption [110]
Ticlopidine	Ticlopidine inhibits the metabolism of phenytoin and can increase plasma phenytoin levels [111]
Tolazamide	Tolazamide does not affect the pharmacokinetics of phenytoin [112]
Tolbutamide	Tolbutamide can cause a transient 45% increase in free nonprotein-bound plasma phenytoin levels and a 10% decrease in total phenytoin plasma levels [112, 113]
Zileuton	Zileuton does not affect the pharmacokinetics of phenytoin [114]

References

1. Neuvonen PJ, Lehtovaara R, Bardy A, Elomaa E. Antipyretic analgesics in patients on antiepileptic drug therapy. Eur J Clin Pharmacol. 1979;15:263–8.
2. Hansen SB, Dam M, Brandt J, Hvidberg EF, Angelo H, Christensen JM, Lous P. Influence of dextropropoxyphene on steady state serum levels and protein binding of three anti-epileptic drugs in man. Acta Neurol Scand. 1980;61:357–67.
3. Solomon HM, Schrogie JJ. The effect of phenyramidol on the metabolism of diphenylhydantoin. Clin Pharmacol Ther. 1967;8:554–6.
4. Bachmann KA, Schwartz JI, Forney RB, Jauregui L, Sullivan TJ. Inability of ibuprofen to alter single dose phenytoin disposition. Br J Clin Pharmacol. 1986;21:165–9.
5. Antoniou T, Gomes T, Mamdani MM, Juurlink DN. Trimethoprim/sulfamethoxazole-induced phenytoin toxicity in the elderly: a population-based study. Br J Clin Pharmacol. 2011;71:544–9.
6. Christensen LK, Skovsted L. Inhibition of drug metabolism by chloramphenicol. Lancet. 1969;1:1397–9.
7. Polak PT, Slayter KL. Hazards of doubling phenytoin dose in the face of an unrecognised interaction with ciprofloxacin. Ann Pharmacother. 1997;31:61–4.
8. Schroeder D, Frye J, Alldredge B, Messing R, Flaherty J. Effect of ciprofloxacin on serum phenytoin in epileptic patients. Pharmacotherapy. 1990;11:275.
9. Burger DM, Meenhorst PL, Mulder JW, Ktaaijeveld CL, Koks CHW, Bult A, Beijnen JH. Therapeutic drug monitoring in patients with acquired immunodeficiency syndrome. Ther Drug Monit. 1994;16:616–20.
10. Randinitis EJ, Alvey CW, Koup JR, Rausch G, Abel R, Bron NJ, Hounslow NJ, Vassos AB, Sedman AJ. Drug interactions with clinafloxacin. Antimicrob Agents Chemother. 2001;45:2543–52.
11. Milne RW, Coulthard K, Nation RL, Penna AC, Roberts G, Sansom LN. Lack of effect of erythromycin on the pharmacokinetics of single oral doses of phenytoin. Br J Clin Pharmacol. 1988;26:330–3.

12. Oo C, Barsanti F, Zhang R. Lack of effect of isotretinoin on the pharmacokinetics of phenytoin at steady-state. Pharm Res. 1997;14(Suppl 11):S–561.
13. Blyden GT, Scavoner JM, Greenblatt DJ. Metronidazole impairs clearance of phenytoin but not alprazolam or lorazepam. J Clin Pharmacol. 1988;28:240–5.
14. Jensen JC, Gugler R. Interaction between metronidazole and drugs eliminated by oxidative metabolism. Clin Pharmacol Ther. 1985;37:407–10.
15. Hansen JM, Kampmann JP, Siersbaek-Nielsen K, Lumholtz IB, Arroe M, Abildgaard U, Skovsted L. The effect of different sulfonamides on phenytoin metabolism in man. Acta Med Scand. 1979;624(Suppl):106–10.
16. Blum RA, Wilton JH, Hilligoss DM, Gardner MJ, Henry EB, Harrison NJ, Schentag JJ. Effect of fluconazole on the disposition of phenytoin. Clin Pharmacol Ther. 1991;49:420–5.
17. Ducharme MP, Slaughter RL, Warbasse LH, Chandrasekar PH, Van de Velde V, Mannens G, Edwards DJ. Itraconazole and hydroxyitraconazole serum concentrations are reduced more than 10-fold by phenytoin. Clin Pharmacol Ther. 1995;58:617–24.
18. Touchette MA, Chandrasekar PH, Milad MA, Edwards DJ. Contrasting effects of fluconazole and ketoconazole on phenytoin and testosterone disposition. Br J Clin Pharmacol. 1992;34:75–8.
19. Rolan PE, Somogyi AA, Drew MJR, Cobain WG, South D, Bochner F. Phenytoin intoxication during treatment with parenteral miconazole. Br Med J. 1983;287:1760.
20. Krishna G, Sansone-Parsons A, Kantesaria B. Drug interaction assessment following concomitant administration of posaconazole and phenytoin in healthy men. Curr Med Res Opin. 2007;23:1415–22.
21. Purkins L, Wood N, Ghahramani P, Love ER, Eve MD, Fielding A. Coadministration of voriconazole and phenytoin: pharmacokinetic interaction, safety, and tolerance. Br J Clin Pharmacol. 2003;56:37–44.
22. Grossman SA, Sheidler VR, Gilbert MR. Decreased phenytoin levels in patients receiving chemotherapy. Am J Med. 1989;87:505–10.
23. Sylvester RK, Lewis FB, Caldwell KC, Lobell M, Perri R, Sawchuk RA. Impaired phenytoin bioavailability secondary to cisplatinum, vinblastine, and bleomycin. Ther Drug Monit. 1984;6:302–5.
24. Sakurai M, Kawahara K, Ueda R, Fukui E, Yamada R. A case of toxicity caused by drug interaction between capecitabine and phenytoin in patient with colorectal cancer. Gan To Kagaku Ryoho. 2011;38:841–3.
25. McGrath C, Munro A, Goel R, Linden K, Dennis K. Phenytoin toxicity during neoadjuvant concurrent capecitabine and radiation therapy and rectal adenocarcinoma: Case report of a drug interaction. Cureus. 2018;10:e3625.
26. Dofferhoff AS, Berenden HH, Naalt J, Haaxma-Reiche H, Smit EF, Postmus PE. Decreased phenytoin level after carboplatin treatment. Am J Med. 1990;89:247–9.
27. Konishi H, Morita K, Minouchi T, Nakajima M, Matsuda M, Yamaji A. Probable metabolic interaction of doxifluridine with phenytoin. Ann Pharmacother. 2002;36:831–4.
28. Ohgami M, Kaburagi T, Kurosawa A, Homma M. Drug interaction between erlotinib and phenytoin for brain metastases in a patient with nonsmall cell lung cancer. Lung Cancer. 2016;101:9–10.
29. Gunes A, Coskun U, Boruban C, Gunel N, Babaoglu MO, Sencan O, Bozkurt A, Rane A, Hassan M, Zengil H, Yasar U. Inhibitory effect of 5-fluorouracil on cytochrome P450 2C9 activity in cancer patients. Basic Clin Pharmacol Toxicol. 2006;98:197–200.
30. Bollini P, Riva R, Albani F, Ida N, Cacciari L, Bollini C, Baruzzi A. Decreased phenytoin level during antineoplastic therapy: a case report. Epilepsia. 1983;24:75–8.
31. Jarosinski PF, Moscow JA, Alexander MS, Lesko LJ, Balis FM, Poplack DG. Altered phenytoin clearance during intensive chemotherapy for acute lymphoblastic leukemia. J Pediatr. 1988;112:996–9.
32. Boruban MC, Yasar U, Babaoglu MO, Sencan O, Bozkurt A. Tamoxifen inhibits cytochrome P450 2C9 activity in breast cancer patients. J Chemother. 2006;18:421–4.

33. Baker DK, Relling MV, Pui CH, Christensen ML, Evans WE, Rodman JH. Increased teniposide clearance with concomitant anticonvulsant therapy. J Clin Oncol. 1992;10:311–5.
34. Wakisaka S, Shimauchi M, Kaji Y, Nonaka A, Kinoshita K. Acute phenytoin intoxication associated with the antineoplastic agent UFT. Fukuoka Igaky Zasshi. 1990;81:192–6.
35. Chapron DJ, Blum MR, Kramer PA. Evidence of trimodal pattern of acetylation of isoniazid in uremic patients. J Pharm Sci. 1978;67:1018–9.
36. Miller RR, Porter J, Greenblatt DJ. Clinical importance of the interaction of phenytoin and isoniazid. Chest. 1979;75:356–8.
37. Kay L, Kampmann JP, Svendsen TL, Vergman B, Hansen JEM, Skovsted L, Kristensen M. Influence of rifampicin and isoniazid on the kinetics of phenytoin. Br J Clin Pharmacol. 1985;20:323–6.
38. Carter BL, Garnett WR, Pellock JM. Effects of antacids on phenytoin bioavailability. Ther Drug Monit. 1981;3:333–40.
39. Smart HL, Somerville KW, Williams J, Richens A, Langman MJS. The effects of sucralfate upon phenytoin absorption in man. Br J Clin Pharmacol. 1985;20:238–40.
40. Frigo GM, Lecchini S, Caravaggi M, Gatti G, Tonini M, D'Angelo L, Perucca E, Crema A. Reduction in phenytoin clearance caused by cimetidine. Eur J Clin Pharmacol. 1983;25:135–7.
41. Sambol NC, Upton RA, Chremos AN, Lin ET, Williams RA. A comparison of the influence of famotidine and cimetidine on phenytoin elimination and hepatic blood flow. Br J Clin Pharmacol. 1989;27:83–7.
42. Bachmann KA, Sullivan TJ, Jauregui L, Reese JH, Miller K, Levine L. Absence of an inhibitory effect of omeprazole and nizatidine on phenytoin disposition. A marker of CYP2C activity. Br J Clin Pharmacol. 1993;36:380–2.
43. Watts RW, Hetzel DL, Bochner F, Hallpike JF, Hann CS, et al. Lack of interaction between ranitidine and phenytoin. Br J Clin Pharmacol. 1983;15:499–500.
44. Bramhall D, Levine M. Possible interaction of ranitidine with phenytoin. Drug Intell Clin Pharm. 1988;22:979–80.
45. Karol MD, Locke CS, Cavanaugh JH. Lack of pharmacokinetic interaction between lansoprazole and intravenously administered phenytoin. J Clin Pharmacol. 1999;39:1283–9.
46. Prichard PJ, Walt RP, Kitchingman GK, Somerville KW, Langman MJS, Williams J, Richens A. Oral phenytoin pharmacokinetics during omeprazole therapy. Br J Clin Pharmacol. 1987;24:543–5.
47. Middle MV, Muller FO, Schall R, Groenewoud G, Hundt HK, Huber R, Bliesath H, Steinijans VW. No influence of pantoprazole on the pharmacokinetics of phenytoin. Int J Clin Pharmacol Ther. 1996;33:304–7.
48. Parmeggiani A, Riva R, Posar A, Rossi PG. Possible interaction between acyclovir and antiepileptic treatment. Ther Drug Monit. 1995;17:312–5.
49. Robertson SM, Penzak SR, Lane J, Pau AK, Mican JM. A potential significant interaction between efavirenz and phenytoin: a case report and review of the literature. Clin Infect Dis. 2005;41:e15–8.
50. Lim ML, Min SS, Eron JJ, Bertz RJ, Robinson M, Gaedigk A, Kashuba AD. Coadministration of lopinavir/ritonavir and phenytoin results in two-way drug interaction through cytochrome P-450 induction. J Acquir Immune Defic Syndr. 2004;36:1034–40.
51. Honda M, Yassuoka A, Aoki M, Oka S. A generalized seizure following initiation of nelfinavir in a patient with human immunodeficiency virus type 1 infection, suspected due to interaction between nelfinavir and phenytoin. Intern Med. 1999;38:302–3.
52. Dasgupta A, Okhuysen PC. Pharmacokinetic and other interactions in patients with AIDS. Ther Drug Monit. 2001;23:591–605.
53. Broderick A, Webb DW, McMenamin J, Butler K. A novel use of ritonavir. AIDS. 1998;12(Suppl 4):S29.
54. Gore JM, Haffajee CI, Alpert JS. Interaction of amiodarone and diphenylhydantoin. Am J Cardiol. 1984;54:1145.

55. McGovern B, Geer VR, LaRaie PJ, Garan H, Ruskin JN. Possible interaction between amiodarone and phenytoin. Ann Intern Med. 1984;101:650–1.
56. Roe TF, Podosin RL, Blaskovics ME. Drug interaction: diazoxide and diphenylhydantoin. J Pediatr. 1975;87:480–4.
57. Bahls FH, Ozuna J, Ritchie DE. Interactions between calcium channel blockers and the anticonvulsants carbamazepine and phenytoin. Neurology. 1991;41:740–2.
58. Fischer TL, Pieper JA, Graff DW, Rodgers JE, Fischer JD, Parnell KJ, Goldstein JA, Greenwood R, Patterson JH. Evaluation of potential losartan-phenytoin drug interactions in healthy volunteers. Clin Pharmacol Ther. 2002;72:238–46.
59. Ahmad S. Nifedipine-phenytoin interaction. J Am Coll Cardiol. 1984;3:1582.
60. Greendyke RM, Gulya A. Effect of pindolol administration on serum levels of thioridazine, haloperidol, phenytoin, and phenobarbital. J Clin Psychiatry. 1988;49:105–7.
61. Macphee GA, McInnes GT, Thompson GG, Brodie MJ. Verapamil potentiates carbamazepine neurotoxicity: a clinically important inhibitory interaction. Lancet. 1986;1:700–3.
62. Rameis H. On the interaction between phenytoin and digoxin. Eur J Clin Pharmacol. 1985;29:49–53.
63. Callaghan JT, Tsuru M, Holtzman JL, Hunninghaka DB. Effect of cholestyramine and colestipol on the absorption of phenytoin. Eur J Clin Pharmacol. 1983;24:675–8.
64. Barzaghi N, Monteleone M, Amione C, Lecchini S, Perucca E, Frigo GM. Lack of effect of cholestyramine on phenytoin bioavailability. J Clin Pharmacol. 1988;28:1112–4.
65. He L, Wickremasingha P, Lee J, Tao B, Mendell-Harary J, Walker J, Wight D. Lack of effect of colesevelam HCl on the single-dose pharmacokinetics of aspirin, atenolol, enalapril, phenytoin, rosiglitazone, and sitagliptin. Diabetes Res Clin Pract. 2014;104:401–9.
66. Hansen JM, Kristensen M, Skovsted L, Christensen LK. Dicoumarol-induced diphenylhydantoin intoxication. Lancet. 1966;2:265–6.
67. Skovsted L, Kristensen M, Molholm Hansen J, Siersbaek-Nielsen K. The effect of different oral anticoagulants on diphenylhydantoin (DPH) and tolbutamide metabolism. Acta Med Scand. 1976;199:513–5.
68. Kumar N, Garg SK, Prabhakar S. Lack of pharmacokinetic interaction between grapefruit juice and phenytoin in healthy male volunteers and epileptic patients. Methods Find Exp Clin Pharmacol. 1999;21:629–32.
69. Kang YC, Chen MH, Lai SL. Potentially unsafe herb-drug interactions between a commercial product of noni juice and phenytoin-A case report. Acta Neurol Taiwanica. 2015;24:43 6.
70. Pattanaik S, Hota D, Prabhakar S, Kharbanda P, Pandhi P. Effect of piperine on the steady-state pharmacokinetics of phenytoin in patients with epilepsy. Phytother Res. 2006;20:683–6.
71. Dandekar UP, Chandra RS, Dalvi SS, Joshi MV, Gokhale PC, Sharma AV, Shah PU, Kshirsagar NA. Analysis of a clinically important interaction between phenytoin and shankhapushpi, an ayurvedic preparation. J Ethnopharmacol. 1992;35:285–8.
72. Perucca E, Richens A. Interaction between phenytoin and imipramine. Br J Clin Pharmacol. 1977;4:485–6.
73. Jalil P. Toxic reaction following the combined administration of fluoxetine and phenytoin: two case reports. J Neurol Neurosurg Psychiatry. 1992;55:412–3.
74. Mamiya K, Kojima K, Yukawa E, Higuchi S, Ieiri I, Ninomiya H, Tashiro N. Phenytoin intoxication induced by fluvoxamine. Ther Drug Monit. 2001;23:75–7.
75. Spaans E, van den Heuvel MW, Schnabel PG, Peeters PAM, Chin-Kon-Sung UG, Colbers EPH, Sitsen JMA. Concomitant use of mirtazapine and phenytoin: a drug-drug interaction study in healthy male subjects. Eur J Clin Pharmacol. 2002;58:423–9.
76. Marino MR, Langenbacher KM, Hammett JL, Nichola P, Uderman HD. The effect of nefazodone on the single-dose pharmacokinetics of phenytoin in healthy male subjects. J Clin Psychopharmacol. 1977;17:27–33.
77. Houghton GW, Richens A. Inhibition of phenytoin metabolism by other drugs used in epilepsy. Int J Clin Pharmacol Biopharm. 1975;12:210–6.

78. Andersen BB, Mikkelsen M, Vesterager A, Dam M, Kristensen HB, Pedersen B, Lund J, Mengel H. No influence of the antidepressant paroxetine on carbamazepine, valproate and phenytoin. Epilepsy Res. 1991;10:201–4.
79. Haselberger MB, Freedman LS, Tolbert S. Elevated serum phenytoin concentrations associated with coadministration of sertraline. J Clin Psychopharmacol. 1997;17:107–9.
80. Repeport WG, Muirhead DC, Williams SA, Cross M, Wesnes K. Absence of effect of sertraline on the pharmacokinetics and pharmacodynamics of phenytoin. J Clin Psychiatry. 1996;57(Suppl 1):24–8.
81. Dorn JM. A case of phenytoin toxicity possibly precipitated by trazodone. J Clin Psychiatry. 1986;47:89–90.
82. Pisani F, Fazio A, Artesi C, Russo M, Trio R, Oteri G, Perucca E, Di Perri R. Elevation of plasma phenytoin by viloxazine in epileptic patients: a clinically significant interaction. J Neurol Neurosurg Psychiatry. 1992;55:126–7.
83. Siris JH, Pippenger CE, Werner WL, Masland RL. Anticonvulsant drug-serum levels in psychiatric patients with seizure disorders. Effects of certain psychotropic drugs. N Y State J Med. 1974;74:1554–6.
84. Kutt H, McDowell F. Management of epilepsy with diphenylhydantoin sodium. Dosage regulation for problem patients. J Am Med Assoc. 1968;203:969–72.
85. Ryan GM, Matthews PA. Phenytoin metabolism stimulated by loxapine. Drug Intell Clin Pharm. 1977;11:428.
86. Sanderson DR. Drug interaction between risperidone and phenytoin resulting in extrapyramidal symptoms. J Clin Psychiatry. 1996;57:177.
87. Vincent FM. Phenothiazine-induced phenytoin intoxication. Ann Intern Med. 1980;93:56–7.
88. Sands CD, Robinson JD, Salem RB, Stewart RB, Muniz C. Effect of thioridazine on phenytoin serum concentration: a retrospective study. Drug Intell Clin Pharm. 1987;21:267–72.
89. Lawson LA, Blouin RA, Smith RB, Rapp RP, Young AB. Phenytoin dexamethasone interaction: a previously unreported observation. Surg Neurol. 1981;16:23–4.
90. Lackner TE. Interaction of dexamethasone with phenytoin. Pharmacotherapy. 1991;11:344–7.
91. Recuenco I, Espinosa E, Garcia B, Carcas A. Effect of dexamethasone on the decrease of serum phenytoin concentrations. Ann Pharmacother. 1995;29:935.
92. Zielinski JJ, Lichten EM, Haidukewych D. Clinically significant danazol-carbamazepine interaction. Ther Drug Monit. 1987;9:24–7.
93. Ogiso T, Ito Y, Iwaki M, Tsunekawa K. Drug interaction between phenytoin and allopurinol. J Pharmacobiodyn. 1990;13:36–43.
94. Davis JD, Dixon R, Khan AZ, Toon S, Rolan PE, Posner J. Atovaquone has no effect on the pharmacokinetics of phenytoin in healthy male volunteers. Br J Clin Pharmacol. 1996;42:246–8.
95. Geaney DP, Carver JG, Davies CL, Aronson JK. Pharmacokinetic investigation of the interaction of azapropazone with phenytoin. Br J Clin Pharmacol. 1983;15:727–34.
96. Ahmad S, Laidlaw J, Houghton GW, Richens A. Involuntary movements caused by phenytoin intoxication in epileptic patients. J Neurol Neurosurg Psychiatry. 1975;38:225–31.
97. Pugh RNH, Geddes AM, Yeoman WB. Interaction of phenytoin with chlorpheniramine. Br J Clin Pharmacol. 1975;2:173–5.
98. Norman H, Maghadam AT, Emami SA, Mohammadpour AH, Johnston TP, Sahebkar A. Drug interactions of cola-containing drinks. Clin Nutr. 2019;38:2545–51.
99. Murphy A, Wilbur K. Phenytoin-diazepam interaction. Ann Pharmacother. 2003;37:559–63.
100. Olesen OV. The influence of disulfiram and calcium carbimide on the serum diphenylhydantoin. Excretion of HPPH in the urine. Arch Neurol. 1967;16:642–4.
101. Svedsen TL, Kristensen M, Hansen JM, Skovsted L. The influence of disulfiram on the half-life and metabolic clearance of diphenylhydantoin and tolbutamide in man. Eur J Clin Pharmacol. 1976;9:439–41.

102. Kapetanovic IM, Torchin CD, Kupferberg HJ, Treiman DM, Di Giorgio C, Barber K, Norton L, Lau M, Whitley L, Cereghino JJ. Pharmacokinetic profile of flunarizine after single and multiple dosing in epileptic patients receiving co-medication. Epilepsia. 1988;29:770–4.
103. Verma R, Tiwari N. Phenytoin intoxication induced by Mandrax (methaqualone). Epilepsy Res. 2012;98:281–2.
104. Garrettson LK, Perel JM, Dayton PG. Methylphenidate interaction with both anticonvulsants and ethyl biscoumacetate. J Am Med Assoc. 1969;207:2053–6.
105. Mirkin BL, Wright F. Drug interactions: effect of methylphenidate on the disposition of diphenylhydantoin in man. Neurology. 1971;21:1123–8.
106. Kupferberg HJ, Jeffery W, Hunninghake DB. Effect of methylphenidate on plasma anticonvulsant levels. Clin Pharmacol Ther. 1972;13:201–4.
107. Melia AT, Mulligan TE, Zhi J. The effect of orlistat on the pharmacokinetics of phenytoin in healthy volunteers. J Clin Pharmacol. 1996;36:654–8.
108. Pedersen AK, Jacobsen P, Kampmann JP, Hansen JM. Clinical pharmacokinetics and potentially important drug interactions of sulphinpyrazone. Clin Pharmacokinet. 1982;7:42–56.
109. Thompson PA, Mosley CA. Tacrolimus-phenytoin interaction. Ann Pharmacother. 1996;30:544.
110. Taylor JW, Hendeles L, Weinberger M, Lyon LW, Wyatt R, Riegelman S. The interaction of phenytoin and theophylline. Drug Intell Clin Pharm. 1980;14:638.
111. Wesseling H, Mols-Thurkow I. Interaction of diphenylhydantoin (DPH) and tolbutamide in man. Eur J Clin Pharmacol. 1975;8:75–8.
112. Kutt H. Interactions between anticonvulsants and other commonly prescribed drugs. Epilepsia. 1984;25(Suppl 2):S118–31.
113. Samara E, Cavanaugh JH, Mukherjee D, Granneman GR. Lack of pharmacokinetic interaction between zileuton and phenytoin in humans. Clin Pharmacokinet. 1995;29(Suppl 2):84–91.
114. Privatera M, Welty TE. Acute phenytoin toxicity followed by seizure breakthrough from a ticlopidine-phenytoin interaction. Acta Neurol. 1996;53:1191–2.

Piracetam

Alcohol	Alcohol does not affect the pharmacokinetics of piracetam [1]

Reference

1. Summary of Product Characteristics: Piracetam (Nootropil). UCB Pharma Ltd. Last update 9th February 2017.

P. N. Patsalos, *Antiseizure Medication Interactions*,
https://doi.org/10.1007/978-3-030-82790-8_55

Pregabalin

Furosemide	Furosemide does not affect the pharmacokinetics of pregabalin [1]
Glibenclamide (glyburide)	Glibenclamide does not affect the pharmacokinetics of pregabalin [1]
Glimepiride	Glimepiride does not affect the pharmacokinetics of pregabalin [1]
Glipizide	Glipizide does not affect the pharmacokinetics of pregabalin [1]
Insulin	Insulin does not affect the pharmacokinetics of pregabalin [1]
Metformin	Metformin does not affect the pharmacokinetics of pregabalin [1]
Oral contraceptives	Oral contraceptives do not affect the pharmacokinetics of pregabalin [2]
Thioctic acid	Thioctic acid does not affect the pharmacokinetics of pregabalin [3]
Tramadol	Tramadol can increase mean plasma pregabalin AUC values by 8% [4]

References

1. Janiczek-Dolphin N, Corrigan BW, Bockbrader HN. Diuretics, oral hypoglycaemic agents and insulin do not alter pregabalin pharmacokinetics. Epilepsia. 2005;46(Suppl 6):115.
2. Bochbrader H, Miller R, Frame B, Lalonde R, Spiegel K, Barrett J. The concomitant use of pregabalin and oral contraceptives does not affect the efficacy of either agent. Epilepsia. 2005;46(Suppl 8):170–1.
3. Rhee SJ, Lee H, Ahn LY, Lim KS, Yu KS. Lack of clinically significant pharmscokinetic intersction between pregabalin and thioctic acid in healthy volunteers. Clin Ther. 2018;40:1720–8e2.
4. Lee S, Kim Y, Sung Lee JJI, Im G, Cho JY, Chung JY, Yoon S. A pharmacokinetic drug-drug interaction study between pregabalin and tramadol in healthy volunteers. Eur J Clin Pharmacol. 2018;74:1605–13.

P. N. Patsalos, *Antiseizure Medication Interactions*,
https://doi.org/10.1007/978-3-030-82790-8_56

Primidone

Bleomycin	Bleomycin does not affect the pharmacokinetics of primidone [1]
Danazol	Danazol does not affect the pharmacokinetics of primidone [2]
Isomazid	Isoniazid inhibits the metabolism of primidone and can increase plasma primidone levels by 83% and decrease plasma phenobarbital levels by 12% [3]
Nicotinamide	Nicotinamide inhibits the metabolism of primidone to phenobarbital and can increase the plasma primidone/phenobarbital ratio [4]
Special note	As primidone is metabolized to phenobarbital, all the interactions highlighted for phenobarbital will also apply to primidone

References

1. Fincham RW, Schottelius DD. Decreased phenytoin levels in antineoplastic therapy. Ther Drug Monit. 1979;1:277–83.
2. Zielinski JJ, Lichten EM, Haidukewych D. Clinically significant danazol-carbamazepine interaction. Ther Drug Monit. 1987;9:24–7.
3. Sutton G, Kupferberg HJ. Isoniazid as an inhibitor of primidone metabolism. Neurology. 1975;25:1179–81.
4. Bourgeois BFD, Dodson WE, Ferrendelli JA. Interactions between primidone, carbamazepine, and nicotinamide. Neurology. 1982;32:1122–6.

P. N. Patsalos, *Antiseizure Medication Interactions*,
https://doi.org/10.1007/978-3-030-82790-8_57

Rufinamide

There have been no reports of the effect of non-ASM drugs on the pharmacokinetics or pharmacodynamics of rufinamide.

P. N. Patsalos, *Antiseizure Medication Interactions*,
https://doi.org/10.1007/978-3-030-82790-8_58

Stiripentol

There have been no reports of the effect of non-ASM drugs on the pharmacokinetics or pharmacodynamics of stiripentol.

P. N. Patsalos, *Antiseizure Medication Interactions*,
https://doi.org/10.1007/978-3-030-82790-8_59

Sulthiame

Antacids	Antacids containing magnesium trisilicate can decrease the oral bioavailability of sulthiame by up to 73%, while antacids containing bismuth oxycarbonate and magnesium oxide can decrease the oral bioavailability of sulthiame by <15%. To avoid problems, administration of sulthiame and antacids should be separated by at least 2 h [1]

Reference

1. Naggar VF, Khalil SA. The in vitro adsorption of some antiepileptics on antacids. Pharmazie. 1978;33:593–5.

P. N. Patsalos, *Antiseizure Medication Interactions*, https://doi.org/10.1007/978-3-030-82790-8_60

Tiagabine

Cimetidine	Cimetidine can increase mean plasma tiagabine AUC values and mean plasma tiagabine levels by 5% [1]
Digoxin	Digoxin does not affect the pharmacokinetics of tiagabine [2]
Erythromycin	Erythromycin does not affect the pharmacokinetics of tiagabine [3]
Gemfibrozil	Gemfibrozil can increase mean plasma tiagabine levels by 59–75% [4]
Theophylline	Theophylline does not affect the pharmacokinetics of tiagabine [1]
Triazolam	Triazolam does not affect the pharmacokinetics of tiagabine [5]
Warfarin	Warfarin does not affect the pharmacokinetics of tiagabine [1]

References

1. Mengel H, Jansen JA, Sommerville K, Jonkman JHG, Wesnes K, Cohen A, Carlson GF, Marshal LR, Snel S, Dirach J, Kastberg H. Tiagabine: evaluation of the risk of interaction with theophylline, warfarin, digoxin, cimetidine, oral contraceptives, triazolam, or ethanol. Epilepsia. 1995;36(Suppl 3):S160.
2. Snel S, Jansen JA, Pedersen PC, Jonkman JH, van Heiningen PN. Tiagabine, a novel antiepileptic agent: lack of pharmacokinetic interaction with digoxin. Eur J Clin Pharmacol. 1998;54:355–7.
3. Thomsen MS, Groes L, Agerso H, Kruse T. Lack of pharmacokinetic interaction between tiagabine and erythromycin. J Clin Pharmacol. 1998;38:1051–6.
4. Burstein AH, Boudreau EA, Theodore WH. Increase in tiagabine serum concentration with coadministration of gemfibrozil. Ann Pharmacother. 2009;43:379–82.
5. Richens A, Marshall RW, Dirach J, Jansen JA, Snel P, Pedersen PC. Absence of interaction between tiagabine, a new antiepileptic drug, and the benzodiazepine triazolam. Drug Metabol Drug Interact. 1998;14:159–77.

P. N. Patsalos, *Antiseizure Medication Interactions*,
https://doi.org/10.1007/978-3-030-82790-8_61

Topiramate

Amitriptyline	Amitriptyline can decrease the plasma clearance of topiramate [1]
Atkins diet (modified)	The modified Atkins diet can decrease mean plasma topiramate levels by 16% [2].
Dihydroergotamine	Dihydroergotamine does not affect the pharmacokinetics of topiramate [1]
Diltiazem	Diltiazem can increase mean plasma topiramate AUC values by 20% [3]
Flunarizine	Flunarizine does not affect the pharmacokinetics of topiramate [3]
Glibenclamide (glyburide)	Glibenclamide does not affect the pharmacokinetics of topiramate [4]
Hydrochlorothiazide	Hydrochlorothiazide can increase mean plasma topiramate Cmax values by 27% and mean plasma topiramate AUC values by 29% [3]
Ketogenic diet	The ketogenic diet can decrease mean plasma topiramate levels [5]
Lithium	Lithium can decrease the clearance of topiramate [1]
Metformin	Metformin can decrease the mean plasma clearance of topiramate by 35% and increase mean plasma topiramate AUC values by 53% [6]
Pioglitazone	Pioglitazone does not affect the pharmacokinetics of topiramate [6]
Pizotifen	Pizotifen does not affect the pharmacokinetics of topiramate [3]
Posaconazole	Posaconazole inhibits topiramate metabolism, probably via an action on CYP3A4, and can increase plasma topiramate levels by 137% [7]
Propranolol	Propranolol can decrease mean plasma topiramate clearance values by 14% and increase mean plasma topiramate AUC values by 17% [1]

P. N. Patsalos, *Antiseizure Medication Interactions*,
https://doi.org/10.1007/978-3-030-82790-8_62

Sumatriptan	Sumatriptan can decrease the plasma clearance of topiramate [1]
Temozolomide	Temozolomide does not affect the pharmacokinetics of topiramate [8]
Venlafaxine	Venlafaxine does not affect the pharmacokinetics of topiramate [1]

References

1. Bialer M, Doose DR, Murthy B, Curtin C, Wang SS, Twyman RE, Schwabe S. Pharmacokinetic interactions of topiramate. Clin Pharmacokinet. 2004;43:763–80.
2. Kvemeland M, Taubull E, Molteberg E, Veierod MB, Selmer KK, Nakken KO, Iversen PO. Pharmacokinetic interaction between modified Atkins diet and antiepileptic drugs in adults with drug-resistant epilepsy. Epilepsia. 2019;60:2235–440.
3. Summary of Product Characteristics: Topiramate (Topamax). Janssen-Cilag Ltd. Last update 14 Jan 2021.
4. Manitpisitkul P, Curtin CR, Shalayda K, Wang SS, Ford L, Heald SL. An open-label drug-drug interaction study of the steady-state pharmacokinetics of topiramate and glyburide in patients with type-2 diabetes mellitus. Clin Drug Invest. 2013;33:929–38.
5. Heo C, Kim SH, Chang MJ. Effect of ketogenic diet and other dietary therapies on anti-epileptic drug comedication in patients with epilepsy. J Clin Pharm Ther. 2017;42:758–64.
6. Manitpisitkul P, Curtin CR, Shalayda K, Wang SS, Ford L, Heald D. Pharmacokinetic interactions between topiramate and pioglitazone and metformin. Epilepsy Res. 2015;108:1519–32.
7. Marriott D, Levy R, Doyle T, Ray J. Posaconazole-induced topiramate toxicity. Ann Intern Med. 2009;151:143.
8. Maschio M, Albani F, Jandolo B, Zarabla A, Contin M, Dinapoli L, Fabi A, Pace A, Baruzzi A. Temozolomide treatment does not affect topiramate and oxcarbazepine plasma concentrations in chronically treated patients with brain tumor-related epilepsy. J Neuro-Oncol. 2008;90:217–21.

Valproic Acid

Analgesics

Aspirin	Salicylic acid displaces valproic acid from plasma protein binding sites (primarily albumin) and can inhibit valproic acid metabolism, via the β-oxidation pathway, by 66%. Concurrent administration of an antipyretic dose of aspirin to children can result in a 23% increase in free nonprotein-bound plasma valproic acid levels. In this setting, clinical management may best be guided by measurement of free phenytoin levels [1, 2]
Diflunisal	Diflunisal can increase the clearance of valproic acid and decrease plasma valproic acid levels. These changes are the consequence of an interaction at the renal level whereby diflunisal interferes with the renal excretion of at least three of the metabolites of valproic acid [3]
Ibuprofen	Ibuprofen can decrease plasma valproic acid levels [4]
Naproxen	Naproxen can decrease mean plasma valproic acid levels by 20%, increase mean plasma valproic acid clearance values by 22%, and increase the mean valproic acid unbound fraction by 20%. These changes are the consequence of valproic acid protein binding displacement by naproxen [5]

Antibacterials

Amikacin	Amikacin can decrease plasma valproic acid levels, probably via an induction of valproic acid metabolism [6]
Doripenem	Doripenem can decrease plasma valproic acid levels by 69%. The mechanism of this interaction is unknown but may involve induction of valproic acid metabolism via an action on UGT1A [7]
Ertapenem	Ertapenem can decrease mean plasma valproic acid levels by 71% (38–98%). The mechanism of this interaction is unknown but may involve induction of metabolism via an action on UGT1A [8]
Erythromycin	Two single cases of an increase in valproic acid plasma levels and toxicity following the addition of erythromycin have been reported [9, 10]

P. N. Patsalos, *Antiseizure Medication Interactions*,
https://doi.org/10.1007/978-3-030-82790-8_63

Imipenem	Imipenem can decrease plasma mean valproic acid levels by 52% (29–73%). The mechanism of this interaction is unknown but may involve induction of valproic acid metabolism via an action on UGT1A [8]
Meropenem	Meropenem can decrease mean plasma valproic acid levels by 77% (34–99%). The mechanism of this interaction is unknown but may involve induction of valproic acid metabolism via an action on UGT1A [8]
Panipenem	Panipenem can decrease plasma valproic acid levels by >99%. The mechanism of this interaction is unknown but may involve induction of valproic acid metabolism via an action on UGT1A [11]
Tebipenem	Tebipenem can decrease plasma valproic acid levels [12]

Antifungal Agents

Posaconazole	Posaconazole does not affect the pharmacokinetics of valproic acid [13]

Antineoplastic Agents

Capecitabine	Capecitabine does not affect the pharmacokinetics of valproic acid [14]
Cisplatin	Cisplatin can decrease plasma valproic acid levels by 50% [15]
Methotrexate	Methotrexate can decrease plasma valproic acid levels by 75%. The exact mechanism is unknown. Possible mechanisms include plasma protein binding displacement or a decrease in valproic acid absorption [16]

Antituberculous Agents

Isoniazid	Isoniazid inhibits the metabolism of valproic acid and can increase plasma valproic acid levels [17, 18]
Rifampicin	Rifampicin enhances the metabolism of valproic acid and can decrease plasma valproic acid levels [9]

Antiulcer Drugs

Antacids and Surface-Acting Drugs

Antacids	A single-dose study in healthy volunteers evaluated the effect of three antacid preparations on valproic acid absorption. While no significant change in extent of absorption occurred with some antacids (e.g., aluminum hydroxide/magnesium trisilicate, or calcium carbonate), concurrent administration of another (aluminum hydroxide/magnesium hydroxide) produced a small (mean 12%; range 3–28%) but statistically significant increase in mean plasma valproic acid AUC values [19]

Histamine H_2-Receptor Antagonists

Cimetidine	Cimetidine can increase plasma valproic acid clearance by 2–17% [20]
Ranitidine	Ranitidine does not affect the pharmacokinetics of valproic acid [20]

Antiviral Agents

Acyclovir	Acyclovir can decrease plasma valproic acid levels by 33%. The exact mechanism of this interaction is not known but is thought to be an effect on gastrointestinal absorption [21]
Efavirenz	Efavirenz can decrease plasma valproic acid levels by >50% [22]
Lopinavir/ritonavir	Lopinavir combined with ritonavir does not affect the pharmacokinetics of valproic acid [23]
Ritonavir	Ritonavir enhances the metabolism of valproic acid, via induction of glucuronyltransferases, and can decrease plasma valproic levels by 48% [24]

Cardioactive Drugs

Propranolol	Propranolol does not affect the pharmacokinetics of valproic acid [25]
Verapamil	Verapamil can increase plasma valproic acid levels by 155% [26]

Psychoactive Drugs

Antidepressants

Bupropion	Bupropion can increase plasma valproic acid levels [27]
Lithium	Lithium can increase plasma valproic acid AUC values by 11% and plasma valproic acid levels by 7% [28]
Fluoxetine	Anecdotal reports in two patients suggest that fluoxetine causes an increase in plasma valproic acid levels. In contrast, two cases of decreased plasma valproic acid levels have also been reported [29–31]
Paroxetine	Paroxetine does not affect the pharmacokinetics of valproic acid [32]
Sertraline	Sertraline can increase plasma valproic acid levels three-fold [33]

Antipsychotics

Aripiprazole	Aripiprazole does not affect the pharmacokinetics of valproic acid [34]
Chlorpromazine	Chlorpromazine can decrease mean plasma valproic acid clearance values by 14%, increase mean plasma elimination half-life values by 14%, and increase mean plasma valproic acid levels by 22% [35]
Haloperidol	Haloperidol does not affect the pharmacokinetics of valproic acid [36]
Quetiapine	It is not known whether quetiapine affects the pharmacokinetics of valproic acid
	Cases of delirium have been reported when quetiapine was added to valproic acid. This effect is probably the consequence of a pharmacodynamic interaction [37]
Zotepine	It is not known whether zotepine affects the pharmacokinetics of valproic acid
	A case of delirium has been reported when zotepine was added to valproic acid. This effect is probably the consequence of a pharmacodynamic interaction [38]

CNS Stimulants and Drugs Used for Attention Deficit Disorders

Methylphenidate	Methylphenidate does not affect the pharmacokinetics of valproic acid [38]
	Adverse effects comprising of dyskinesia and bruxism can occur during methylphenidate and valproic acid combination therapy which is considered to be the consequence of a pharmacodynamic interaction [38]

Steroids

Danazol	The effects of danazol on the pharmacokinetics of valproic acid are conflicting with both an increase and a decrease in plasma valproic acid levels observed [39]
Oral contraceptives	Oral contraceptives enhance the metabolism of valproic acid and can decrease plasma total and free valproic acid levels by 18% and 29%, respectively [40]

Miscellanea

Atkins diet (modified)	The modified Atkins diet can decrease mean plasma valproic acid levels by 20% [41]
Cholestyramine	Cholestyramine decreases the absorption of valproic acid and decrease mean plasma valproic acid AUC values by 15%. This interaction can be avoided by separating the administration of valproic acid and cholestyramine by at least 3 h [42, 43]
Guanfacine	Guanfacine inhibits the metabolism of valproic acid, via an action on glucuronidation, and can increase plasma valproic acid levels by 68% [44]
Ketogenic diet	The ketogenic diet can decrease plasma valproic acid levels [45]
Oxiracetam	Oxiracetam does not affect the pharmacokinetics of valproic acid [46]

Paeoniae radix (Chinese medicine)	Paeoniae radix does not affect the pharmacokinetics of valproic acid [47]
Protein supplement	Enteral co-administered protein supplementation and valproic acid can substantially decrease valproic acid absorption and decrease plasma valproic acid levels [48]
Theophylline	Theophylline does not affect the pharmacokinetics of valproic acid [49]

References

1. Orr JM, Abbot FS, Farrell K, Ferguson S, Sheppard I, Godolphin W. Interaction between valproic acid and aspirin in epileptic children: serum protein binding and metabolic effects. Clin Pharmacol Ther. 1982;31:642–9.
2. Abbott FS, Kassam J, Orr JM, Farrell K. The effect of aspirin on valproic acid metabolism. Clin Pharmacol Ther. 1986;40:94–100.
3. Addison RS, Parker-Scott SL, Eadie MJ, Hooper WD, Dickinson RG. Steady-state dispositions of valproate and diflunisal alone and coadministered to healthy volunteers. Eur J Clin Pharmacol. 2000;56:715–21.
4. Lana F, Marti-Bonany J, Fuster J. deLeon J. Reduction in serum concentrations of valproic acid secondary to the intake of ibuprofen as an example of valproic acid auto-induction metabolism. Actas Esp Psiquiatr. 2016;44:136–44.
5. Addison RS, Parker-Scott SL, Hooper WD, Eadie MJ, Dickinson RG. Effect of naproxen co-administration on valproate disposition. Biopharm Drug Dispos. 2000;21:235–42.
6. De Turck BJ, Diltoer MW, Cornelis PJ, Maes V, Spapen HD, Camu F, Huyghens LP. Lowering of plasma valproic acid concentrations during concomitant therapy with meropenem and amikacin. J Antimicrob Chemother. 1998;42:563–4.
7. Hellwig TR, Onisk ML, Chapman BA. Potential interaction between valproic acid and doripenem. Curr Drug Saf. 2011;6:54–8.
8. Huang CR, Lin CH, Hsioa SC, Chen SD, Tsui WC, Chen SD, Lu YT, Chung YC. Drug interactions between valproic acid and carbapenems in patients with epilepsy. Kaohsiung Med Sci. 2017;33:130–6.
9. Redington K, Wells C, Petito F. Erythromycin and valproate interaction. Ann Intern Med. 1992;116:877.
10. Desai J. Perspectives on interactions between antiepileptic drugs (AEDs) and antimicrobials. Epilepsia. 2008;49(Suppl 6):47–9.
11. Nagai K, Shimizu T, Togo A, Takeya M, Yokomizo Y, Sakata Y, Matsuishi T, Kato H. Decrease in serum levels of valproic acid during treatment with carbapenem, panipenem/betamipron. J Antimicrob Chemother. 1997;39:295–6.
12. Shihyakugari A, Miki A, Nakamoto N, Satoh H, Sawada Y. First case report of suspected onset of convulsive seizures due to co-administration of valproic acid and tebipenem. Int J Clin Pharmacol Ther. 2015;53:92–6.
13. Marriott D, Levy R, Doyle T, Ray J. Posaconazole-induced topiramate toxicity. Ann Intern Med. 2009;151:143.
14. Tanaka H, Jotoku H, Takasaki M, Ibayashi Y, Watanabe K, Takahashi M. Effect of capecitabine therapy on the blood levels of antiepileptic drugs-report of two cases. Gan To Kagaku Ryoho. 2014;41:527–30.
15. Ikeda H, Murakami T, Takan M, Usai T, Kihira K. Pharmacokinetic interaction on valproic acid and recurrence of epileptic seizures during chemotherapy in an epileptic patient. Br J Clin Pharmacol. 2005;59:592–7.

16. Schroder H, Ostergaard JR. Interference of high-dose methotrexate in the metabolism of valproate? Pediatr Hematol Oncol. 1994;11:445–9.
17. Jonville AP, Gauchez AS, Autret E, Billard C, Barbier P, Nsabiyumva F, Breteau M. Interaction between isoniazid and valproate: a case of valproate overdosage. Eur J Clin Pharmacol. 1991;40:197–8.
18. Stewaet JT, Nesmith MW, Mattox KM. A case of valproate toxicity related to isoniazid. J Clin Psychopharmacol. 2012;32:840–1.
19. May CA, Garnett WR, Small RE, Pellock JM. Effects of three antacids on the bioavailability of valproic acid. Clin Pharm. 1982;1:244–7.
20. Webster LK, Mihaly GW, Jones DB, Smallwood RA, Philips JA, Vajda FJ. Effect of cimetidine and ranitidine on carbamazepine and sodium valproate pharmacokinetics. Eur J Clin Pharmacol. 1984;27:341–3.
21. Parmeggiani A, Riva R, Posar A, Rossi PG. Possible interaction between acyclovir and antiepileptic treatment. Ther Drug Monit. 1995;17:312–5.
22. Saraga M, Preisig M, Zullini DF. Reduced valproate plasma levels possible after introduction of efavirenz in a bipolar patient. Bipolar Disord. 2006;8:415–7.
23. DiCenzo R, Peterson DR, Cruttenden K, Morse G, Riggs G, Gelbard H, Schifitto G. Effects of valproic acid coadministration on plasma efavirenz and lopinavir concentrations in human immunodeficiency virus-infected adults. Antimicrob Agents Chemother. 2004;48:4328–31.
24. Sheehan NL, Brouillette MJ, Delisle MS, Allan J. Possible interaction between lopinavir/ritonavir and valproic acid exacerbates bipolar disorder. Ann Pharmacother. 2006;40:147–50.
25. Nemire RE, Toledo CA, Ramsey RE. A pharmacokinetic study to determine the drug interaction between valproate and propranolol. Pharmacotherapy. 1996;16:1059–62.
26. Macphee GA, McInnes GT, Thompson GG, Brodie MJ. Verapamil potentiates carbamazepine neurotoxicity: a clinically important inhibitory interaction. Lancet. 1986;1:700–3.
27. Popli AP, Tanquary J, Lamparella V, Masand PS. Bupropion and anticonvulsant drug interaction. Ann Clin Psychiatry. 1995;7:99–101.
28. Granneman GR, Schneck DW, Cavanagh JH, Witt GF. Pharmacokinetic interactions and side effects resulting from concomitant administration of lithium and divalproex sodium. J Clin Psychiatry. 1996;57:204–6.
29. Sovner R, Davis JM. A potential drug interaction between fluoxetine and valproic acid. J Clin Psychopharmacol. 1991;11:389.
30. Lucena MI, Blanco E, Corrales MA, Berthier ML. Interaction of fluoxetine and valproic acid. Am J Psychiatry. 1998;155:575.
31. Droulers A, Bodak N, Oudjhani M, Lefevre des Noettes V, Bodak A. Decrease of valproic acid concentration in blood when coprescribed fluoxetine. J Clin Psychopharmacol. 1997;17:139–40.
32. Andersen BB, Mikkelsen M, Vesterager A, Dam M, Kristensen HB, Pedersen B, Lund J, Mengel H. No influence of the antidepressant paroxetine on carbamazepine, valproate and phenytoin. Epilepsy Res. 1991;10:201–4.
33. Berigan TR, Harazin J. A sertraline/valproic acid drug interaction. Int J Psychiat Clin Pract. 1999;3:287–8.
34. Boulton DW, Kollia GD, Mallikaarjun S, Kornhauser DM. Lack of pharmacokinetic drug-drug interaction between lithium and valproate when co-administered with aripiprazole. J Clin Pharm Ther. 2012;37:565–70.
35. Ishizaki T, Chiba K, Saito M, Kobayashi K, Iizuka R. The effects of neuroleptics (haloperidol and chlorpromazine) on the pharmacokinetics of valproic acid in schizophrenic patients. J Clin Psychopharmacol. 1984;4:254–61.
36. Huang CC, Wei IH. Unexpected interaction between quetiapine and valproate in patients with bipolar disorder. Gen Hosp Psychiatry. 2010;32:446.e1–2.
37. Hsu WY, Kuo SY, Huang SS, Chang TG, Chiu NY. Valproate and high dosage of zotepine induced delirium: a case report. Br J Clin Pharmacol. 2011;73:486–8.

38. Gara L, Roberts W. Adverse response to methylphenidate in combination with valproic acid. J Child Adolesc Psychopharmacol. 2000;10:39–43.
39. Zielinski JJ, Lichten EM, Haidukewych D. Clinically significant danazol-carbamazepine interaction. Ther Drug Monit. 1987;9:24–7.
40. Galimberti CA, Mazzucchelli I, Arbasino C, Canevini MP, Fattore C, Perucca E. Increased apparent oral clearance of valproic acid during intake of combined contraceptive steroids in women with epilepsy. Epilepsia. 2006;47:1569–72.
41. Kvemeland M, Taubull E, Molteberg E, Veierod MB, Selmer KK, Nakken KO, Iversen PO. Pharmacokinetic interaction between modified Atkins diet and antiepileptc drugs in adults with drug-resistant epilepsy. Epilepsia. 2019;60:2235–440.
42. Pennell AT, Ravis WR, Malloy MJ, Sead A, Diskin C. Cholestyramine decreases valproic acid serum concentrations. J Clin Pharmacol. 1992;32:755.
43. Malloy MJ, Ravis WR, Pennell AT, Diskin CJ. Effect of cholestyramine resin on single dose valproate pharmacokinetics. Int J Clin Pharmacol Ther. 1996;34:208–11.
44. Ambrosini PJ, Sheikh RM. Increased plasma valproate concentrations when coadministered with guanfacine. J Child Adolesc Psychopharmacol. 1998;8:143–7.
45. Heo C, Kim SH, Chang MJ. Effect of ketogenic diet and other dietary therapies on antiepileptic drug comedication in patients with epilepsy. J Clin Pharm Ther. 2017;42:758–64.
46. van Wieringen A, Meijer JWA, van Emde BW, Vermeij TAC. Pilot study to determine the interaction of oxiracetam with antiepileptics. Clin Pharmacokinet. 1990;18:332–8.
47. Chen LC, Chou MH, Lin MF, Yang LL. Lack of pharmacokinetic interaction between valproic acid and a traditional Chinese medicine, Paeoniae radix, in healthy volunteers. J Clin Pharm Ther. 2000;25:453–9.
48. VandenBerg A, Broadway J. Enteral administration of protein supplement and valproate: a potential pharmacokinetic interaction. Ment Health Clin. 2017;7:10–2.
49. Kulkarni C, Vaz J, David J, Joseph T. Aminophylline alters pharmacokinetics of carbamazepine but not that of sodium valproate–a single dose pharmacokinetic study in human volunteers. Indian J Physiol Pharmacol. 1995;39:122–6.

Vigabatrin

There have been no reports on the effects of non-ASM drugs on the pharmacokinetics or pharmacodynamics of vigabatrin.

P. N. Patsalos, *Antiseizure Medication Interactions*,
https://doi.org/10.1007/978-3-030-82790-8_64

Zonisamide

Atkins diet (modified)	The modified Atkins diet can decrease plasma zonisamide levels [1]
Cimetidine	Cimetidine does not affect the pharmacokinetics of zonisamide [2]
Risperidone	Risperidone can decrease plasma zonisamide levels by 55% [3]
Ritonavir	Ritonavir does not affect the pharmacokinetics of zonisamide [4]

References

1. Kvemeland M, Taubull E, Molteberg E, Veierod MB, Selmer KK, Nakken KO, Iversen PO. Pharmacokinetic interaction between modified Atkins diet and antiepileptc drugs in adults with drug-resistant epilepsy. Epilepsia. 2019;60:2235–440.
2. Groves L, Wallace J, Shellenberger K. Effect of cimetidine on zonisamide pharmacokinetics in healthy volunteers. Epilepsia. 1998;39(Suppl 6):191.
3. Okumura K. Decrease in plasma zonisamide concentrations after coadministration of risperidone in a patient with schizophrenia receiving zonisamide therapy. Int Clin Psychopharmacol. 1999;14:55.
4. Kato Y, Fujii T, Mizoguchi N, Takata N, Ueda K, Feldman MD, Kayser SR. Potential interaction between ritonavir and carbamazepine. Pharmacotherapy. 2000;20:851–4.

P. N. Patsalos, *Antiseizure Medication Interactions*,
https://doi.org/10.1007/978-3-030-82790-8_65

Part III
Drug Interactions Between ASMs and Non-ASMs: Interactions Affected by ASMs

Analgesics

Codeine

Carbamazepine	Carbamazepine enhances the metabolism of codeine and decreases plasma codeine levels [1]

Diflunisal

Valproic acid	Valproic acid does not affect the pharmacokinetics of diflunisal [2]

Fentanyl

Carbamazepine	Carbamazepine enhances the metabolism of fentanyl so that a higher fentanyl dosage is required in order to maintain anesthesia [3]
Phenobarbital	Phenobarbital enhances the metabolism of fentanyl so that a higher fentanyl dosage is required in order to maintain anesthesia [3]
Phenytoin	Phenytoin enhances the metabolism of fentanyl so that a higher fentanyl dosage is required in order to maintain anesthesia [3]
Primidone	Primidone enhances the metabolism of fentanyl so that a higher fentanyl dosage is required in order to maintain anesthesia [3]

P. N. Patsalos, *Antiseizure Medication Interactions*,
https://doi.org/10.1007/978-3-030-82790-8_66

Meperidine (Pethidine)

Phenobarbital	Phenobarbital enhances the metabolism of meperidine so that plasma meperidine levels are decreased while plasma levels of normeperidine, its pharmacologically active metabolite that has a lower analgesic potency but greater toxicity than meperidine, are increased [4]
	An increase in meperidine toxicity may be attributable to the increased plasma levels of normeperidine, its pharmacologically active metabolite [5]
Phenytoin	Phenytoin enhances the metabolism of meperidine and can increase mean plasma meperidine clearance values by 20% and decrease mean plasma meperidine AUC values by 50% [6]

Methadone

Carbamazepine	Carbamazepine enhances the metabolism of methadone and can decrease plasma methadone levels [7]
Phenobarbital	Phenobarbital enhances the metabolism of methadone and can decrease plasma methadone levels [8]
Phenytoin	Phenytoin enhances the metabolism of methadone and can decrease plasma methadone levels [9]
Valproic acid	Valproic acid does not affect the pharmacokinetics of methadone [10]

Morphine

Gabapentin	Gabapentin does not affect the pharmacokinetics of morphine [11]
	A pharmacodynamic interaction occurs whereby gabapentin enhances the analgesic effect of morphine [11]
Pregabalin	Pregabalin does not affect the pharmacokinetics of morphine [12]

Naproxen

Gabapentin	Gabapentin does not affect the pharmacokinetics of naproxen [13]
Valproic acid	Valproic acid inhibits the metabolism of naproxen, via an action on glucuronidation, and can decrease mean plasma naproxen clearance values by 7% and increase mean plasma naproxen AUC values by 7% [14]

Oxycodone

Phenytoin	Phenytoin can enhance the metabolism of oxycodone, via an action on CYP3A4, and decrease the analgesic effect of oxycodone [15]
Pregabalin	Pregabalin does not affect the pharmacokinetics of oxycodone [16] Pregabalin appears to be assistive in the impairment of cognitive and gross motor function caused by oxycodone. This is considered to be a consequence of a pharmacodynamic interaction [16]

Paracetamol

Carbamazepine	Carbamazepine enhances the metabolism of paracetamol, probably via an action on CYP1A2, and can increase mean plasma paracetamol clearance by 52% and decrease mean plasma paracetamol AUC values by 39% [17]
Phenobarbital	Phenobarbital enhances the metabolism of paracetamol, probably via an action on CYP1A2, and can increase mean plasma paracetamol clearance by 52% and decrease mean plasma paracetamol AUC values by 39% [18]
Phenytoin	Phenytoin enhances the metabolism of paracetamol, probably via an action on CYP1A2, and can decrease plasma paracetamol AUC values by 40%, increase plasma paracetamol clearance by 52% and can decrease plasma paracetamol levels by up to 75% [18]
Primidone	Primidone enhances the metabolism of paracetamol, probably via an action on CYP1A2, and can increase mean plasma paracetamol clearance by 52% and decrease mean plasma paracetamol AUC values by 39% [17]

Thioctic Acid

Pregabalin	Pregabalin does not affect the pharmacokinetics of thioctic acid [19]

Tramadol

Pregabalin	Pregabalin does not affect the pharmacokinetics of tramadol [20]

References

1. Yue QY, Tomson T, Sawe J. Carbamazepine and cigarette smoking induce differentially the metabolism of codeine in man. Pharmacogenetics. 1994;4:193–8.
2. Addison RS, Parker-Scott SL, Eadie MJ, Hooper WD, Dickinson RG. Steady-state dispositions of valproate and diflunisal alone and coadministered to healthy volunteers. Eur J Clin Pharmacol. 2000;56:715–21.
3. Templefoff R, Modica PA, Spitznagel EL. Anticonvulsant therapy increases fentanyl requirements during anaesthesia for craniotomy. Can J Anaesth. 1990;37:327–32.
4. Dundee JW. Alterations in response to somatic pain associated with anaesthesia. II. The effect of thiopentone and pentobarbital. Br J Anaesth. 1960;32:407–14.
5. Stambaugh JE, Wainer IW, Hemphill DM, Schwartz I. A potential toxic drug interaction between pethidine (meperidine) and phenobarbital. Lancet. 1977;1:398–9.
6. Pond SM, Kretschzmar KM. Effect of phenytoin on meperidine clearance and normeperidine formation. Clin Pharmacol Ther. 1981;30:680–6.
7. Bell J, Seres V, Bowron P, Lewis J, Batey R. The use of serum methadone levels in patients receiving methadone maintenance. Clin Pharmacol Ther. 1988;43:623–9.
8. Liu SJ, Wang RIH. Case report of barbiturate-induced enhancement of methadone metabolism and withdrawal syndrome. Am J Psychiatry. 1984;141:1287–8.
9. Tong TG, Pond SM, Kteek MJ, Jaffery NF, Benowitz NL. Phenytoin-induced methadone withdrawal. Ann Intern Med. 1981;94:349–51.

10. Saxon AJ, Whittaker S, Hawker CS. Valproic acid unlike other anti-convulsants, has no effect on methadone metabolism: two cases. J Clin Psychiatry. 1989;50:1287–8.
11. Eckhardt K, Ammon S, Hofmann U, Riebe A, Gugler N, Mikus G. Gabapentin enhances the analgesic effect of morphine in healthy volunteers. Anesth Analg. 2000;91:185–91.
12. Mercadante S, Porzio G, Aielli F, Ferrera P, Codipietro L, Lo Presti C, Cascuccio A. The effects of low doses of pregabalin on morphine analgesia in advanced cancer patients. Clin J Pain. 2013;29:15–9.
13. Lal R, Sukbuntherng J, Luo W, Vicente V, Blumenthal R, Ho J, Cundy KC. Clinical pharmacokinetic drug interaction studies of gabapentin enacarbil, a novel transporter prodrug of gabapentin, with naproxen and cimetidine. Br J Clin Pharmacol. 2010;69:498–507.
14. Addison RS, Parker-Scott SL, Hooper WD, Eadie MJ, Dickinson RG. Effect of naproxen co-administration on valproate disposition. Biopharm Drug Dispos. 2000;21:235–42.
15. Pon D, Hwang J, Zyl CV. Decreased responsiveness to oxycodone: a case of a pharmacokinetic drug interaction? J Opioid Manag. 2015;11:357–61.
16. Summary of Product Characteristics: Pregabalin (Lyrica). Upjohn UK Ltd; Last update November 2020.
17. Perucca E, Richens A. Paracetamol disposition in normal subjects and in patients treated with antiepileptic drugs. Br J Clin Pharmacol. 1979;7:201–6.
18. Cunningham JL, Price Evans DA. Acetanilide and paracetamol pharmacokinetics before and during phenytoin administration: genetic control of induction? Br J Clin Pharmacol. 1981;11:591–5.
19. Rhee SJ, Lee H, Ahn LY, Lim KS, Yu KS. Lack of clinically significant pharmacokinetic interaction between pregabalin and thioctic acid in healthy volunteers. Clin Ther. 2018;40:1720–8e2.
20. Lee S, Kim Y, Sung Lee JJI, Im G, Cho JY, Chung JY, Yoon S. A pharmacokinetic drug-drug interaction study between pregabalin and tramadol in healthy volunteers. Eur J Clin Pharmacol. 2018;74:1605–13.

Antimicrobials

Antibacterials

Chloramphenicol

Phenobarbital	Phenobarbital enhances the metabolism of chloramphenicol and can decrease plasma chloramphenicol levels by 70–95% [1]
Phenytoin	Phenytoin inhibits the metabolism of chloramphenicol and can increase mean plasma chloramphenicol half-life values by 14% and mean plasma chloramphenicol levels by 15% [2]

Clinafloxacin

Phenytoin	Phenytoin does not affect the pharmacokinetics of clinafloxacin [3]

Doxycycline

Carbamazepine	Carbamazepine enhances the metabolism of doxycycline and can decrease mean plasma doxycycline half-life values by 44% [4]
Phenobarbital	Phenobarbital enhances the metabolism of doxycycline and can decrease plasma doxycycline levels [5]
Phenytoin	Phenytoin enhances the metabolism of doxycycline and can decrease mean plasma doxycycline half-life values by 52% [4]

P. N. Patsalos, *Antiseizure Medication Interactions*,
https://doi.org/10.1007/978-3-030-82790-8_67

Metronidazole

Phenobarbital	Phenobarbital enhances the metabolism of metronidazole and can increase plasma metronidazole clearance by 50% and decrease plasma metronidazole AUC values by 33% [6]

Rifampicin

Phenobarbital	Phenobarbital enhances the metabolism of rifampicin and can decrease plasma rifampicin levels by 20–40% [7]

Antifungal Agents

Fluconazole

Phenytoin	Phenytoin does not affect the pharmacokinetics of fluconazole [8]

Griseofulvin

Phenobarbital	Phenobarbital can decrease plasma griseofulvin levels consequent to a possible impairment of gastrointestinal absorption [9]

Itraconazole

Carbamazepine	Carbamazepine enhances the metabolism of itraconazole, probably via an action on CYP3A4, and can decrease plasma itraconazole levels so that they are not detectable [10]
Phenobarbital	Phenobarbital enhances the metabolism of itraconazole, probably via an action on CYP3A4, and can decrease plasma itraconazole levels [11]
Phenytoin	Phenytoin enhances the metabolism of itraconazole, probably via an action on CYP3A4, and can decrease mean plasma itraconazole AUC values by 93% and decrease mean plasma itraconazole half-life values by 83% [12]

Ketoconazole

Carbamazepine	Carbamazepine enhances the metabolism of ketoconazole, probably via an action on CYP3A4, and can decrease plasma ketoconazole levels so that they are not detectable [10]
Phenytoin	Phenytoin enhances the metabolism of ketoconazole, probably via an action on CYP3A4, and can decrease plasma ketoconazole levels so that they are not detectable [10]

Posaconazole

Phenytoin	Phenytoin enhances the metabolism of posaconazole, probably via an action on UGT1A4, and can decrease mean plasma posaconazole AUC values by 52% [13]

Voriconazole

Carbamazepine	Carbamazepine can enhance the metabolism of voriconazole and can decrease plasma voriconazole levels [14]
Phenobarbital	Phenobarbital can enhance the metabolism of voriconazole and can decrease plasma voriconazole levels [15]
Phenytoin	Phenytoin enhances the metabolism of voriconazole, via an action on CYP2C9 and possibly CYP2C19, and can decrease mean plasma voriconazole AUC values by ~70% [16]

Antihelmintics

Albendazole

Carbamazepine	Carbamazepine enhances the metabolism of albendazole, probably via an action on CYP3A4, and can decrease mean plasma albendazole AUC values by 50%, plasma albendazole half-life values by 50% and can decrease plasma albendazole levels by 50% [17]
Phenobarbital	Phenobarbital enhances the metabolism of albendazole, probably via an action on CYP3A4, and can decrease mean plasma albendazole AUC values by 71%, plasma albendazole half-life values by 39% and can decrease plasma albendazole levels by 63% [17]
Phenytoin	Phenytoin enhances the metabolism of albendazole, probably via an action on CYP3A4, and can decrease mean plasma albendazole AUC values by 66%, decrease plasma albendazole half-life values by 53% and can decrease plasma albendazole levels by 63% [17]

Mebendazole

Carbamazepine	Carbamazepine enhances the metabolism of mebendazole and can decrease plasma mebendazole levels [18]
Phenytoin	Phenytoin enhances the metabolism of mebendazole and can decrease plasma mebendazole levels [18]

Praziquantel

Carbamazepine	Carbamazepine enhances the first-pass metabolism of praziquantel and can decrease plasma praziquantel half-life values by 88% and can decrease plasma praziquantel levels by 90% [19]
Phenytoin	Phenytoin enhances the first-pass metabolism of praziquantel and can decrease plasma praziquantel half-life values by 86% and can decrease plasma praziquantel levels by 74% [19]

Antituberculous Agents

Isoniazid

Carbamazepine	Carbamazepine enhances the metabolism of acetylhydrazine, a major metabolite of isoniazid, to a reactive intermediate, thereby contributing to isoniazid-associated hepatotoxicity [20]

Antiviral Agents

Atazanavir

Carbamazepine	Carbamazepine enhances the metabolism of atazanavir and can decrease plasma atazanavir levels [21]
Oxcarbazepine	Oxcarbazepine enhances the metabolism of atazanavir and can decrease plasma atazanavir levels [21]
Valproic acid	Valproic acid does not affect the pharmacokinetics of atazanavir [22]

Daclatasvir

Oxcarbazepine	Oxcarbazepine can enhance the metabolism of daclatasvir [23]

Delavirdine

Phenytoin	Phenytoin enhances the metabolism of delavirdine and can decrease plasma delavirdine levels [24]
Phenobarbital	Phenobarbital enhances the metabolism of delavirdine and can decrease plasma delavirdine levels [24]

Dolutegravir

Carbamazepine	Carbamazepine can enhance the metabolism of dolutegravir and decrease plasma dolutegravir levels [21]
Oxcarbazepine	Oxcarbazepine can enhance the metabolism of dolutegravir and decrease plasma dolutegravir levels [21, 43]
Phenobarbital	Phenobarbital enhances the metabolism of dolutegravir, probably via an action on UGT1A1, and can decrease plasma dolutegravir levels by 82% [25]
Valproic acid	Valproic acid can decrease plasma dolutegravir levels via an unknown mechanism [26]

Efavirenz

Carbamazepine	Carbamazepine enhances the metabolism of efavirenz, via an action on CYP3A4, and can decrease mean plasma efavirenz Cmax values by 21% and mean plasma efavirenz AUC values by 36% [27]
Phenytoin	Phenytoin enhances the metabolism of efavirenz, via an action on CYP3A4, and can decrease plasma efavirenz levels [28]
Valproic acid	Valproic acid does not affect the pharmacokinetics of efavirenz [29]

Indinavir

Carbamazepine	Carbamazepine enhances the metabolism of indinavir, via an action on CYP3A4, and can decrease plasma indinavir levels by 25% [30]

Lersivirine

Valproic acid	Valproic acid inhibits the metabolism of lersivirine, via an action on UGT2B7, and can increase mean plasma lersivirine AUC values by 25% [31]

Lopinavir

Lamotrigine	Lamotrigine does not affect the pharmacokinetics of lopinavir and low-dose ritonavir [32]
Phenytoin	Phenytoin enhances the metabolism of lopinavir and can decrease mean plasma lopinavir AUC values by 33% [33, 34]
Valproic acid	Valproic acid can increase mean plasma lopinavir AUC values by 38% [29]

Nevirapine

Carbamazepine	Carbamazepine enhances the metabolism of nevirapine, via an action on CYP3A4, and can decrease mean plasma nevirapine half-life values by 37% and decreases plasma nevirapine levels [35]
Phenytoin	Phenytoin enhances the metabolism of nevirapine, via an action on CYP3A4, and can decrease nevirapine half-life by 60%, and can decrease plasma nevirapine levels by up to 85% [36]
Phenobarbital	Phenobarbital does not affect the pharmacokinetics of nevirapine [37]

Raltegravir

Lamotrigine	Lamotrigine does not affect the pharmacokinetics of raltegravir [38]

Ritonavir

Lamotrigine	Lamotrigine does not affect the pharmacokinetics of low-dose ritonavir when administered in combination with lopinavir [32]
Phenytoin	Phenytoin enhances the metabolism of ritonavir and can decrease mean plasma ritonavir AUC values by 28% [33, 34]
Valproic acid	Valproic acid does not affect the pharmacokinetics of ritonavir [22]

Saquinavir

Stiripentol	Stiripentol does not affect the pharmacokinetics of saquinavir [39, 40]

Sofosbuvir

Oxcarbazepine	Oxcarbazepine does not affect the pharmacokinetics of sofosbuvir [23]

Zidovudine

Phenytoin	Phenytoin does not affect the pharmacokinetics of zidovudine [41]
Valproic acid	Valproic acid inhibits the metabolism of zidovudine, via an action on glucuronidation, and can increase plasma zidovudine levels by 100% [42]

References

1. Bloxham RA, Durbin GM, Johnson T, Winterborn MH. Chloramphenicol and phenobarbitone–a drug interaction. Arch Dis Childhood. 1979;54:76–7.
2. Krasinski K, Kusmiesz H, Nelson JD. Pharmacologic interactions among chloramphenicol, phenytoin and phenobarbital. Pediatr Infect Dis. 1982;1:232–5.
3. Randinitis EJ, Alvey CW, Koup JR, Rausch G, Abel R, Bron NJ, Hounslow NJ, Vassos AB, Sedman AJ. Drug interactions with clinafloxacin. Antimicrob Agents Chemother. 2001;45:2543–52.
4. Penttila O, Neuvonen PJ, Aho K, Lehtovaara R. Interaction between doxycycline and some antiepileptic drugs. Br Med J. 1974;2:470–2.
5. Neuvonen PJ, Penttila O, Lehtovaara R, Aho K. Effects of antiepileptic drugs on the elimination of various tetracycline derivatives. Eur J Clin Pharmacol. 1975;9:147–54.
6. Eradiri O, Jamali F, Thomson ABR. Interaction of metronidazole with phenobarbital, cimetidine, prednisone, and sulfasalazine in Crohn's disease. Biopharm Drug Dispos. 1988;9:219–27.
7. Acocella G, Bonollo L, Mainardi M, Margaroli P, Nicolis FB. Kinetic studies on rifampicin. III. Effect of phenobarbital on the half-life of the antibiotic. Tijdschr Gastroenterol. 1974;17:151–8.
8. Blum RA, Wilton JH, Hilligoss DM, Gardner MJ, Henry EB, Harrison NJ, Schentag JJ. Effect of fluconazole on the disposition of phenytoin. Clin Pharmacol Ther. 1991;49:420–5.
9. Reigelman S, Rowland M, Epstein WL. Griseofulvin-phenobarbital interaction in man. J Am Med Assoc. 1970;213:426–31.

10. Tucker RM, Denning DW, Hanson LH, Rinaldi MG, Graybill JR, Sharkey PK, Pappagianis D, Stevens DA. Interaction of azoles with rifampin, phenytoin, and carbamazepine: in vitro and clinical observations. Clin Infect Dis. 1992;14:165–74.
11. Bonay M, Jonville-Bera AP, Diot P, Lemarie E, Lavendier M, Autret E. Possible interaction between phenobarbital, carbamazepine and itraconazole. Drug Saf. 1993;9:309–11.
12. Ducharme MP, Slaughter RL, Warbasse LH, Chandrasekar PH, Van de Velde V, Mannens G, Edwards DJ. Itraconazole and hydroxyitraconazole serum concentrations are reduced more than 10-fold by phenytoin. Clin Pharmacol Ther. 1995;58:617–24.
13. Krishna G, Sansone-Parsons A, Kantesaria B. Drug interaction assessment following concomitant administration of posaconazole and phenytoin in healthy men. Curr Med Res Opin. 2007;23:1415–22.
14. Malingre MM, Godschalk PCR, Klein SK. A case report of voriconazole therapy failure in a homozygous ultrarapid CYP19*19/*17 patient comedicated with carbamazepine. Br J Clin Pharmacol. 2011;74:205–6.
15. Cojutti P, Candoni A, Forghieri F, Isola M, Zannier ME, Bigliardi S, Luppi M, Fanin R, Pea F. Variability of voriconazole trough levels in haematological patients: influence of comedication with cytochrome P450 (CYP) inhibitors and/or with CYP inhibitors plus CYP inducers. Basic Clin Pharmacol Toxicol. 2015;118:474–9.
16. Purkins L, Wood N, Ghahramani P, Love ER, Eve MD, Fielding A. Coadministration or voriconazole and phenytoin: pharmacokinetic interaction, safety, and tolerance. Br J Clin Pharmacol. 2003;56(Suppl 1):37–44.
17. Lanchote VL, Garcia FS, Dreossi SAC, Takayanagui OM. Pharmacokinetic interaction between albendazole sulfoxide enantiomers and antiepileptic drugs in patients with neurocysticercosis. Ther Drug Monit. 2002;24:338–45.
18. Luder PJ, Siffert B, Witassek F, Meister F, Bircher J. Treatment of hydatid disease with high oral doses of mebendazole. Long-term follow-up of plasma mebendazole levels and drug interactions. Eur J Clin Pharmacol. 1986;31:443–8.
19. Bittencourt PRM, Garcia CM, Martins R, Fernandes AG, Dieckmann HW, Jung W. Phenytoin and carbamazepine decrease oral bioavailability of praziquantel. Neurology. 1992;42:492–6.
20. Wright JM, Stokes EF, Sweeney VP. Isoniazid-induced carbamazepine toxicity and vice versa. A double drug interaction. N Engl J Med. 1982;307:1325–7.
21. Catteneo D, Baldelli S, Cozzi V, Fuci M, Atzori C, Micheli V, Felice C, Gervasoni C. Drug-drug interactions between antiretrovirals and carbamazepine/oxcarbazepine: a real-life investigation. Ther Drug Monit. 2020;42:330–4.
22. DiCenzo R, Peterson DR, Cruttenden K, Mariuz P, Rezk NL, Hochreiter J, Gelbard H, Schifitto G. Effects of minocycline and valproic acid coadministration on atazanavir plasma concentrations in human immunodeficiency virus-infected adults receiving atazanavir-ritonavir. Antimicrob Agents Chemother. 2008;52:3035–9.
23. Smoulders EJ, de Kanter CTMM, van't Veer N, D'avolio A, Di Perri G, Burger DM, van Wijngaarden P. Effective treatment of hepatitis C virus infection with sofosbuvir and daclatasvir 90 mg in a patient with severe epilepsy on oxcarbazepine. Int J Antimicrob Agents. 2016;48:347–8.
24. Dasgupta A, Okhuysen PC. Pharmacokinetic and other interactions in patients with AIDS. Ther Drug Monit. 2001;23:591–605.
25. Hikasa S, Sawada A, Seino H, Shimabukuro S, Hideta K, Uwa N, Higasa S, Tokugawa T, Kimura T. A potential interaction between phenobarbital and dolutegravir: a case report. J Infect Chemother. 2018;24:476–8.
26. Ji P, Damle B, Xie J, Unger SE, Grasela DM, Kaul S. Pharmacokinetic interaction between efavirenz and carbamazepine after multiple-dose administration in healthy subjects. J Clin Pharmacol. 2008;48:948–56.
27. Robertson SM, Penzak SR, Lane J, Pau AK, Mican JM. A potential significant interaction between efavirenz and phenytoin: a case report and review of the literature. Clin Infect Dis. 2005;41:e15–8.

28. Calcagno A, Cusato J, Ferrara M, De Nicolo A, Lazzaro S, Manca A, D'Avolio A, DiPerri G, Bonora S. Antiviral concentrations in the presence and absence of valproic acid. J Antimicrob Chemother. 2020;75:1969–71.
29. DiCenzo R, Peterson DR, Cruttenden K, Morse G, Riggs G, Gelbard H, Schifitto G. Effects of valproic acid coadministration on plasma efavirenz and lopinavir concentrations in human immunodeficiency virus-infected adults. Antimicrob Agents Chemother. 2004;48:4328–31.
30. Hugen PWH, Burger DM, Brinkman K, ter Hofstede HJM, Schuuman R, Koopmans PP, Hekster YA. Carbamazepine-indinavir interaction causes antiretroviral failure. Ann Pharmacother. 2000;34:465–70.
31. Langdon G, Davis J, Layton G, Chong C, Weissgerber G, Vourvahis M. Effects of ketoconazole and valproic acid on the pharmacokinetics of the next-generation NNRTI lersivirine (UK-453,061) in healthy adult subjects. Br J Clin Pharmacol. 2012;73:768–75.
32. Van der Lee MJ, Dawood L, ter Hofstede HJM, de Graaff-Teulen MJA, van Ewijk-Beneken-Kolmer EWJ, Caliskan-Yassen N, Koopmans PP, Burger DM. Lopinavir/ritonavir reduces lamotrigine plasma concentrations in healthy volunteers. Clin Pharmacol Ther. 2006;80:159–68.
33. Wong MC, Suite ND, Labar DR. Seizures in human immunodeficiency virus infection. Arch Neurol. 1990;47:640–2.
34. Lim ML, Min SS, Eron JJ, Bertz RJ, Robinson M, Gaedigk A, Kashuba AD. Coadministration of lopinavir/ritonavir and phenytoin results in two-way drug interaction through cytochrome P-450 induction. J Acquir Immune Defic Syndr. 2004;36:1034–40.
35. Muro EP, Fillekes Q, Kisanga ER, L'homme R, Aitken SC, Mariki G, Van der Ven AJ, Dolmans W, Schuurman R, Walker AS, Gibb DM, Burger DM. Intrapartum single-dose carbamazepine reduces nevirapine levels faster and may decrease resistance after single dose nevirapine for perinatal HIV prevention. J Acquir Immune Defic Syndr. 2012;59:266–73.
36. Fillekes Q, Muro EP, Chunda C, Aitken S, Kisanga ER, Kankasa C, Thomason MJ, Gibb DM, Walker AS, Burger DM. Effect of 7 days of phenytoin on the pharmacokinetics of and the development of resistance to single-dose nevirapine for perinatal HIV prevention: a randomized pilot trial. J Antimicrob Chemother. 2013;68:2609–15.
37. L'Homme RF, Dijkema T, van der Ven AJ, Burger DM. Brief report: enzyme inducers reduce the elimination half-life after a single dose of nevirapine in healthy women. J Acquir Immune Defic Syndr. 2006;43:193–6.
38. van Luin M, Colbers A, Verwey-van Wissen CP, van Ewijk-Beneken-Kolmer EW, van der Kolk M, Hoitsama A, da Silva HG, Burger DM. The effect of raltegravir on the glucuronidation of lamotrigine. J Clin Pharmacol. 2009;49:1220–7.
39. Cazali N, Tran A, Treluyer JM, Rey E, d'Athis P, Vincent J, Pons G. Inhibitory effect of stiripentol on carbamazepine and saquinavir metabolism in human. Br J Clin Pharmacol. 2003;56:526–36.
40. Kellinghaus C, Engbrine C, Kovac S, Moddel G, Boesebeck F, Fischera M, Anneken K, Klonne K, Reichelt D, Evers S, Husstedt IW. Frequency of seizures and epilepsy in neurological HIV-infected patients. Seizure. 2008;17:27–33.
41. Burger DM, Meenhorst PL, Mulder JW, Kraaijeveld CL, Koks CH, Bult A, Beijnen JH. Therapeutic drug monitoring of phenytoin in patients with acquired immunodeficiency syndrome. Ther Drug Monit. 1994;16:616–20.
42. Lertora JJ, Rege AB, Greenspan DL, Akula S, George WJ, Hyslop NE, Agrawal KC. Pharmacokinetic interaction between zidovudine and valproic acid in patients infected with human immunodeficiency virus. Clin Pharmacol Ther. 1994;56:272–8.
43. Kandil MM, Badowski ME, Schriever CA. Sustained viral suppression with co-administration of oxcarbazepine and dolutegravir. Int J STD AIDS. 2018;29:831–3.

Antineoplastic Agents

9-Aminocamptothecin

Carbamazepine	Carbamazepine enhances the mean plasma clearance of 9-aminocamptothecin by 68% and can decrease median plasma 9-aminocamptothecin levels by 67% [1]
Phenobarbital	Phenobarbital enhances the mean plasma clearance of 9-aminocamptothecin by 68% and can decrease median plasma 9-aminocamptothecin levels by 67% [1]
Phenytoin	Phenytoin enhances the mean plasma clearance of 9-aminocamptothecin by 68% and can decrease median plasma 9-aminocamptothecin levels by 67% [1]

Busulfan

Phenytoin	Phenytoin enhances the metabolism of busulfan and can increase mean plasma busulfan clearance by 19%, decrease mean plasma busulfan elimination half-life values by 23% and decrease mean plasma busulfan AUC values by 16% [2]

CCNU (1-(2-Chloroethyl)-3-Cyclohexyl-1-Nitrosourea)

Carbamazepine	Carbamazepine enhances the metabolism of CCNU [3]
Lamotrigine	Lamotrigine does not affect the pharmacokinetics of CCNU [3]
Levetiracetam	Levetiracetam does not affect the pharmacokinetics of CCNU [3]
Phenytoin	Phenytoin enhances the metabolism of CCNU [3]
Valproic acid	Valproic acid does not affect the pharmacokinetics of CCNU [3]

P. N. Patsalos, *Antiseizure Medication Interactions*, https://doi.org/10.1007/978-3-030-82790-8_68

Celecoxib

Levetiracetam	Levetiracetam does not affect the pharmacokinetics of celecoxib [4]
Phenytoin	Phenytoin does not affect the pharmacokinetics of celecoxib [4]

Cisplatin

Valproic acid	Valproic acid in combination with cisplatin is associated with a threefold higher incidence of reversible thrombopenia, neutropenia, or both. This is considered to be a consequence of a pharmacodynamic interaction, and this interaction may also occur with etoposide and fotemustine [5]

Cyclophosphamide

Carbamazepine	Carbamazepine enhances the metabolism of cyclophosphamide, a pharmacologically inactive prodrug, to the pharmacologically active metabolite 4-hydroxycyclophosphamide. Plasma 4-hydroxycyclophosphamide AUC values can increase by 58%, while plasma cyclophosphamide AUC values can decrease by 40% [6]
Phenytoin	Phenytoin enhances the metabolism of cyclophosphamide, a pharmacologically inactive prodrug, to the pharmacologically active metabolite 4-hydroxycyclophosphamide. Plasma 4-hydroxycyclophosphamide AUC values can increase by 51%, while plasma 4-hydroxycyclophosphamide Cmax values can increase by sixfold [7]

Cytarabine

Carbamazepine	Carbamazepine does not affect the pharmacokinetics of cytarabine [8]
Phenobarbital	Phenobarbital does not affect the pharmacokinetics of cytarabine [8]
Phenytoin	Phenytoin does not affect the pharmacokinetics of cytarabine [8]

Dolutegravir

Carbamazepine	Carbamazepine enhances the metabolism of dolutegravir, via an action on UGT1A1 and CYP3A4, and can decrease mean plasma etoposide AUC values by 49% [9]

Erlotinib

Phenytoin	Phenytoin enhances the metabolism of erlotinib and can decrease erlotinib plasma levels by 79–92% [10]

Etoposide

Phenobarbital	Phenobarbital enhances the metabolism of etoposide and can increase mean plasma etoposide clearance by 77% and decrease mean plasma etoposide half-life values by 18% [11]
Phenytoin	Phenytoin enhances the metabolism of etoposide and can increase mean plasma etoposide clearance by 77% and decrease mean plasma etoposide half-life values by 18% [11]

Gefitinib

Phenytoin	Phenytoin enhances the metabolism of gefitinib and can decrease plasma gefitinib clearance by 2.3-fold and mean plasma gefitinib Cmax and AUC values by 36% and 52%, respectively [12]

Glufosfamide

Carbamazepine	Carbamazepine enhances the plasma clearance of glufosfamide by up to 15% and can decrease plasma glufosfamide AUC values by up to 15% [13]
Oxcarbazepine	Oxcarbazepine enhances the plasma clearance of glufosfamide by up to 15% and can decrease plasma glufosfamide AUC values by up to 15% [13]
Phenobarbital	Phenobarbital enhances the plasma clearance of glufosfamide by up to 15% and can decrease plasma glufosfamide AUC values by up to 15% [13]
Phenytoin	Phenytoin enhances the plasma clearance of glufosfamide by up to 15% and can decrease plasma glufosfamide AUC values by up to 15% [13]

Ifosfamide

Phenobarbital	Phenobarbital does not affect the pharmacokinetics of ifosfamide [14]
	A pharmacodynamic interaction between phenytoin and ifosfamide, resulting in encephalopathy, may occur [15]
Phenytoin	Phenytoin enhances the metabolism of ifosfamide. In general, this interaction would be expected to result in decreased efficacy of ifosfamide. However, because the metabolism of ifosfamide results in a pharmacologically active metabolite, enzyme induction could theoretically potentiate drug effects by stimulating bioactivation processes [16]

Imatinib

Carbamazepine	Carbamazepine enhances the metabolism of imatinib and can decrease mean plasma imatinib levels by 66% [17]
Lamotrigine	Lamotrigine does not affect the pharmacokinetics of imatinib [17]
Levetiracetam	Levetiracetam does not affect the pharmacokinetics of imatinib [17]
Oxcarbazepine	Oxcarbazepine enhances the metabolism of imatinib and can decrease mean plasma imatinib levels by 62% [17]

Topiramate	Topiramate enhances the metabolism of imatinib and can decrease mean plasma imatinib levels by 49% [17]
Phenytoin	Phenytoin enhances the metabolism of imatinib and can decrease mean plasma imatinib levels by 73% [17]
Primidone	Primidone enhances the metabolism of imatinib and can decrease plasma imatinib levels [18]
Valproic acid	Valproic acid does not affect the pharmacokinetics of imatinib [17]

Irinotecan

Phenytoin	Phenytoin enhances the metabolism of irinotecan, a prodrug that is metabolized to a pharmacologically active metabolite 7-ethyl-10-hydroxy-camptothecin, via carboxylesterases, and to an inactive metabolite APC, via an action on CYP3A4. 7-ethyl-10-hydroxy-camptothecin is further metabolized by glucuronidation, primarily via UGT1A1. Mean plasma irinotecan AUC values decrease by 26%, while mean plasma 7-ethyl-10-hydroxy-camptothecin and APC AUC values decrease by 53% and increase by 17%, respectively [19]
Phenobarbital	Phenobarbital enhances the metabolism of irinotecan, a prodrug that is metabolized to a pharmacologically active metabolite 7-ethyl-10-hydroxy-camptothecin, via carboxylesterases, and to an inactive metabolite APC, via an action on CYP3A4. 7-ethyl-10-hydroxy-camptothecin is further metabolized by glucuronidation, primarily via UGT1A1. Mean plasma 7-ethyl-10-hydroxy-camptothecin AUC values decrease by 75% [20]
Primidone	Primidone enhances the metabolism of irinotecan, a prodrug that is metabolized to a pharmacologically active metabolite 7-ethyl-10-hydroxy-camptothecin, via carboxylesterases, and to an inactive metabolite APC, via an action on CYP3A4. 7-ethyl-10-hydroxy-camptothecin is further metabolized by glucuronidation, primarily via UGT1A1. Mean plasma 7-ethyl-10-hydroxy-camptothecin clearance values decrease by 37% [21]
Valproic acid	Valproic acid interacts with irinotecan, a prodrug that is metabolized to a pharmacologically active metabolite 7-ethyl-10-hydroxy-camptothecin, via carboxylesterases, and to an inactive metabolite APC, via an action on CYP3A4. 7-ethyl-10-hydroxy-camptothecin is further metabolized by glucuronidation, primarily via UGT1A1. Mean plasma irinotecan, 7-ethyl-10-hydroxy-camptothecin, and glucuronide metabolite AUC values decrease by 16%, 43% and 33%, respectively. The exact mechanism of these effects is not known but may be due to a combination of induction of UGT1A1 metabolism and a plasma protein binding displacement interaction involving 7-ethyl-10-hydroxy-camptothecin [22]

Lapatinib

Carbamazepine	Carbamazepine enhances the metabolism of lapatinib, via an action on CYP3A4, and decreases mean plasma AUC lapatinib values by 72%. A concurrent 28% mean decrease in lapatinib absorption also occurs, probably via an action on the ABCB2 transporter [23]

Methotrexate

Carbamazepine	Carbamazepine enhances the metabolism of methotrexate and can increase plasma methotrexate clearance by up to 55% [8]
Levetiracetam	Levetiracetam does not affect the plasma elimination of methotrexate [24, 25]
Phenobarbital	Phenobarbital enhances the metabolism of methotrexate and can increase plasma methotrexate clearance by up to 55% [8]
Phenytoin	Phenytoin enhances the metabolism of methotrexate and can increase plasma methotrexate clearance by up to 55% [8]
Topiramate	Topiramate does not affect the pharmacokinetics of methotrexate [26]

Paclitaxel

Carbamazepine	Carbamazepine enhances the metabolism of paclitaxel and can increase mean plasma paclitaxel clearance by 101% and decrease mean plasma paclitaxel AUC values by 52% [27]
Phenobarbital	Phenobarbital enhances the metabolism of paclitaxel and can increase mean plasma paclitaxel clearance by 101% and decrease mean plasma paclitaxel AUC values by 52% [27]
Phenytoin	Phenytoin enhances the metabolism of paclitaxel and can increase mean plasma paclitaxel clearance by 101% and decrease mean plasma paclitaxel AUC values by 52% [27]
Valproic acid	Valproic acid inhibits the metabolism of paclitaxel and can decrease plasma paclitaxel clearance by 26% and increase plasma paclitaxel AUC values by 40% [27]

Pomalidomide

Carbamazepine	Carbamazepine enhances the metabolism of pomalidomide and can decrease mean plasma pomalidomide AUC and Cmax values by 20% and 25%, respectively [28]

Procarbazine

Carbamazepine	Carbamazepine enhances the metabolism of procarbazine and increases procarbazine hypersensitivity reactions, possibly through an intermediate metabolite generated by the induction of a CYP3A isoform [29]
Gabapentin	Gabapentin does not affect the pharmacokinetics of procarbazine [30]
Lamotrigine	Lamotrigine does not affect the pharmacokinetics of procarbazine [30]
Levetiracetam	Levetiracetam does not affect the pharmacokinetics of procarbazine [30]
Phenobarbital	Phenobarbital enhances the metabolism of procarbazine and increases procarbazine hypersensitivity reactions, possibly through an intermediate metabolite generated by the induction of a CYP3A isoform [29]
Phenytoin	Phenytoin enhances the metabolism of procarbazine and increases procarbazine hypersensitivity reactions, possibly through an intermediate metabolite generated by the induction of a CYP3A isoform [29]

Topiramate	Topiramate does not affect the pharmacokinetics of procarbazine [30]
Valproic acid	Valproic acid does not affect the pharmacokinetics of procarbazine [30]

Tamoxifen

Phenytoin	Phenytoin can enhance the metabolism of tamoxifen and can decrease plasma levels of the pharmacologically active metabolite endoxifen [31]

Temozolomide

Carbamazepine	Carbamazepine enhances the metabolism of temozolomide and can decrease plasma temozolomide levels [3]
Lamotrigine	Lamotrigine does not affect the pharmacokinetics of temozolomide [3]
Levetiracetam	Levetiracetam does not affect the pharmacokinetics of temozolomide [3]
Phenytoin	Phenytoin enhances the metabolism of temozolomide and can decrease plasma temozolomide levels [3]
Valproic acid	Valproic acid does not affect the pharmacokinetics of temozolomide [3]

Temsirolimus

Carbamazepine	Carbamazepine enhances the metabolism of temsirolimus so that after IV administration, mean plasma Cmax values are decreased by 36%. Additionally, mean plasma Cmax and AUC values for the pharmacologically active metabolite, sirolimus, are decreased by 67% and 43%, respectively [32]
Phenytoin	Phenytoin enhances the metabolism of temsirolimus so that after IV administration, mean plasma Cmax values are decreased by 36%. Additionally, mean plasma Cmax and AUC values for the pharmacologically active metabolite, sirolimus, are decreased by 67% and 43%, respectively [32]

Teniposide

Carbamazepine	Carbamazepine enhances the metabolism of teniposide, via an action on CYP3A4, and can increase plasma teniposide clearance by 100% and decrease plasma teniposide levels [8]
Phenobarbital	Phenobarbital enhances the metabolism of teniposide, via an action on CYP3A4, and can increase mean plasma teniposide clearance by 146% and decrease plasma teniposide levels [33]
Phenytoin	Phenytoin enhances the metabolism of teniposide, via an action on CYP3A4, and can increase plasma teniposide clearance by 217% and decrease plasma teniposide levels [33]

Thiotepa

Carbamazepine	Carbamazepine enhances the metabolism of thiotepa, via an action on CYP2B6 and CYP3A4, resulting in an increase in the equipotent pharmacologically active metabolite tepa. Plasma tepa AUC values are increased by 75%, while plasma thiotepa AUC values are decreased by 43% [6]
Phenytoin	Phenytoin enhances the metabolism of thiotepa, via an action on CYP2B6 and CYP3A4, resulting in an increase in the equipotent pharmacologically active metabolite tepa. Mean plasma tepa AUC values are increased by 115% [7]

Topotecan

Phenytoin	Phenytoin enhances the metabolism of topotecan and can increase mean plasma topotecan clearance by 47%. This interaction is complicated by the fact that mean plasma AUC values of the N-desmethyl metabolite of topotecan, which is pharmacologically equipotent to that of topotecan, can be increased by 117% [34]

Vincristine

Carbamazepine	Carbamazepine enhances the metabolism of vincristine, via an action on CYP3A4, and can increase mean plasma vincristine clearance values by 63%, decrease mean plasma vincristine half-life values by 35%, and decrease mean plasma vincristine AUC values by 43% [35]
Gabapentin	Gabapentin does not affect the pharmacokinetics of vincristine [35]
Oxcarbazepine	Oxcarbazepine does not affect the pharmacokinetics of vincristine [34]
Phenytoin	Phenytoin enhances the metabolism of vincristine, via an action on CYP3A4, and can increase mean plasma vincristine clearance values by 63%, decrease mean plasma vincristine half-life values by 35%, and decrease mean plasma vincristine AUC values by 43% [35]
Vigabatrin	Vigabatrin does not affect the pharmacokinetics of vincristine [35]

References

1. Grossman SA, Hochberg F, Fisher J, Chen TL, Kim L, Gregory R, Grochow LB, Piantadosi S. Increased 9-aminocamptothecin dose requirements in patients with anticonvulsants. Cancer Chemother Pharmacol. 1998;42:118–26.
2. Hassan M, Oberg G, Bjorkholm M, Wallin I, Lindgren M. Influence of prophylactic anticonvulsant therapy on high-dose busulphan kinetics. Cancer Chemother Pharmacol. 1993;33:181–6.
3. Oberndorfer S, Piribauer M, Marosi C, Lahrmann H, Hitzenberger P, Grisold W. P450 Enzyme inducing and non-enzyme inducing antiepileptics in glioblastoma patients treated with standard chemotherapy. J Neuro-Oncol. 2005;72:255–60.
4. Grossman SA, Olson J, Batchelor T, Peereboom D, Lesser G, Desideri S, Ye X, Hammour T, Supko JG. Effect of phenytoin on celecoxib pharmacokinetics in patients with glioblastoma. Neuro-Oncology. 2008;10:190–8.

5. Bourg V, Lebrun C, Chichmanian RM, Thomas P, Frenay M. Nitrosourea-cisplatine-based chemotherapy associated with valproate: increase of haematologic activity. Ann Oncol. 2001;12:217–9.
6. Ekhart C, Rodenhuis S, Beijnen JH, Huitema ADR. Carbamazepine induces bioactivation of cyclophosphamide and thiotepa. Cancer Chemother Pharmacol. 2009;63:543–7.
7. de Jong ME, Huitema ADR, van Dam AM, Beijnen JH, Rodenhuis S. Significant induction of cyclophosphamide and thiotepa metabolism by phenytoin. Cancer Chemother Pharmacol. 2005;55:507–10.
8. Relling MV, Pui CH, Sandlund JT, Rivera GK, Hancock ML, Boyett JM, Schuetz EG. Adverse effect of anticonvulsants on efficacy of chemotherapy for acute lymphoblastic leukemia. Lancet. 2000;356:285–90.
9. Song I, Weller S, Patel J, Borland J, Wynne B, Choukour M, Jerva F, Piscitelli S. Effect of carbamazepine on dolutegravir pharmacokinetics and dosing recommendation. Eur J Clin Pharmacol. 2016;72:665–70.
10. Ohgami M, Kaburagi T, Kurosawa A, Homma M. Drug interaction between erlotinib and phenytoin for brain metastases in a patient with nonsmall cell lung cancer. Lung Cancer. 2016;101:9–10.
11. Rodman JH, Murry DJ, Madden T, Santana VM. Altered etoposide pharmacokinetics and time to engraftment in pediatric patients undergoing autologous bone marrow transplantation. J Clin Oncol. 1994;12:2390–7.
12. Chhun S, Verstuyft C, Rizzo-Padoin N, Simoneau G, Becquemont L, Peretti I, Swaisland A, Wortelboer R, Bergmann JF, Mouly S. Gefitinib-phenytoin interaction is not correlated with the 14C-erythromycin breath test in healthy male volunteers. Br J Clin Pharmacol. 2009;68:226–37.
13. van den Bent MJ, Grisold W, Frappaz D, Stupp R, Desir JP, Lesimple T, Dittrich CV, de Jong MJA, Brandes A, Frenay M, Carpentier AF, Chollet P, Oliveira J, Baron B, Lacombe D, Schuessler M, Fumoleau P. European Organisation for Research and Treatment of Cancer (EORTC) open label phase II study on glufosfamide administered as a 60-minute infusion every 3 weeks in recurrent glioblastoma multiforme. Ann Oncol. 2003;14:1732–4.
14. Lokiec F, Santoni J, Weill S, Tubiana-Hulin M. Phenobarbital administration does not affect high-dose ifosfamide pharmacokinetics in humans. Anti-Cancer Drugs. 1996;7:893–6.
15. Ghosn M, Carde P, Leclerq B, Flamant F, Friedman S, Droz JP, Hayat M. Ifosfamide/mesa related encephalopathy: a case report with possible role of phenobarbital in enhancing neurotoxicity. Bull Cancer. 1988;74:391–2.
16. Ducharme MP, Bernstein ML, Granvil CP, Gehrcke B, Wainer IW. Phenytoin-induced alteration in the N-dechloroethylation of ifosfamide stereoisomers. Cancer Chemother Pharmacol. 1997;40:531–2.
17. Pursche S, Schleyer E, von Bonin M, Ehningger G, Said SM, Prondzinsky R, Illmer T, Wang Y, Hosius C, Nikolova Z, Bornhauser M, Dresemann G. Influence of enzyme-inducing antiepileptic drugs on trough level of imatinib in glioblastoma patients. Curr Clin Pharmacol. 2008;3:198–203.
18. Reardon DA, Egorin MJ, Quinn JA, Rich JN, Gururangan I, Vredenburgh JJ, Desjardins A, Sathornsumetee S, et al. Phase II study of imatinib mesylate plus hydroxyurea in adults with recurrent glioblastoma multiforme. J Clin Oncol. 2005;23:9359–68.
19. Gajjar A, Chintagumpala MM, Bowers DC, Jones-Wallace D, Stewart CF, Crews KR. Effect of intrapatient dosage escalation of irinotecan on its pharmacokinetics in patients who have high-grade gliomas receiving enzyme-inducing anticonvulsant therapy. Cancer. 2003;95(Suppl):2374–80.
20. Innocenti F, Undevia SD, Ramirez J, Mani S, Schilsky RL, Vogelzang NJ, Prado M, Ratain MJ. A phase I trial of pharmacological modulation or irinotecan with cyclosporine and phenobarbital. Clin Pharmacol Ther. 2004;76:490–502.

21. Gilbert MR, Supko JG, Batchelor T, Lesser G, Fisher JD, Piantadosi S, Grossman S. Phase I clinical and pharmacokinetic study of irinotecan in adults with recurrent malignant glioma. Clin Cancer Res. 2003;9:2940–9.
22. de Jong FA, van der Bol JM, Mathijssen RHJ, Loos WJ, Mathot RAA, Kitzen JJEM, van den Bent MJ, Verweij J. Irinotecan chemotherapy during valproic acid treatment. Pharmacokinetic interaction and hepatotoxicity. Cancer Biol Ther. 2007;6:1368–74.
23. Smith DA, Koch KM, Arya N, Bowen CJ, Herendeen JM, Beelen A. Effects of ketoconazole and carbamazepine on lapatinib pharmacokinetics in healthy subjects. Br J Clin Pharmacol. 2009;67:421–6.
24. Reeves D, DiDominick S, Finn S, Kim HJ. Shake A Methotrexate elimination when coadministered with levetiracetam. Annals Pharmacother. 2016;50:1016–22.
25. Lou U, Kwok J, Nguyen TA, Zhou A, Luk SO. Effect of levetiracetam on time to high-dose methotrexate clearance in patients with hematologic malignances. J Clin Pharmacol. 2020;60:324–30.
26. Riva M, Landonio G, Defanti CA, Siena S. The effect of anticonvulsant drugs on blood levels of methotrexate. J Neuro-Oncol. 2000;48:249–50.
27. Chang SM, Kuhn JG, Rizzo J, Robins HA, Schold SC, Spence AM, Berger MS, Mehta MP, Bozik ME, Pollack I, Gilbert M, Fulton D, Rankin C, Malec M, Prados MD. Phase I study of paclitaxel in patients with recurrent malignant glioma: a North American brain tumor consortium report. J Clin Oncol. 1998;16:2188–94.
28. Kasserra C, Assaf M, Hoffmann M, Li Y, Liu L, Wang X, Kumar G, Palmisano M. Pomalidomide: evaluation of cytochrome P450 and transporter-mediated drug-drug interaction potential in vitro and healthy subjects. J Clin Pharmacol. 2015;55:168–78.
29. Lehmann DF, Hurteau TE, Newman N, Coyle TE. Anticonvulsant usage is associated with increased risk of procarbazine hypersensitivity reactions in patients with brain tumors. Clin Pharmacol Ther. 1997;62:225–9.
30. Grossman SA, Carson KA, Batchelo TT, Lesser G, Mikkelsen T, Alavi JB, Phuphanich S, Hammour T, Fisher JD, Supko JG. The effect of enzyme-inducing antiseizure drugs on the pharmacokinetics and tolerability of procarbazine hydrochloride. Clin Cancer Res. 2006;12:5174–81.
31. Gryn SE, Teft WA, Kim RB. Profound reduction in the tamoxifen active metabolite endoxifen in a patient on phenytoin for epilepsy compared with a CYP2D6 genotype matched cohort. Pharmacogenet Genomics. 2014;24:367–9.
32. Boni J, Leister C, Burns J, Cincotta M, Hug B, Moore L. Pharmacokinetic profile of temsirolimus with concomitant administration of cytochrome P450-inducing medication. J Clin Pharmacol. 2007;47:1430–9.
33. Baker DK, Relling MV, Pui CH, Christensen ML, Evans WE, Rodman JH. Increased teniposide clearance with concomitant anticonvulsant therapy. J Clin Oncol. 1992;10:311–5.
34. Zamboni WC, Gajja AJ, Heideman RL, Beijnen JH, Rosing H, Houghton PJ, Stewart CF. Phenytoin alters the disposition of topotecan and N-desmethyl topotecan in a patient with medulloblastoma. Clin Cancer Res. 1998;4:783–9.
35. Villikka K, Kivisto KT, Maenpaa H, Joensuu H, Neuvonen PJ. Cytochrome P450-inducing antiepileptics increase the clearance of vincristine in patients with brain tumors. Clin Pharmacol Ther. 1999;66:589–93.

Antiulcer Drugs

Histamine H_2-Receptor Antagonists

Cimetidine

Gabapentin	Gabapentin does not affect the pharmacokinetics of cimetidine [1]
Phenobarbital	Phenobarbital decreases mean plasma cimetidine AUC values by 15% [2]

Proton-Pump Inhibitors

Omeprazole

Carbamazepine	Carbamazepine enhances the metabolism of omeprazole, via an action on CYP3A4, and can decrease plasma omeprazole AUC values by 40% [3]
Cenobamate	Cenobamate inhibits the metabolism of omeprazole, via an action on CYP2C19, and can increase plasma omeprazole AUC values by 107% [4]
Lacosamide	Lacosamide does not affect the pharmacokinetics of omeprazole [5]

References

1. Lal R, Sukbuntherng J, Luo W, Vicente V, Blumenthal R, Ho J, Cundy KC. Clinical pharmacokinetic drug interaction studies of gabapentin enacarbil, a novel transporter prodrug of gabapentin, with naproxen and cimetidine. Br J Clin Pharmacol. 2010;69:498–507.
2. Somogyi A, Thielscher S, Gugler R. Influence of phenobarbital treatment on cimetidine kinetics. Eur J Clin Pharmacol. 1981;19:343–7.

P. N. Patsalos, *Antiseizure Medication Interactions*,
https://doi.org/10.1007/978-3-030-82790-8_69

3. Bertilsson L, Tybring G, Widen J, Chang M, Tomson T. Carbamazepine treatment induces the CYP3A4 catalysed sulphoxidation of omeprazole, but has no or less effect on hydroxylation via CYP2C19. Br J Clin Pharmacol. 1997;44:186–9.
4. Bialer M, Johannessen SI, Koepp MJ, Levy RH, Perucca E, Perucca P, Tomson T, White HS. Progress report on new antiepileptic drugs: A summary of the fifteenth Eilat conference on new antiepileptic drugs and devices (EILAT XV). II Drugs in more advanced clinical development. Epilepsia. 2020;61:2365–85.
5. Cawello W, Mueller-Voessing C, Fichtner A. Pharmacokinetics of omeprazole coadministration in healthy volunteers: results from a phase I randomized, crossover trial. Clin Drug Investig. 2014;34:317–25.

Cardiovascular Drugs

Antianginals

Ivabradine

Carbamazepine	Carbamazepine enhances the metabolism of ivabradine, via an action on CYP3A4, and can decrease mean plasma ivabradine C_{max} and AUC values by 77% and 80%, respectively [1]
Phenytoin	Phenytoin enhances the metabolism of ivabradine and can decrease mean plasma ivabradine C_{max} and AUC values by 65% and 69%, respectively [2]

Antiarrhythmics

Amiodarone

Phenytoin	Phenytoin enhances the metabolism of amiodarone and can decrease mean plasma amiodarone levels by 32–49% [3]

Disopyramide

Phenytoin	Phenytoin enhances the metabolism of disopyramide and can decrease mean plasma disopyramide AUC values by 53% and decrease mean plasma disopyramide elimination half-life values by 51%. That there is a concurrent increase (up to 150%) in the AUC values of the pharmacologically active metabolite (mono-*N*-dealkyl disopyramide) of disopyramide complicates the interpretation of this interaction [4, 5]

P. N. Patsalos, *Antiseizure Medication Interactions*,
https://doi.org/10.1007/978-3-030-82790-8_70

Mexiletine

Phenytoin	Phenytoin enhances the metabolism of mexiletine and can decrease mean plasma mexiletine AUC values by 55% and decrease mean plasma mexiletine elimination half-life values by 51% [6]

Quinidine

Phenobarbital	Phenobarbital enhances the metabolism of quinidine, via an action on CYP3A4, and can decrease mean plasma quinidine elimination half-life values by 50% and increase mean plasma quinidine clearance values by 60% [7]
Phenytoin	Phenytoin enhances the metabolism of quinidine, via an action on CYP3A4, and can decrease mean plasma quinidine elimination half-life values by 50% and increase mean plasma quinidine clearance values by 60% [7]
Primidone	Primidone enhances the metabolism of quinidine, via an action on CYP3A4, and can decrease plasma quinidine levels [7]

Antihypertensive Agents

Atenolol

Phenobarbital	Phenobarbital can enhance the metabolism of atenolol and can decrease mean plasma AUC values by 24% [8]

Diazoxide

Phenytoin	Phenytoin enhances the metabolism of diazoxide and can decrease plasma diazoxide levels [9]

Digoxin

Eslicarbazepine acetate	Eslicarbazepine acetate can decrease mean plasma digoxin C_{max} values by 19% and mean plasma digoxin AUC values by 8% [10]
Lacosamide	Lacosamide does not affect the pharmacokinetics of digoxin [11]
Levetiracetam	Levetiracetam does not affect the pharmacokinetics of digoxin [12]
Phenytoin	Phenytoin enhances the metabolism of digoxin and can decrease mean plasma digoxin half-life values by 30%, decrease mean plasma digoxin AUC values by 23% and decrease plasma digoxin levels by 22% [13]
Tiagabine	Tiagabine does not affect the pharmacokinetics of digoxin [14]
Topiramate	Topiramate can increase plasma digoxin clearance by 13%, decrease plasma digoxin C_{max} values by 16%, and decrease plasma digoxin AUC values by 12% [15]

Diltiazem

Topiramate	Topiramate can increase mean plasma diltiazem AUC values by 20% [16]

Felodipine

Carbamazepine	Carbamazepine enhances the metabolism of felodipine and can decrease mean plasma felodipine AUC values by 94% and mean plasma felodipine levels by 82% [17]
Phenobarbital	Phenobarbital enhances the metabolism of felodipine and can decrease mean plasma felodipine AUC values by 94% and mean plasma felodipine levels by 82% [17]
Phenytoin	Phenytoin enhances the metabolism of felodipine and can decrease mean plasma felodipine AUC values by 94% and mean plasma felodipine levels by 82% [17]
Oxcarbazepine	Oxcarbazepine enhances the metabolism of felodipine and can decrease mean plasma felodipine C_{max} values by 34% and mean felodipine AUC values by 28% [18]

Flunarizine

Topiramate	Topiramate does not affect the pharmacokinetics of flunarizine [16]

Losartan

Phenytoin	Phenytoin can increase mean plasma losartan AUC values by 17% and can decrease mean plasma AUC values of the pharmacologically active carboxylic acid metabolite (E3174) of losartan by 63%. The mechanism of the interaction is via an inhibition of CYP2C9-mediated conversion of losartan to E3174 [19]

Nifedipine

Phenobarbital	Phenobarbital enhances the metabolism of nifedipine and can decrease plasma nifedipine AUC values by 60% [20]
Phenytoin	Phenytoin does not affect the pharmacokinetics of nifedipine [21]

Nilvadipine

Carbamazepine	Carbamazepine enhances the metabolism of nilvadipine and can decrease plasma nilvadipine levels [22]

Nimodipine

Carbamazepine	Carbamazepine enhances the metabolism of nimodipine and can decrease mean plasma nimodipine AUC values by 86% [23]
Phenobarbital	Phenobarbital enhances the metabolism of nimodipine and can decrease mean plasma nimodipine AUC values by 86% [23]
Phenytoin	Phenytoin enhances the metabolism of nimodipine and can decrease mean plasma nimodipine AUC values by 86% [23]
Valproic acid	Valproic acid inhibits the metabolism of nimodipine and can increase mean plasma nimodipine AUC values by 54% [23]

Nisoldipine

Phenytoin	Phenytoin enhances the metabolism of nisoldipine and can decrease mean plasma nisoldipine AUC values by 90% [24]

Propranolol

Phenobarbital	Phenobarbital enhances the metabolism of propranolol and can decrease plasma propranolol levels [25]
Phenytoin	Phenytoin enhances the metabolism of propranolol and can decrease plasma propranolol levels [25]
Topiramate	Topiramate inhibits the metabolism of propranolol and can increase mean plasma propranolol AUC values by 17% [26]

Verapamil

Phenobarbital	Phenobarbital enhances the metabolism of verapamil and can increase mean verapamil plasma clearance by 4.3-fold and decrease mean plasma verapamil AUC values by 70% [27]
Phenytoin	Phenytoin enhances the metabolism of verapamil and can decrease plasma verapamil levels [28]

Diuretics

Furosemide (Frusemide)

Phenytoin	Phenytoin delays and reduces the magnitude of the diuretic effect of furosemide. It is thought that the mechanism of this interaction is a phenytoin-induced decrease in the spontaneous activity of gastrointestinal smooth muscle leading to reduced furosemide absorption [29]
	Additionally, a pharmacodynamic interaction might occur since renal responsiveness to furosemide is also impaired [29]

Hydrochlorothiazide

Topiramate	Topiramate does not affect the pharmacokinetics of hydrochlorothiazide [16]

Oral Anticoagulants

Apixaban

Phenobarbital	Phenobarbital can decrease plasma apixaban levels [30]
Phenytoin	Phenytoin increases the incidence of a serious bleed by 93% [31]

Dabigatran

Carbamazepine	Carbamazepine can decrease plasma dabigatran levels, probably via enhancement of PgP activity [32]
Phenobarbital	Phenobarbital can decrease plasma dabigatran levels, probably via enhancement of PgP activity [33]
Phenytoin	Phenytoin can decrease plasma dabigatran levels, probably via enhancement of CYP3A4 and PgP activities [34]

Dicoumarol

Phenytoin	Phenytoin enhances the metabolism of dicoumarol, possibly via an action on CYP2C9, and can reduce the anticoagulant effects of dicoumarol [35]

Phenprocoumon

Carbamazepine	Carbamazepine reduces the anticoagulant effects of phenprocoumon, possibly by increasing its metabolism [36]
Valproic acid	Valproic acid does not affect the anticoagulant effect of phenprocoumon [36]

Rivaroxaban

Carbamazepine	Carbamazepine can decrease plasma rivaroxaban levels, probably via enhancement of PgP activity [37]
Levetiracetam	Levetiracetam can decrease rivaroxaban plasma levels [38]
Oxcarbazepine	Oxcarbazepine can decrease plasma rivaroxaban levels, probably via induction of CYP3A4 [39]
Phenytoin	Phenytoin can decrease plasma rivaroxaban levels, probably via enhancement of CYP3A4 and PgP activities [40]
Valproic acid	Valproic acid can increase plasma rivaroxaban levels [41]

Warfarin

Carbamazepine	Carbamazepine enhances the metabolism of warfarin resulting in a decrease in plasma warfarin half-life values, a decrease in plasma warfarin levels, and a decrease in the prothrombin time response to warfarin. Typically, a twofold increase in warfarin dosage is required so as to maintain an appropriate international normalized ratio (INR). Because enzyme induction may take several weeks to fully develop or subside, frequent monitoring of INR with appropriate dosage adjustment is advised for at least 4 weeks after starting or stopping carbamazepine [42, 43]
	Upon carbamazepine discontinuation, warfarin levels will increase and may lead to potentially fatal hemorrhage [44]
Cannabidiol	Cannabidiol inhibits the metabolism of warfarin resulting in an increased INR [45]
Cenobamate	Cenobamate does not affect the pharmacokinetics of warfarin [46]
Eslicarbazepine acetate	Eslicarbazepine acetate has no effect on the pharmacokinetics of R-warfarin, but decreases mean plasma S-warfarin C_{max} and AUC values by 20% and 21%, respectively. INR values are increased by 4% but are not accompanied by a change in bleeding time [47]
Felbamate	Felbamate inhibits the metabolism of warfarin resulting in an increased INR [48]
Lacosamide	Lacosamide does not affect the pharmacokinetics of warfarin [49]
Levetiracetam	Levetiracetam does not affect the pharmacokinetics of warfarin [50]
Oxcarbazepine	Oxcarbazepine does not affect the pharmacokinetics of warfarin [51]
Perampanel	Perampanel does not affect the plasma protein binding of warfarin [52]
Phenobarbital	Phenobarbital enhances the metabolism of warfarin and decreases the prothrombin time response to warfarin. Typically, a 25–50% increase in warfarin dosage is required. Because enzyme induction may take several weeks to fully develop or subside, frequent monitoring of INR with appropriate dosage adjustment is advised for at least 4 weeks after starting or stopping phenobarbital [53]
Phenytoin	Despite an expected induction of warfarin metabolism by phenytoin, several cases of hypoprothrombinemia and severe bleeding complications have been reported after the addition of phenytoin to warfarin. Proposed mechanisms for an enhanced anticoagulant response are displacement of warfarin from plasma protein binding sites or inhibition of its metabolism by phenytoin [54, 55]
	Because of potential induction and inhibition of warfarin metabolism via CYP 2C9 by phenytoin, the occurrence of a biphasic interaction has been suggested, with warfarin plasma levels initially increasing due to inhibition and then decreasing after 1–2 weeks as enzyme induction predominates. Thus, the interaction between phenytoin and warfarin is complex in that after an initial enhancement in anticoagulant action, the latter can be subsequently decreased [56]
	Due to the unpredictability of this interaction, frequent monitoring of INR with appropriate dosage adjustment is advised for at least 4 weeks after starting or stopping phenytoin
Primidone	Primidone may enhance the metabolism of warfarin, resulting in a decreased INR value [57]

Tiagabine	Tiagabine does not affect the pharmacokinetics of warfarin [58]
Valproic acid	Valproic acid can displace warfarin from its plasma protein binding sites, increase free pharmacologically active plasma warfarin levels, and lead to an increase in INR [59]

Statins

Atorvastatin

Lamotrigine	Lamotrigine increases mean plasma atorvastatin C_{max} values by 14% and mean plasma 2OH-atorvastatin and 4OH-atorvastatin (pharmacologically active metabolites) levels by 20% and 21%, respectively. Inhibition through an effect on UGT1A1 and UGT1A3 is considered to be the mechanism of this interaction [60]
Phenytoin	Phenytoin decreases mean plasma atorvastatin C_{max} values by 24% and mean plasma 2OH-atorvastatin and 4OH-atorvastatin (pharmacologically active metabolites) levels by 22% and 52%, respectively. Induction through an effect on CYP3A4 is considered to be the mechanism of this interaction [60]

Rosuvastatin

Oxcarbazepine	Oxcarbazepine decreases the bioavailability of rosuvastatin, possibly via an action on uptake transporters, and can decrease mean AUC values by 36–39% [61]

Simvastatin

Carbamazepine	Carbamazepine enhances the metabolism of simvastatin, probably via an action on CYP3A4, and decreases mean plasma simvastatin and simvastatin acid AUC values by 75% and 82%, respectively [62]
Eslicarbazepine acetate	Eslicarbazepine acetate enhances the metabolism of simvastatin, probably via an action on CYP3A4, and decreases mean plasma simvastatin, and its pharmacologically active metabolite simvastatin-β-hydroxy acid, AUC values by up to 54% [63]
Phenytoin	Phenytoin enhances the metabolism of simvastatin, probably via an action on CYP3A4, and decreases plasma simvastatin levels [64]

References

1. Vlase L, Neag M, Popa A, Muntean D, Baldea I, Leucuta SE. Pharmacokinetic interaction between ivabradine and carbamazepine in healthy volunteers. J Clin Pharm Ther. 2011;36:225–9.

2. Vlase L, Popa A, Neag M, Muntean D, Leucuta SE. Pharmacokinetic interaction between ivabradine and phenytoin in healthy subjects. Clin Drug Investig. 2012;32:533–8.
3. Nolan PE, Marcus FI, Karol MD, Hoyer GL, Gear K. Effect of phenytoin on the clinical pharmacokinetics of amiodarone. J Clin Pharmacol. 1990;30:1112–9.
4. Aitio ML, Mansuri L, Tala E, Haataja M, Aitio A. The effect of enzyme induction on the metabolism of disopyramide in man. Br J Clin Pharmacol. 1981;11:279–85.
5. Nightingale J, Nappi JM. Effect of phenytoin on serum disopyramide concentrations. Clin Pharm. 1987;6:46–50.
6. Begg EJ, Chinwah PM, Webb C, Day RO, Wade DN. Enhanced metabolism of mexiletine after phenytoin administration. Br J Clin Pharmacol. 1982;14:219–23.
7. Data JL, Wilkinson GR, Nies AS. Interaction of quinidine with anticonvulsant drugs. N Engl J Med. 1976;294:699–702.
8. Mantyla R, Mannisto P, Nykanen S, Koponen A, Lamminsivu U. Pharmacokinetic interactions of timolol with vasodilating drugs, food and phenobarbital in healthy human volunteers. Eur J Clin Pharmacol. 1983;24:227–30.
9. Petro TF, Vannucci RC, Kulin HE. Diazoxide-diphenylhydantoin interaction. J Pediatr. 1976;89:331–2.
10. Vaz-da-Silva M, Costa R, Soares E, Maia J, Falcao A, Almeida L, Soares-da-Silva P. Effect of eslicarbazepine acetate on the pharmacokinetics of digoxin in healthy subjects. Fundam Clin Pharmacol. 2009;23:509–14.
11. Cawello W, Mueller-Voessing C, Andreas JO. Effect of lacosamide on steady-state pharmacokinetics of digoxin: results from a phase I, multiple-dose, double-blind, randomised, placebo-controlled, crossover trial. Clin Drug Investig. 2014;34:327–34.
12. Patsalos PN. Pharmacokinetic profile of levetiracetam: toward ideal characteristics. Pharmacol Ther. 2000;85:77–85.
13. Rameis H. On the interaction between phenytoin and digoxin. Eur J Clin Pharmacol. 1985;29:49–53.
14. Snel S, Jansen JA, Pedersen PC, Jonkman JH, van Heiningen PN. Tiagabine, a novel antiepileptic agent: lack of pharmacokinetic interaction with digoxin. Eur J Clin Pharmacol. 1998;54:355–7.
15. Liao S, Palmer M. Digoxin and topiramate drug interaction study in male volunteers. Pharm Res. 1993;10(Suppl):S405.
16. Summary of Product Characteristics: Topiramate (Topamax). Janssen-Cilag Ltd. Last update 14th January 2021.
17. Capewell S, Freestone S, Critchley JAJH, Pottage A, Prescott LF. Reduced felodipine bioavailability in patients taking anticonvulsants. Lancet. 1988;2(8609):480–2.
18. Zaccara G, Gangemi PF, Bendoni L, Menge GP, Schwabe S, Monza GC. Influence of single and repeated doses of oxcarbazepine on the pharmacokinetic profile of felodipine. Ther Drug Monit. 1993;15:39–42.
19. Fischer TL, Pieper JA, Graff DW, Rodgers JE, Fischer JD, Parnell KJ, Goldstein JA, Greenwood R, Patterson JH. Evaluation of potential losartan-phenytoin drug interactions in healthy volunteers. Clin Pharmacol Ther. 2002;72:238–46.
20. Schellens JHM, van der Wart JHF, Brugman M, Breimer DD. Influence of enzyme induction and inhibition on the oxidation of nifedipine, sparteine, mephenytoin and antipyrine in humans as assessed by a "cocktail" study design. J Pharmacol Exp Ther. 1989;249:638–45.
21. Schellens JHM, Soons PA, van der Wart JHF, Hoevers JW, Breimer DD. Lack of pharmacokinetic interaction between nifedipine, sparteine and phenytoin in man. Br J Clin Pharmacol. 1991;31:175–8.
22. Yasui-Furukori N, Tateishi T. Carbamazepine decreases antihypertensive effect of nilvadipine. J Clin Pharmacol. 2002;42:100–3.
23. Tartara A, Galimberti CA, Manni R, Parietti L, Zucca C, Baasch H, Caresia L, Muck W, Barzaghi N, Gatti G, Perucca E. Differential effects of valproic acid and enzyme-inducing anticonvulsants on nimodipine pharmacokinetics in epileptic patients. Br J Clin Pharmacol. 1991;32:335–40.

24. Michelucci R, Cipolla G, Passarelli D, Gatti G, Ochan M, Heinig R, Tassinari CA, Perucca E. Reduced plasma nisoldipine concentrations in phenytoin-treated patients with epilepsy. Epilepsia. 1996;37:1107–10.
25. Wood AJ, Feely J. Pharmacokinetic drug interactions with propranolol. Clin Pharmacokinet. 1983;8:253–62.
26. Bialer M, Doose DR, Murthy B, Curtin C, Wang SS, Twyman RE, Schwabe S. Pharmacokinetic interactions of topiramate. Clin Pharmacokinet. 2004;43:763–80.
27. Rutledge DR, Pieper JA, Mirvis DM. Effects of chronic phenobarbital on verapamil disposition in humans. J Pharmacol Exp Ther. 1988;246:7–13.
28. Woocock BG, Kirsten R, Nelson K, Rietbrock S, Hopf R, Kaltenbach M. A reduction in verapamil concentrations with phenytoin. N Engl J Med. 1991;325:1179.
29. Fine A, Henderson IA, Morgan DR. Malabsorption of frusemide caused by phenytoin. Br Med J. 1977;2:1061–2.
30. King PK, Stump TA, Walkama AM, Ash BM, Bowling SM. Management of phenobarbital and apixaban interaction in recurrent cardioembolic stroke. Ann Pharmacother. 2018;52:605–6.
31. Chang SH, Chou IJ, Yeh YH. Association between use of non-vitamin K oral anticoagulants with and without concurrent medications and risk of major bleeding in nonvalvular atrial fibrillation. J Am Med Assoc. 2017;318:1250–9.
32. Laureano M, Crowther M, Eikelboom J, Boonywat K. Measurement of dabigatran drug levels to manage patients taking interacting drugs: A case report. Am J Med. 2016;129:E247–8.
33. Chin PKL, Wright DFB, Xhang M, Wallace MC, Robert RL, Paterson DM, et al. Correlation between trough plasma dabigatran concentrations and estimates of glomerular filtration rate based on creatinine and cystatin C. Drugs R D. 2014;14:113–23.
34. Hager N, Bolt J, Albers L, Wojcik W, Duffy P, Semichuk W. Development of left atrial thrombus after coadministration of dabigatran elexilate and phenytoin. Can J Cardiol. 2017;33:554e13–4.
35. Hansen JM, Siersboeck-Nielsen K, Kristensen M, Skovsted L, Christensen LK. Effect of diphenylhydantoin on the metabolism of dicoumarol in man. Acta Med Scand. 1971;189:15–9.
36. Schlienger R, Kurmann M, Drewe J, Muller-Spahn F, Seifritz E. Inhibition of phenprocoumon anticoagulation by carbamazepine. Eur Neuropsychopharmacol. 2000;10:219–21.
37. Stollberger C, Finsterer J. Recurrent venous thrombosis under rivaroxaban and carbamazepine for symptomatic epilepsy. Neurol Neurochir Pol. 2017;51:194–6.
38. Paciullo F, Costa C, Gresele P. Rivaroxaban plasma levels and levetiracetam. Ann Intern Med. 2020;173:71–2.
39. Serra W, Li Calzi K, Coruzzi P. Left atrial appendage thrombosis during therapy with rivaroxaban in elective cardioversion for permanent atrial fibrillation. Clin Pract. 2015;5:788.
40. Becerra AE, Amuchastegui T, Tabares AH. Decreased rivaroxaban levels in a patient with cerebral vein thrombosis receiving phenytoin. Case Rep Hematol. 2017:4760612.
41. Stollberger C, Finsterer J, Stollberger C, Finsterer J. Prolonged anticoagulant activity of rivaroxaban in a polymorbid elderly female with non-convulsive epileptic state. Hear Lung. 2014;43:262–3.
42. Hansen JM, Siersboeck-Nielsen K, Skovsted L. Carbamazepine induced acceleration of diphenylhydantoin and warfarin metabolism in man. Clin Pharmacol Ther. 1971;12:539–43.
43. Clark NP, Hoang K, Delate T, Horn JR, Witt DM. Warfarin interaction with hepatic cytochrome P-450 enzyme-inducing anticonvulsants. Clin Applied Thrombo Hemostas. 2018;24:172–8.
44. Denbow CE, Fraser HS. Clinically significant hemorrhage due to warfarin-carbamazepine interaction. South Med J. 1990;83:981.
45. Grayson L, Brannon V, Nichol K, Szaflarski JP. for the UAB CBD program. An interaction between warfarin and cannabidiol, a case report. Epilepsy Behav Case Reports. 2019;9:10–1.
46. Summary of Product Characteristics: Cenobamate (XCopri). SK Life Science Inc. Last update August 2020.
47. Vaz-da-Silva M, Almeida L, Falcao A, Soares E, Maia J, Nunes T, Soares-da-Silva P. Effect of eslicarbazepine acetate on the steady-state pharmacokinetics and pharmacodynamics of

warfarin in healthy subjects during a three-stage, open-label, multiple-dose, single-period study. Clin Ther. 2010;32:179–92.
48. Tisdel KA, Israel DS, Kolb KW. Warfarin-felbamate interaction: first report. Ann Pharmacother. 1994;28:805.
49. Stockis A, van Lier JJ, Cawello W, Kumke T, Eckhardt K. Lack of effect of lacosamide on the pharmacokinetic and pharmacodynamic profiles of warfarin. Epilepsia. 2013;54:1161–6.
50. Ragueneau-Majlessi I, Levy RH, Meyerhoff C. Lack of effect of repeated administration of levetiracetam on the pharmacodynamic and pharmacokinetic profiles of warfarin. Epilepsy Res. 2001;47:55–63.
51. Kramer G, Tettenborn B, Klosterskov Jense P, Menge GP, Stoll KD. Oxcarbazepine does not affect the anticoagulant activity of warfarin. Epilepsia. 1992;33:1145–8.
52. Gidal BE, Ferry J, Laurenza A, Ueno T. Potential protein-binding displacement interactions with perampanel: An in vitro analysis. Epilepsy Res. 2019;149:102–6.
53. MacDonald MG, Robinson DS. Clinical observation of possible barbiturate interference with anticoagulants. J Am Med Assoc. 1968;204:97–100.
54. Nappi JM. Warfarin and phenytoin interaction. Ann Intern Med. 1979;90:852.
55. Panegyres PK, Rischbieth RH. Fatal phenytoin warfarin interaction. Postgrad Med J. 1991;67:98.
56. Levine M, Sheppard I. Biphasic interaction of phenytoin with warfarin. Clin Pharm. 1984;3:200–3.
57. Rindone JP, Mellen CK. Warfarin resistance from primidone in patient with essential tremor. Eur J Clin Pharmacol. 2018;74:377–8.
58. Mengel H, Jansen JA, Sommerville K, Jonkman JHG, Wesnes K, Cohen A, Carlson GF, Marshall R, Snel S, Dirach J, Kastberg H. Tiagabine: evaluation of the risk of interaction with theophylline, warfarin, digoxin, cimetidine, oral contraceptives, triazolam, or ethanol. Epilepsia. 1995;36(Suppl 3):S160.
59. Yoon HW, Giraldo EA, Wijdicks EF. Valproic acid and warfarin: an under recognised drug interaction. Neurocrit Care. 2011;15:182–5.
60. Bullman J, Nichols A, Van Landingham K, Fleck R, Vuong A, Miller J, Alexander S, Messenheimer J. Effects of lamotrigine and phenytoin on the pharmacokinetics of atorvastatin in healthy volunteers. Epilepsia. 2011;52:1351–8.
61. Gidal BE, Mintzer S, Schwab M, Schutz R, Kharidia J, Blum D, Grinnell T, Sunkaraneni S. Evidence for a pharmacokinetic interaction between eslicarbazepine and rosuvastatin: Potential effects on xenobiotic transporters. Epilepsy Res. 2017;135:64–70.
62. Ucar M, Neuvonen M, Luurial H, Dahlqvist R, Neuvonen PJ, Mjorndal T. Carbamazepine markedly reduces serum concentrations of simvastatin and simvastatin acid. Eur J Clin Pharmacol. 2004;59:879–82.
63. Falcao A, Pinto R, Nunes T, Soares-da-Silva P. Effect of repeated administration of eslicarbazepine acetate on the pharmacokinetics of simvastatin in healthy subjects. Epilepsy Res. 2013;106:244–9.
64. Murphy MJ, Dominiczak MH. Efficacy of statin therapy: possible effect of phenytoin. Postgrad Med J. 1999;75:359–60.

Immunosuppressants

Cyclosporine A

Acetazolamide	Acetazolamide can increase plasma cyclosporine levels [1]
Carbamazepine	Carbamazepine enhances the metabolism of cyclosporine, via an action on CYP3A4, and can decrease plasma cyclosporine levels by >75% [2, 3]
Levetiracetam	Levetiracetam does not affect the pharmacokinetics of cyclosporine [4]
Oxcarbazepine	Oxcarbazepine can decrease plasma cyclosporine levels by up to 25% [5]
Phenobarbital	Phenobarbital enhances the metabolism of cyclosporine, via an action on CYP3A4, and can decrease plasma cyclosporine levels by up to 95% [6]
Phenytoin	Phenytoin enhances the metabolism of cyclosporine, via an action on CYP3A4, and can decrease mean plasma cyclosporine and mean whole blood cyclosporine AUC values by 47% and 44%, respectively [7]
Primidone	Primidone enhances the metabolism of cyclosporine, via an action on CYP3A4, and can decrease plasma cyclosporine levels [8]
Valproic acid	Valproic acid does not affect the pharmacokinetics of cyclosporine. However, its use, particularly in renal transplant recipients, should be weighed out against possible risks of hepatotoxicity consequent to its pharmacologically active metabolite(s) [2]

Everolimus

Cannabidiol	Cannabidiol inhibits the metabolism of everolimus and can increase plasma everolimus levels [9]

Lamivudine

Levetiracetam	Levetiracetam does not affect the pharmacokinetics of lamivudine [10]

P. N. Patsalos, *Antiseizure Medication Interactions*,
https://doi.org/10.1007/978-3-030-82790-8_71

Mycophenolate

Levetiracetam	Levetiracetam does not affect the pharmacokinetics of mycophenolate [10]

Sirolimus

Cannabidiol	Cannabidiol inhibits the metabolism of sirolimus and can increase plasma sirolimus levels [9]
Levetiracetam	Levetiracetam does not affect the pharmacokinetics of sirolimus [10]
Phenytoin	Phenytoin enhances the metabolism of sirolimus, via an action on CYP3A4/5, and can decrease plasma sirolimus levels by 74% [11]

Tacrolimus

Carbamazepine	Carbamazepine enhances the metabolism of tacrolimus, via induction of CYP3A, and can decrease plasma tacrolimus levels [12]
Levetiracetam	Levetiracetam does not affect the pharmacokinetics of tacrolimus [10, 13]
Phenytoin	Phenytoin enhances the metabolism of tacrolimus, via induction of CYP3A, and can decrease plasma tacrolimus levels [14]
Phenobarbital	Phenobarbital enhances the metabolism of tacrolimus, via induction of CYP3A, and can decrease plasma tacrolimus levels [13]

References

1. Keogh A, Esmore D, Spratt P, Savdie E, McCluskey P. Acetazolamide and cyclosporine. Transplantation. 1988;46:478–9.
2. Hillebrand G, Castro LA, Van Scheidt W, Beukelmann D, Land W, Schmidt D. Valproate for epilepsy in renal transplant recipients receiving cyclosporine. Transplantation. 1987;43:915–6.
3. Alvarez JS, Del Castillo JAS, Oriz MJA. Effect of carbamazepine on cyclosporine blood level. Nephron. 1991;58:235–6.
4. Franzoni E, Sarajlija J, Garone C, Malaspina E, Marchiani V. No kinetic interaction between levetiracetam and cyclosporine: a case report. J Child Neurol. 2007;22:440–2.
5. Rosche J, Froscher W, Abendroth D, Liebel J. Possible oxcarbazepine interaction with cyclosporine serum levels: a single case study. Clin Neuropharmacol. 2001;24:113–6.
6. Carstensen H, Jacobsen N, Dieperink H. Interaction between cyclosporine A and phenobarbitone. Br J Clin Pharmacol. 1986;21:550–1.
7. Freeman DJ, Laupacis A, Keown PA, Stiller CR, Carruthers SG. Evaluation of cyclosporine-phenytoin interaction with observation on cyclosporine metabolites. Br J Clin Pharmacol. 1984;18:887–93.
8. Klintmalm G, Sawe J, Ringden O, von Bahr C, Magnusson A. Cyclosporine plasma levels in renal transplant patients. Association with renal toxicity and allograft rejection. Transplantation. 1985;39:132–7.
9. Ebrahim-Fakhari D, Agricola KD, Tudor C, Krueger D, Franz DN. Cannabidiol elevates mechanistic target of rapamycin inhibitor levels in patients with tuberous sclerosis complex. Pediatr Neurol. 2020;105:59–61.

10. Lin CH, Chen CL, Lin TK, Chen NC, Tsai MH, Chuang YC. Levetiracetam in the treatment of epileptic seizures after liver transplantation. Medicine. 2015;94:e1350–3.
11. Fridell JA, Jain AKB, Patel K, Virji M, Rao KN, Fung JJ, Venkataramanan R. Phenytoin decreases the blood concentrations of sirolimus in a liver transplant recipient: a case report. Ther Drug Monit. 2003;25:117–9.
12. Wada K, Takada M, Sakai M, Ochi H, Kotake T, Okada H, Morishita H, Oda N, Mano A, Kato TS, Komamura K, Nakatani T. Drug interaction between tacrolimus and carbamazepine in a Japanese heart transplant recipient: a case report. J Heart Lung Transplant. 2009;28:409–11.
13. Siddiqi N, Marfo K. Clinically significant drug-drug interaction between tacrolimus and phenobarbital: the price we pay. J Pharm Pract. 2010;23:585–9.
14. Wada K, Takada M, Ueda T, Ochi H, Kotake T, Morishita H, Hanatani A, Nakatami T. Drug interaction between tacrolimus and phenytoin in Japanese heart transplant recipients: 2 case reports. Int J Clin Pharmacol Ther. 2007;45:524–8.

10. Lin CH, Chen CL, Lin TK, Chen NC, Tsai MH, Chuang YC. Levetiracetam in the treatment of epileptic seizures after liver transplantation. Medicine. 2015;94:e1350–3.
11. Fridell JA, Jain AKB, Patel K, Virji M, Rao KN, Fung JJ, Venkataramanan R. Phenytoin decreases the blood concentrations of sirolimus in a liver transplant recipient: a case report. Ther Drug Monit. 2003;25:117–9.
12. Wada K, Takada M, Sakai M, Ochi H, Kotake T, Okada H, Morishita H, Oda N, Mano A, Kato TS, Komamura K, Nakatani T. Drug interaction between tacrolimus and carbamazepine in a Japanese heart transplant recipient: a case report. J Heart Lung Transplant. 2007;26:409–11.
13. Siddiqi N, Marfo K. Clinically significant drug-drug interaction between tacrolimus and phenobarbital: the price we pay. J Pharm Pract. 2010;23:585–9.
14. Wada K, Takada M, Ueda T, Ochi H, Kotake T, Morishita H, Hanatani A, Nakatani T. Drug interactions between tacrolimus and phenytoin in Japanese heart transplant recipients: 2 case reports. Int J Clin Pharmacol Ther. 2007;45:524–8.

Neuromuscular Blocking Agents

Atracurium

Carbamazepine	Carbamazepine has been reported not to affect the pharmacokinetics of atracurium and also to enhance the metabolism of atracurium resulting in decreased duration of neuromuscular blockade and higher atracurium dosage requirements [1, 2]
Phenytoin	Phenytoin has been reported not to affect the pharmacokinetics of atracurium and also to enhance the metabolism of atracurium resulting in decreased duration of neuromuscular blockade and higher atracurium dosage requirements [1, 3]

Cisatracurium

Carbamazepine	Carbamazepine enhances the metabolism of cisatracurium and can increase plasma cisatracurium clearance by 25%. Patients receiving chronic therapy with carbamazepine show a decreased duration of neuromuscular blockade and higher cisatracurium dosage requirements. Both pharmacokinetic (enzyme induction) and pharmacodynamic (upregulation of acetylcholine receptors) mechanisms may explain this interaction [4]
Phenytoin	Phenytoin enhances the metabolism of cisatracurium and can increase plasma cisatracurium clearance by 25%. Patients receiving chronic therapy with phenytoin show a decreased duration of neuromuscular blockade and higher cisatracurium dosage requirements. Both pharmacokinetic (enzyme induction) and pharmacodynamic (upregulation of acetylcholine receptors) mechanisms may explain this interaction [4]

P. N. Patsalos, *Antiseizure Medication Interactions*,
https://doi.org/10.1007/978-3-030-82790-8_72

Doxacurium

Carbamazepine	Carbamazepine enhances the metabolism of doxacurium. Patients receiving chronic therapy with carbamazepine show a decreased duration of neuromuscular blockade and higher doxacurium dosage requirements. Both pharmacokinetic (enzyme induction) and pharmacodynamic (upregulation of acetylcholine receptors) mechanisms may explain this interaction [5]
Phenytoin	Phenytoin enhances the metabolism of doxacurium. Patients receiving chronic therapy with phenytoin show a decreased duration of neuromuscular blockade and higher doxacurium dosage requirements. Both pharmacokinetic (enzyme induction) and pharmacodynamic (upregulation of acetylcholine receptors) mechanisms may explain this interaction [5]

Mivacurium

Carbamazepine	Carbamazepine does not affect the pharmacokinetics of mivacurium [6]
Phenytoin	Phenytoin does not affect the pharmacokinetics of mivacurium [7]
Valproic acid	Valproic acid does not affect the pharmacokinetics of mivacurium [7]

Pancuronium

Carbamazepine	Carbamazepine enhances the metabolism of pancuronium. Patients receiving chronic therapy with carbamazepine show a decreased duration of neuromuscular blockade and higher pancuronium dosage requirements. Both pharmacokinetic (enzyme induction) and pharmacodynamic (upregulation of acetylcholine receptors) mechanisms may explain this interaction [8]
Phenytoin	Phenytoin enhances the metabolism of pancuronium. Patients receiving chronic therapy with phenytoin show a decreased duration of neuromuscular blockade and higher pancuronium dosage requirements. Both pharmacokinetic (enzyme induction) and pharmacodynamic (upregulation of acetylcholine receptors) mechanisms may explain this interaction [9]

Pipecuronium

Carbamazepine	Carbamazepine enhances the metabolism of pipecuronium. Patients receiving chronic therapy with carbamazepine show a decreased duration of neuromuscular blockade and higher pancuronium dosage requirements. Both pharmacokinetic (enzyme induction) and pharmacodynamic (upregulation of acetylcholine receptors) mechanisms may explain this interaction [10]

Rapacuronium

Carbamazepine	Carbamazepine enhances the metabolism of rapacuronium. Patients receiving chronic therapy with carbamazepine show a decreased duration of neuromuscular blockade and higher rapacuronium dosage requirements. Both pharmacokinetic (enzyme induction) and pharmacodynamic (upregulation of acetylcholine receptors) mechanisms may explain this interaction [11]
Phenytoin	Phenytoin enhances the metabolism of rapacuronium. Patients receiving chronic therapy with phenytoin show a decreased duration of neuromuscular blockade and higher rapacuronium dosage requirements. Both pharmacokinetic (enzyme induction) and pharmacodynamic (upregulation of acetylcholine receptors) mechanisms may explain this interaction [11]

Rocuronium

Carbamazepine	Carbamazepine enhances the metabolism of rocuronium. Patients receiving chronic therapy with carbamazepine show a decreased duration of neuromuscular blockade and higher rocuronium dosage requirements. Both pharmacokinetic (enzyme induction) and pharmacodynamic (upregulation of acetylcholine receptors) mechanisms may explain this interaction [12]
Phenytoin	Phenytoin does not affect the pharmacokinetics of rocuronium when administered acutely and instead results in a potentiation of neuromuscular block. However, when administered chronically, phenytoin enhances the metabolism of rocuronium. Patients receiving chronic therapy with phenytoin show a decreased duration of neuromuscular blockade and higher rocuronium dosage requirements. Both pharmacokinetic (enzyme induction) and pharmacodynamic (upregulation of acetylcholine receptors) mechanisms may explain this interaction [13, 14]
Primidone	Primidone enhances the metabolism of rocuronium. Patients receiving chronic therapy with primidone show a decreased duration of neuromuscular blockade and higher rocuronium dosage requirements. Both pharmacokinetic (enzyme induction) and pharmacodynamic (upregulation of acetylcholine receptors) mechanisms may explain this interaction [15]
Valproic acid	Valproic acid enhances the elimination of rocuronium, possibly via an action on P-glycoprotein [16]

Vecuronium

Carbamazepine	Carbamazepine enhances the metabolism of vecuronium and can decrease plasma vecuronium half-life values by 62% and can increase vecuronium clearance values by two-fold. Patients receiving chronic therapy with carbamazepine show a decreased duration of neuromuscular blockade and higher vecuronium dosage requirements. Both pharmacokinetic (enzyme induction) and pharmacodynamic (upregulation of acetylcholine receptors) mechanisms may explain this interaction [17]

Phenytoin	Phenytoin does not affect the pharmacokinetics of vecuronium when administered acutely and instead can result in a potentiation of neuromuscular block. However, when administered chronically, phenytoin enhances the metabolism of vecuronium and can decrease plasma vecuronium half-life values by 51% and can increase plasma vecuronium clearance values by 68%. Patients receiving chronic therapy with phenytoin show a decreased duration of neuromuscular blockade and higher vecuronium dosage requirements. Both pharmacokinetic (enzyme induction) and pharmacodynamic (upregulation of acetylcholine receptors) mechanisms may explain this interaction [18, 19]

References

1. Tempelhoff R, Modica PA, Jellish WS, Spitznagel EL. Resistance to atracurium-induced neuromuscular blockade in patients with intractable seizure disorders treated with anticonvulsants. Anesth Analg. 1990;71:665–9.
2. Spacek A, Neiger FX, Spiss CK, Kress HG. Atracurium-induced neuromuscular block is not affected by chronic anticonvulsant therapy with carbamazepine. Acta Anaesthesiol Scand. 1997;41:1308–11.
3. Ornstein E, Matteo RS, Schwartz AE, Silverberg PA, Young WL, Diaz J. The effect of phenytoin on the magnitude and duration of neuromuscular block after atracurium or vecuronium. Anesthesiology. 1987;67:191–6.
4. Richard A, Girard F, Girard DC, Boudreault D, Chouinard P, Moumdjian R, Bouthilier A, Ruel M, Couture J, Varin F. Cisatracurium-induced neuromuscular blockade is affected by chronic phenytoin or carbamazepine treatment in neurosurgical patients. Anesth Analg. 2005;100:538–44.
5. Ornstein E, Matteo RS, Weinstein JA, Halevy J, Young WL, Abou-Donia MM. Accelerated recovery from doxacurium-induced neuromuscular blockade in patients receiving chronic anticonvulsant therapy. J Clin Anesth. 1991;3:108–11.
6. Spacek A, Neiger FX, Spiss CK, Kress HG. Chronic carbamazepine therapy does not influence mivacurium-induced neuromuscular block. Br J Anaesth. 1996;77:500–2.
7. Jellish WS, Thalji Z, Brundidge PK, Tempelhoff R. Recovery from mivacurium-induced neuromuscular blockade is not affected by anticonvulsant therapy. J Neurosurg Anesthesiol. 1996;8:4–8.
8. Roth S, Ebrahim ZY. Resistance to pancuronium in patients receiving carbamazepine. Anesthesiology. 1987;66:691–3.
9. Liberman BA, Norman P, Hardy BG. Pancuronium-phenytoin interaction: a case of decreased duration of neuromuscular blockade. Int J Clin Pharmacol Ther Toxicol. 1988;26:371–4.
10. Jellish WS, Modica PA, Tempelhoff R. Accelerated recovery from pipecuronium in patients treated with chronic anticonvulsant therapy. J Clin Anesth. 1993;5:105–8.
11. Tobias JD, Johnson JO. Rapacuronium administration to patients receiving phenytoin or carbamazepine. J Neurolsurg Anesthesiol. 2001;13:240–2.
12. Spacek A, Neiger FX, Krenn CG, Hoerauf K, Kress HG. Rocuronium-induced neuromuscular block is affected by chronic carbamazepine therapy. Anesthesiology. 1999;90:109–12.
13. Spacek A, Nickl S, Neiger FX, Nigrovic V, Ullrich OW, Weindlmayr-Goettel M, Schwall B, Taeger K, Kress HG. Augmentation of the rocuronium-induced neuromuscular block of the acutely administered phenytoin. Anesthesiology. 1999;90:1551–5.
14. Fernandez-Candil J, Gambus PL, Troconiz IF, Valero R, Carrero E, Bueno L, Fabregas N. Pharmacokinetic-pharmacodynamic modelling of the influence of chronic phenytoin therapy on the rocuronium bromide response in patients undergoing brain surgery. Eur J Clin Pharmacol. 2008;64:795–806.

15. Dreissen JJ, Robertson EN, Booij LHDJ, Vree TB. Accelerated recover and disposition from rocuronium in an end-stage renal failure patient on chronic anticonvulsant therapy with sodium valproate and primidone. Br J Anaesth. 1998;80:386–8.
16. Kim MH, Hwang JW, Jeon YT, Do SH. Effects of valproic acid and magnesium sulphate on rocuronium requirement in patients undergoing craniotomy for cerebrovascular surgery. Br J Anaesthes. 2012;109:407–12.
17. Alloul K, Whalley DG, Shutway F, Ebrahim Z, Varin F. Pharmacokinetic origin of carbamazepine-induced resistance to vecuronium neuromuscular blockade in anesthetized patients. Anesthesiology. 1996;84:330–9.
18. Wright PMC, McCarthy G, Szenohradazky J, Sharma ML, Caldwell JE. Influence of chronic phenytoin administration on the pharmacokinetics and pharmacodynamics of vecuronium. Anesthesiology. 2004;100:626–33.
19. Soriano SG, Sullivan LJ, Venkatakrishnan K, Greenblatt DJ, Martyn JAJ. Pharmacokinetics and pharmacodynamics of vecuronium in children receiving phenytoin or carbamazepine for chronic anticonvulsant therapy. Br J Anaesth. 2001;86:223–9.

References

15. Driessen JJ, Robertson EN, Booij LHDJ, Vree TB. Accelerated recovery and disposition from rocuronium in an end-stage renal failure patient on chronic anticonvulsant therapy with sodium valproate and primidone. Br J Anaesth. 1997;78:328–9.
16. Kim MH, Hwang JW, Jeon YT, Do SH. Effects of valproic acid and magnesium sulphate on rocuronium requirement in patients undergoing craniotomy for cerebrovascular surgery. Br J Anaesth. 2012;109:407–12.
17. Alloul K, Whalley DG, Shutway F, Ebrahim Z, Varin F. Pharmacokinetic origin of carbamazepine-induced resistance to vecuronium neuromuscular blockade in anesthetized patients. Anesthesiology. 1996;84:330–9.
18. Wright PMC, McCarthy G, Szenohradszky J, Sharma ML, Caldwell JE. Influence of chronic phenytoin administration on the pharmacokinetics and pharmacodynamics of vecuronium. Anesthesiology. 2004;100:626–33.
19. Soriano SG, Sullivan LJ, Venkatakrishnan K, Greenblatt DJ, Martyn JAJ. Pharmacokinetics and pharmacodynamics of vecuronium in children receiving phenytoin or carbamazepine for chronic anticonvulsant therapy. Br J Anaesth. 2001;86:223–9.

Psychotropic Drugs

Antidepressants

Amitriptyline

Carbamazepine	Carbamazepine enhances the metabolism of amitriptyline and can decrease mean plasma amitriptyline levels by 59% [1]
Topiramate	Topiramate enhances the metabolism of amitriptyline and can increase mean plasma amitriptyline clearance by 8% and increase mean plasma amitriptyline and nortriptyline (the pharmacologically active metabolite of amitriptyline) AUC values by 8% and 19%, respectively. Mean steady-state plasma amitriptyline levels can decrease by 23–33% [2]
Valproic acid	Valproic acid inhibits the metabolism of amitriptyline and can increase mean plasma amitriptyline levels by 67% and mean plasma nortriptyline levels by 87% [3]

Bupropion

Carbamazepine	Carbamazepine enhances the metabolism of bupropion and can decrease mean plasma bupropion AUC values by 90% and can increase mean plasma hydroxybupropion, the pharmacologically active metabolite of bupropion, values by 50% [4]
Cenobamate	Cenbamate enhances the metabolism of bupropion, via an action on CYP3A, and can decrease mean plasma bupropion AUC values by 39% [5]
Valproic acid	Valproic acid does not affect the metabolism of bupropion, but it can increase mean plasma hydroxybupropion, the pharmacologically active metabolite of bupropion, values by 94% [4]

P. N. Patsalos, *Antiseizure Medication Interactions*,
https://doi.org/10.1007/978-3-030-82790-8_73

Citalopram

Carbamazepine	Carbamazepine enhances the metabolism of citalopram, probably via an action on CYP3A4, and can decrease mean plasma citalopram levels by 27–31% [6]
Oxcarbazepine	Oxcarbazepine does not affect the pharmacokinetics of citalopram [7]

Clomipramine

Carbamazepine	Carbamazepine inhibits the metabolism of clomipramine and can increase plasma clomipramine levels [8]
Valproic acid	Valproic acid inhibits the metabolism of clomipramine and can increase plasma clomipramine levels [9, 10]

Desipramine

Carbamazepine	Carbamazepine enhances the metabolism of desipramine and can increase mean plasma desipramine clearance values by 31%, and decreases mean plasma desipramine half-life values by 20% and can decrease plasma desipramine levels [11]
Fenfluramine	Fenfluramine inhibits the metabolism of desipramine, probably via an action on CYP2D6, and can increase plasma desipramine levels ~twofold [12]
Phenobarbital	Phenobarbital enhances the metabolism of desipramine and can decrease mean plasma desipramine levels by 31% [13]
Phenytoin	Phenytoin enhances the metabolism of desipramine and can decrease plasma desipramine levels [14]

Doxepin

Carbamazepine	Carbamazepine enhances the metabolism of doxepin and can decrease mean plasma doxepin levels by 55% [1]
Valproic acid	Valproic acid inhibits the metabolism of doxepin and can increase the mean plasma doxepin/N-doxepin ratio by 124% [15]

Fluoxetine

Carbamazepine	It is not known whether carbamazepine affects the pharmacokinetics of fluoxetine
	A pharmacodynamic interaction (toxic serotonin syndrome) can occur between the two drugs [16]

Imipramine

Carbamazepine	Carbamazepine enhances the metabolism of imipramine and can decrease plasma imipramine levels by 42% [17]
Phenobarbital	Phenobarbital enhances the metabolism of imipramine and can decrease plasma imipramine levels [18]

Mianserin

Carbamazepine	Carbamazepine enhances the metabolism of mianserin, via an action on CYP3A4, and can decrease plasma mianserin (unconjugated and total (S)-mianserin—the more potent enantiomer) levels by 56% [19]
Phenobarbital	Phenobarbital enhances the metabolism of mianserin and can decrease plasma mianserin levels [20, 21]
Phenytoin	Phenytoin enhances the metabolism of mianserin and can decrease plasma mianserin levels [20, 21]

Mirtazapine

Carbamazepine	Carbamazepine enhances the metabolism of mirtazapine and can increase mean plasma mirtazapine clearance values by 137% and can decrease mean plasma mirtazapine AUC values by 61% [22]
Phenytoin	Phenytoin enhances the metabolism of mirtazapine and can decrease mean plasma mirtazapine AUC values by 47% and mean plasma mirtazapine levels by 33% [23]

Moclobemide

Carbamazepine	Carbamazepine enhances the metabolism of moclobemide, probably via an action on CYP2C19, and can increase mean plasma moclobemide clearance values by 1.4-fold and decrease mean plasma moclobemide AUC values by 36% and mean plasma moclobemide levels by 52% [24]
Valproic acid	Valproic acid can increase mean plasma moclobemide clearance values by 6% and decrease mean plasma moclobemide AUC values by 11% and mean plasma moclobemide levels by 19% [24]

Nefazodone

Carbamazepine	Carbamazepine enhances the metabolism of nefazodone and can decrease mean plasma AUC values by 92% [25]

Nortriptyline

Carbamazepine	Carbamazepine enhances the metabolism of nortriptyline and can decrease plasma nortriptyline levels by 62% [26]
Phenobarbital	Phenobarbital enhances the metabolism of nortriptyline and can decrease plasma nortriptyline levels [27]
Phenytoin	Phenytoin enhances the metabolism of nortriptyline and can decrease plasma nortriptyline levels [28]
Primidone	Primidone enhances the metabolism of nortriptyline and can decrease plasma nortriptyline levels [27]
Valproic acid	Valproic acid inhibits the metabolism of nortriptyline and can increase plasma nortriptyline levels [28]

Paroxetine

Phenobarbital	Phenobarbital enhances the metabolism of paroxetine and can decrease mean plasma paroxetine levels by 25% [29]
Phenytoin	Phenytoin enhances the metabolism of paroxetine and can decrease plasma paroxetine levels [30]

Sertraline

Carbamazepine	Carbamazepine enhances the metabolism of sertraline and can decrease plasma sertraline levels. However, plasma levels of its metabolite, desmethyl sertraline, are increased concurrently [31, 32]
Phenytoin	Phenytoin enhances the metabolism of sertraline and can decrease plasma sertraline levels [32]

Venlafaxine

Topiramate	Topiramate does not affect the pharmacokinetics of venlafaxine [33]
Valproic acid	Valproic acid does not affect the pharmacokinetics of venlafaxine [15]

Viloxazine

Carbamazepine	Carbamazepine does not affect the pharmacokinetics of viloxazine [34]
Phenobarbital	Phenobarbital does not affect the pharmacokinetics of viloxazine [34]
Phenytoin	Phenytoin does not affect the pharmacokinetics of viloxazine [34]

Antipsychotics

Amisulpride

Carbamazepine	It is not known whether carbamazepine affects the pharmacokinetics of amisulpride
	A pharmacodynamic interaction between carbamazepine and amisulpride has been suggested [35]
Oxcarbazepine	It is not known whether oxcarbazepine affects the pharmacokinetics of amisulpride
	A pharmacodynamic interaction between oxcarbazepine and amisulpride has been suggested [36]

Aripiprazole

Carbamazepine	Carbamazepine can decrease mean plasma aripiprazole C_{max} and AUC values by 66% and 71%, respectively, while values of its pharmacologically active metabolite, dehydroaripiprazole, are decreased by 68% and 69%, respectively. The mechanism of this interaction is considered to be the induction of aripiprazole metabolism, mediated via CYP3A4, and induction of dehydroaripiprazole metabolism, also mediated via CYP3A4 [37]
	A pharmacodynamic interaction between carbamazepine and aripiprazole has also been suggested [38]
Clonazepam	Clonazepam does not affect the pharmacokinetics of aripiprazole [39]
Lamotrigine	Lamotrigine inhibits the metabolism of aripiprazole to its pharmacologically active metabolite dehydroaripiprazole so that the plasma dehydroaripiprazole/aripiprazole ratio decreases by 17% [39]
Oxcarbazepine	Oxarbazepine can decrease plasma aripiprazole by 68% [40]
Valproic acid	Valproic can decrease mean plasma aripiprazole C_{max} and AUC values by 25% and 24%, respectively, while values for its pharmacologically active metabolite, dehydroaripiprazole, are only decreased by 8% and 7%, respectively
	The mechanism of this interaction is considered to be by either induction of aripiprazole metabolism, mediated via CYP3A4 and CYP2D6, or by displacement of aripiprazole from its protein binding sites by valproic acid [41]

Asenapine

Valproic acid	Valproic acid does not affect the pharmacokinetics of asenapine [42]

Bromperidol

Carbamazepine	Carbamazepine enhances the metabolism of bromperidol and can decrease mean plasma bromperidol levels by 37% [43]

Chlorpromazine

Carbamazepine	Carbamazepine enhances the metabolism of chlorpromazine and can decrease plasma chlorpromazine levels [44]
Phenobarbital	Phenobarbital enhances the metabolism of chlorpromazine and can decrease plasma chlorpromazine levels by ~25% [45]

Clozapine

Carbamazepine	Carbamazepine enhances the metabolism of clozapine and can decrease plasma clozapine levels by 31–63% [46]
	Combining carbamazepine with clozapine is generally contraindicated due to concerns about potential additive adverse hematological effects [47]
Lamotrigine	Lamotrigine does not affect the pharmacokinetics of clozapine [48, 49]
Oxcarbazepine	Oxcarbazepine enhances the metabolism of clozapine and can decrease mean plasma clozapine levels by 24% [50]
Phenytoin	Phenytoin enhances the metabolism of clozapine and can decrease plasma clozapine levels by 75–84% [51]
Phenobarbital	Phenobarbital enhances the metabolism of clozapine, via the enhancement of N-oxidation and demethylation pathways, and can decrease mean plasma clozapine levels by 35% [52]
Pregabalin	Pregabalin can increase plasma clozapine levels by 30–60% [53]
Topiramate	Topiramate does not affect the pharmacokinetics of clozapine [54]
Valproic acid	There are conflicting reports on the potential effects of valproic acid on plasma clozapine levels. One study observed a 57% increase in plasma clozapine levels with the addition of valproic acid, while a second study found a 15% decrease. A third study reported an 11% increase in plasma clozapine levels via an action on CYP1A2 and CYP3A4. All studies observed a decrease in plasma levels of norclozapine, the pharmacologically active metabolite of clozapine [55, 56]

Fluphenazine

Carbamazepine	Carbamazepine enhances the metabolism of fluphenazine and can decrease plasma fluphenazine levels by 49% [57]

Haloperidol

Carbamazepine	Carbamazepine enhances the metabolism of haloperidol and can decrease plasma haloperidol levels by 59–61% [58]
Phenobarbital	Phenobarbital enhances the metabolism of haloperidol and can decrease plasma haloperidol levels by 50–60% [59]
Phenytoin	Phenytoin enhances the metabolism of haloperidol and can decrease plasma haloperidol levels by 50–60% [59]

Topiramate	Topiramate can increase plasma haloperidol AUC values by up to 28%. The AUC values of the pharmacologically active metabolite of haloperidol are concurrently increased by up to 50% [60]
Valproic acid	Valproic acid does not affect the pharmacokinetics of haloperidol [61]

Olanzapine

Carbamazepine	Carbamazepine enhances the metabolism of olanzapine, via induction of UGT1A4, and can decrease median plasma olanzapine levels by 59% [62]
Gabapentin	Gabapentin does not affect the pharmacokinetics of olanzapine [63]
Lamotrigine	Lamotrigine does not affect the pharmacokinetics of olanzapine [64]
Levetiracetam	Levetiracetam does not affect the pharmacokinetics of olanzapine [63]
Oxcarbazepine	Oxcarbazepine does not affect the pharmacokinetics of olanzapine [65]
Rufinamide	Rufinamide does not affect the pharmacokinetics of olanzapine [66]
Topiramate	Topiramate does not affect the pharmacokinetics of olanzapine [54]
Valproic acid	Valproic acid can decrease mean plasma olanzapine levels by 30% [62]

Paliperidone

Carbamazepine	Carbamazepine can decrease mean plasma paliperidone levels by up to 35% [67]

Quetiapine

Carbamazepine	Carbamazepine enhances the metabolism of quetiapine, via an action on CYP3A4, and can increase plasma quetiapine clearance by 7.5-fold and decrease mean plasma quetiapine C_{max} values by 80% or to undetectable levels [68, 69]
Lamotrigine	Lamotrigine enhances the metabolism of quetiapine and decreases quetiapine plasma levels [70]
Oxcarbazepine	Oxcarbazepine can enhance the metabolism of quetiapine and decrease quetiapine plasma levels [71]
Phenytoin	Phenytoin enhances the metabolism of quetiapine, probably via an action on CYP3A4, and can increase plasma quetiapine clearance by fivefold and can decrease mean plasma quetiapine C_{max} and AUC values by 27% and 19%, respectively [72]
Topiramate	Topiramate does not affect the pharmacokinetics of quetiapine [54]
Valproic acid	Valproic acid inhibits the metabolism of quetiapine, probably via an action on CYP3A4, and can increase plasma quetiapine levels by 77% [73]

Risperidone

Carbamazepine	Carbamazepine enhances the metabolism of risperidone and its pharmacologically active metabolite 9-hydroxyrisperidone, probably via an action on CYP3A4, and can decrease mean plasma risperidone and 9-hydroxyrisperidone levels by 68% and 64%, respectively [74]
Lamotrigine	Lamotrigine does not affect the pharmacokinetics of risperidone [49]
Oxcarbazepine	Oxcarbazepine does not affect the pharmacokinetics of risperidone [63]
Phenytoin	Phenytoin inhibits the metabolism of risperidone and can increase plasma risperidone levels [75]
Topiramate	Topiramate can increase mean risperidone clearance values by 51% and decrease mean plasma risperidone AUC values by 23%. Mean plasma 9-hydroxyrisperidone (the pharmacologically active metabolite of risperidone) AUC values are concurrently decreased by 8% [2]
Valproic acid	Valproic acid does not affect the pharmacokinetics of risperidone [73, 76]

Thioridazine

Carbamazepine	Carbamazepine does not affect the plasma levels of thioridazine but decreases plasma levels of the pharmacologically active metabolite, mesoridazine [59]
Phenobarbital	Phenobarbital enhances the metabolism of thioridazine and can decrease plasma thioridazine levels by 10%. However, phenobarbital also enhances the metabolism of the pharmacologically active metabolite, mesoridazine, and can decrease plasma mesoridazine levels by 25% [59]
Phenytoin	Phenytoin enhances the metabolism of thioridazine and can decrease plasma thioridazine levels by 10%. However, phenytoin also enhances the metabolism of the pharmacologically active metabolite of thioridazine (mesoridazine) and can decrease plasma mesoridazine levels by 25% [59]

Trazodone

Carbamazepine	Carbamazepine enhances the metabolism of trazodone and can decrease mean plasma trazodone levels by 24% and decrease mean plasma m-chlorophenylpiperazine levels, the pharmacologically active metabolite, by 40% [77]

Ziprasidone

Carbamazepine	Carbamazepine enhances the metabolism of ziprasidone, probably via an action on CYP3A4, and can decrease mean plasma ziprasidone AUC values by 36% and mean plasma ziprasidone levels by 27% [78]

Benzodiazepines

Alprazolam

Carbamazepine	Carbamazepine enhances the metabolism of alprazolam, probably via an action on CYP3A4, and can increase mean plasma alprazolam clearance values by 137% and decrease mean plasma alprazolam half-life values by 55%. Mean plasma alprazolam levels are decreased by >50% [79, 80]

Clobazam

Carbamazepine	Carbamazepine enhances the metabolism of clobazam. Plasma levels of the pharmacologically active metabolite of clobazam, *N*-desmethylclobazam, are increased during comedication with carbamazepine. The mean plasma *N*-desmethylclobazam/clobazam ratio is increased by 117% [81]
Eslicarbazepine Acetate	Eslicarbazepine acetate does not affect the pharmacokinetics of clobazam [82]
Felbamate	Felbamate inhibits the metabolism of clobazam. Plasma levels of the pharmacologically active metabolite of clobazam, *N*-desmethylclobazam, are increased during comedication with felbamate. Typically, the plasma level to weight-adjusted dose ratio of *N*-desmethylclobazam and clobazam can be expected to be fivefold lower and twofold higher, respectively. The interaction may be the consequence of inhibition of *N*-desmethylclobazam metabolism through CYP2C19 [83]
Lamotrigine	Lamotrigine does not affect the pharmacokinetics of clobazam [81]
Levetiracetam	Levetiracetam does not affect the pharmacokinetics of clobazam [84]
Phenobarbital	Phenobarbital enhances the metabolism of clobazam. Plasma levels of the pharmacologically active metabolite of clobazam, *N*-desmethylclobazam, are increased during comedication with phenobarbital. The mean plasma *N*-desmethylclobazam/clobazam ratio is increased by 90% [81]
Phenytoin	Phenytoin enhances the metabolism of clobazam. Plasma levels of the pharmacologically active metabolite of clobazam, *N*-desmethylclobazam, are increased during comedication with phenytoin. The mean plasma *N*-desmethylclobazam/clobazam ratio is increased by 294% [81]
Rufinamide	Rufinamide does not affect the pharmacokinetics of clobazam [85]
Stiripentol	Stiripentol inhibits the metabolism of clobazam. Plasma levels of clobazam and the pharmacologically active metabolite of clobazam, *N*-desmethylclobazam, are increased during co-medication with stiripentol
	Typically, the plasma levels of clobazam and *N*-desmethylclobazam can be expected to be twofold higher and threefold higher, respectively. The interaction is the consequence of inhibition of *N*-demethylation of clobazam through CYP3A4 and the inhibition of the hydroxylation of *N*-desmethylclobazam by CYP2C19 [86]
Valproic acid	Valproic acid does not affect the pharmacokinetics of clobazam [81]

Clonazepam

Carbamazepine	Carbamazepine enhances the metabolism of clonazepam and can decrease plasma clonazepam levels by 19–37% [87]
Felbamate	Felbamate inhibits the metabolism of clonazepam. Mean plasma clonazepam levels and AUC values can be increased by 17% and 24%, respectively [88]
Lacosamide	Lacosamide does not affect the pharmacokinetics of clonazepam [89]
Lamotrigine	Lamotrigine enhances the metabolism of clonazepam and can decrease plasma clonazepam levels by 20–38% [90]
Levetiracetam	Levetiracetam does not affect the pharmacokinetics of clonazepam [84]
Phenobarbital	Phenobarbital enhances the metabolism of clonazepam. Mean plasma clonazepam clearance can be increased by 19–24%, and mean plasma clonazepam levels can be decreased by 11% [91]
Phenytoin	Phenytoin enhances the metabolism of clonazepam. Mean plasma clonazepam clearance can be increased by 46–58%, and mean plasma clonazepam levels can be decreased by 28% [91]
Primidone	Primidone enhances the metabolism of clonazepam and can decrease plasma clonazepam levels [92]

Diazepam

Carbamazepine	Carbamazepine enhances the metabolism of diazepam, so mean plasma diazepam half-life values are decreased by 62%, and mean plasma diazepam clearance values are increased by 158%. A concurrent increase in plasma *N*-desmethyldiazepam, the pharmacologically active metabolite of diazepam, levels also occurs [93]
Phenobarbital	Phenobarbital enhances the metabolism of diazepam, so that mean plasma diazepam half-life values are decreased by 62% and mean plasma diazepam clearance values are increased by 158%. A concurrent increase in plasma *N*-desmethyldiazepam, the pharmacologically active metabolite of diazepam, levels also occurs [93]
Phenytoin	Phenytoin enhances the metabolism of diazepam, so mean plasma diazepam half-life values are decreased by 62% and mean plasma diazepam clearance values are increased by 158%. A concurrent increase in plasma *N*-desmethyldiazepam, the pharmacologically active metabolite of diazepam, levels also occurs [92]
Primidone	Primidone enhances the metabolism of diazepam, so that mean plasma diazepam half-life values are decreased by 62% and mean plasma diazepam clearance values are increased by 158%. A concurrent increase in plasma *N*-desmethyldiazepam, the pharmacologically active metabolite of diazepam, levels also occurs [92]
Valproic acid	Valproic acid displaces diazepam from its plasma protein binding (albumin) sites, so that mean free plasma diazepam levels are increased by 92% [94]

Lorazepam

Pregabalin	Pregabalin does not affect the pharmacokinetics of lorazepam
Valproic acid	Valproic acid can decrease the mean plasma clearance of lorazepam by 31% and increase mean plasma lorazepam levels by 31% [95]

Midazolam

Brivaracetam	Brivaracetam does not affect the pharmacokinetics of midazolam [96]
Cannabidiol	Cannabidiol enhances the metabolism of midazolam and can increase the mean clearance of midazolam by 7%, and can decrease its mean half-life value by 9%. Cannabidiol concurrently increases the mean half-life value of the pharmacologically active metabolite, 1-hydroxymidazolam, by 35% [97]
Carbamazepine	Carbamazepine enhances the metabolism of midazolam and can decrease plasma midazolam levels. Because the mean decrease in plasma midazolam AUC values of orally administered midazolam in patients taking carbamazepine is so marked (94%), the loss of efficacy of the hypnotic can be readily anticipated. However, since midazolam clearance after intravenous administration is more dependent on liver blood flow than on enzyme activity, this interaction would be expected to be far less important when midazolam is given parenterally [98]
Cenobamate	Cenobamate enhances the metabolism of midazolam, via an action on CYP3A, and can decrease plasma midazolam AUC values by 72% [5]
Everolimus	Everolimus inhibits the metabolism of midazolam, probably via an action on CYP3A4, and increases mean midazolam AUC values by 30% [99]
Perampanel	Perampanel enhances the metabolism of midazolam and can decrease mean plasma midazolam Cmax and AUC values by 15% and 13%, respectively [100]
Phenytoin	Phenytoin enhances the metabolism of midazolam and can decrease plasma midazolam levels. Because the mean decrease in plasma midazolam AUC values of orally administered midazolam in patients taking phenytoin is so marked (94%), the loss of efficacy of the hypnotic can be readily anticipated. However, since midazolam clearance after intravenous administration is more dependent on liver blood flow than on enzyme activity, this interaction would be expected to be far less important when midazolam is given parenterally [98]

Lithium

Acetazolamide	Acetazolamide can increase plasma lithium levels by fivefold. This may be the consequence of carbonic anhydrase inhibition by acetazolamide resulting in a decrease in lithium renal clearance [101]
Carbamazepine	Carbamazepine can increase plasma lithium levels by 3.5-fold, resulting in lithium toxicity consequent to carbamazepine-induced acute renal failure [102]
	A pharmacodynamic interaction between lithium and carbamazepine has been described whereby patients develop a syndrome characterized by somnolence, confusion, disorientation, and ataxia and other cerebella symptoms [103, 104]
Clonazepam	Clonazepam can increase plasma lithium levels by 33–61% [105]
Gabapentin	Gabapentin does not affect the pharmacokinetics of lithium [106]
Lamotrigine	Lamotrigine can decrease mean plasma lithium AUC values by 8% [107]
Topiramate	The effects of topiramate in the pharmacokinetics of lithium are controversial. Topiramate has been reported to increase mean plasma lithium clearance by 36% and to decrease mean plasma lithium AUC values by 12%. Topiramate has also been reported to increase plasma lithium levels by up to 140%. Both these effects are considered to be the consequence of carbonic anhydrase inhibition by topiramate which in turn affects lithium renal clearance [2, 108]
Valproic acid	Valproic acid does not affect the pharmacokinetics of lithium [109]

References

1. Leinonen E, Lillsunde P, Laukkanen V, Ylitalo P. Effects of carbamazepine on serum antidepressant concentrations in psychiatric patients. J Clin Psychopharmacol. 1991;11:313–8.
2. Bialer M, Doose DR, Murthy B, Curtin C, Wang SS, Twyman RE, Schwabe S. Pharmacokinetic interactions of topiramate. Clin Pharmacokinet. 2004;43:763–80.
3. Unterecker S, Burger R, Hohage A, Deckert J, Pfuhlmann B. Interaction of valproic acid and amitriptyline-analysis of therapeutic drug monitoring data under naturalistic conditions. J Clin Psychopharmacol. 2013;33:561–4.
4. Ketter TA, Jenkins JB, Schroeder DH, Pazzaglia PJ, Marangell LB, George MS, Callahan AM, Hinton ML, Chao J, Post RM. Carbamazepine but not valproate induces bupropion metabolism. J Clin Psychopharmacol. 1995;15:327–33.
5. Bialer M, Johannessen SI, Koepp MJ, Levy RH, Perucca E, Perucca P, Tomson T, White HS. Progress report on new antiepiletis drugs: A summary of the Fifteenth Eilat Conference on New Antiepileptic Drugs and Devices (EILAT XV). II Drugs in more advanced clinical development. Epiepsia. 2020;61:2365–85.
6. Steinacher L, Vandel P, Zullino DF, Eap CB, Brawand-Amey M, Baumann P. Carbamazepine augmentation in depressive patients non-responding to citalopram: a pharmacokinetic and clinical pilot study. Eur Neuropsychopharmacol. 2002;12:255–60.
7. Leinonen E, Lepola U, Koponen H. Substituting carbamazepine with oxcarbazepine increases citalopram levels. A report of two cases. Pharmacopsychiatry. 1996;29:156–8.
8. Gerson GR, Jones RB, Luscombe DK. Studies on the concomitant use of carbamazepine and clomipramine for the relief of post-herpetic neuralgia. Postgrad Med J. 1977;53(Suppl 4):104–9.
9. DeToledo JC, Haddad H, Ramsey RE. Status epilepticus associated with the combination of valproic acid and clomipramine. Ther Drug Monit. 1997;19:71–3.
10. Fehr C, Grunder G, Hiemke C, Dahman N. Increase in serum clomipramine concentrations caused by valproate. J Clin Psychopharmacol. 2000;20:493–4.
11. Spina E, Avenoso A, Campo GM, Caputi AP, Perucca E. The effect of carbamazepine on the 2-hydroxylation of desipramine. Psychopharmacology. 1995;117:413–6.
12. Summary of Product Characteristics: Fenfluramine (Fintepla). Zogenlix Int. Ltd. Last update 6th January 2021.
13. Spina E, Avenoso A, Campo GM, Caputi AP, Perucca E. Phenobarbital induces the 2-hydroxylation of desipramine. Ther Drug Monit. 1996;18:60–4.
14. Fogel BS, Haltzman S. Desipramine and phenytoin: a potential drug interaction of therapeutic relevance. J Clin Psychiatry. 1987;48:387–9.
15. Unterecker S, Reif A, Hempel S, Proft F, Riederer P, Deckert J, Pfuhlmann B. Interaction of valproic acid and the antidepressants doxepin and venlafaxine: analysis of therapeutic drug monitoring data under naturalistis conditions. Int Clin Psychopharmacol. 2014;29:206–11.
16. Dursum SM, Natthew VM, Reveley MA. Toxic serotonin syndrome after fluoxetine plus carbamazepine. Lancet. 1993;342:442–3.
17. Szymura-Oleksiak J, Wyska E, Wasieczko A. Pharmacokinetic interaction between imipramine and carbamazepine in patients with major depression. Psychopharmacology. 2001;154:38–42.
18. Hewick DS, Sparks RG, Stevenson IH, Watson ID. Induction of imipramine metabolism following barbiturate administration. Br J Clin Pharmacol. 1977;4:339P.
19. Eap CB, Yasui N, Kaneko S, Baumann P, Powell K, Otani K. Effects of carbamazepine coadministration on plasma concentrations of enantiomers of mianserin and its metabolites. Ther Drug Monit. 1999;21:166–70.
20. Nawishy S, Hathway N, Turner P. Interactions of anticonvulsant drugs with mianserin and nomifensine. Lancet. 1981;2(8251):871–2.
21. Richens A, Nawishy S, Trimble M. Antidepressant drugs, convulsions and epilepsy. Br J Clin Pharmacol. 1983;15:295S–8.

22. Sitsen JMA, Maris FA, Timmer CJ. Drug-drug interaction studies with mirtazapine and carbamazepine in healthy male subjects. Eur J Drug Metab Pharmacokinet. 2001;26:109–21.
23. Spaans E, van den Heuvel MW, Schnabel PG, Peeters PAM, Chin-Kon-Sung UG, Colbers EPH, Sitsen JMA. Concomitant use of mirtazapine and phenytoin: a drug-drug interaction study in healthy male subjects. Eur J Clin Pharmacol. 2002;58:423–9.
24. Ignjatovic AR, Miljkovic B, Todorovic D, Timotijevic I, Pokrajac M. Moclobemide monotherapy vs. combined therapy with valproic acid or carbamazepine in depressive patients: a pharmacokinetic interaction study. Br J Clin Pharmacol. 2008;67:199–208.
25. Laroudie C, Salazar DE, Cosson JP, Cheuvart B, Istin B, Girault J, Ingrand I, Decourt JP. Carbamazepine-nefazodone interaction in healthy subjects. J Clin Psychopharmacol. 2000;20:46–53.
26. Bronson K, Kragh-Sorensen P. Concomitant intake of nortriptyline and carbamazepine. Ther Drug Monit. 1993;15:258–60.
27. Braithwaite RA, Flanagan RJ, Richens A. Steady-state plasma nortriptyline concentrations in epileptic patients. Br J Clin Pharmacol. 1975;2:469–71.
28. Fu C, Katzman M, Goldblooom DS. Valproate/nortriptyline interaction. J Clin Psychopharmacol. 1994;14:205–6.
29. Greb WH, Buscher G, Dierdof HD, Koster FE, Wolf D, Mellows G. The effect of liver enzyme inhibition by cimetidine and enzyme induction by phenobarbitone on the pharmacokinetics of paroxetine. Acta Psychiatr Scand. 1989;350(Suppl):95–8.
30. Andersen BB, Mikkelsen M, Vesterager A, Dam M, Kristensen HB, Pedersen B, Lund J, Mengel H. No influence of the antidepressant paroxetine on carbamazepine, valproate and phenytoin. Epilepsy Res. 1991;10:201–4.
31. Rosenqvist U, Tornqbvist M, Bengtsson F. An interaction between sertraline and carbamazepine which resulted in sub-therapeutic concentrations of sertraline and N-desmethylsertraline in serum. Ther Drug Monit. 2003;25:527.
32. Pihlsgard M, Eliasson E. Significant reduction of sertraline plasma levels by carbamazepine and phenytoin. Eur J Clin Pharmacol. 2002;57:915–6.
33. Summary of Product Characteristics: Topiramate (Topamax). Janssen-Cilag Ltd. Last update 14th January 2021.
34. Pisani F, Fazio A, Spina E, Artesi C, Pisani B, Russo M, Trio R, Perucca E. Pharmacokinetics of the antidepressant viloxazine in normal subjects and in epileptic patients receiving chronic anticonvulsant therapy. Psychopharmacology. 1986;90:295–8.
35. van Amelsvoort T. Neuroleptic malignant syndrome and carbamazepine? Br J Psychiatry. 1994;164:269–70.
36. Angelopoulos P, Markopoulou M, Kyamidis K, Bobotas K. Neuroleptic malignant syndrome without fever after addition of oxcarbazepine to long-term treatment with amisulpride. Gen Hosp Psychiatry. 2008;30:482–5.
37. Citrome L, Macher JP, Salazar DE, Mallikaarjun S, Boulton SW. Pharmacokinetics of aripiprazole and concomitant carbamazepine. J Clin Psychopharmacol. 2007;27:279–83.
38. Nakamura A, Mihara K, Nagai G, Suzuki T, Kondo T. Pharmacokinetic and pharmacodynamic interactions between carbamazepine and aripiprazole in patients with schizophrenia. Ther Drug Monit. 2009;31:575–8.
39. Waade RB, Christensen H, Rudberg I, Refsum H, Hermann M. Influence of comedication on serum concentrations of aripiprazole and dehydroaripiprazole. Ther Drug Monit. 2009;31:233–8.
40. McGrane IR, Loveland JG, de Leon J. Possible oxcarbazepine inductive effects on aripiprazole metabolism: A case report. J Pharm Pract. 2018;31:361–3.
41. Citrome L, Josiassen R, Bark N, Salazar DE, Mallikaarjun S. Pharmacokinetics of aripiprazole and concomitant lithium and valproate. J Clin Pharmacol. 2005;45:89–93.
42. Gerrits MG, de Greef R, Dogterom P, Peeters PA. Valproate reduces the glucuronidation of asenapine without affecting asenapine plasma concentrations. J Clin Pharmacol. 2012;52:757–65.

43. Otani K, Ishida M, Yasui N, Kondo T, Mihara K, Suzuki A, Furukori H, Kanneko S, Inoue Y. Interaction between carbamazepine and bromperidol. Eur J Clin Pharmacol. 1997;52:219–22.
44. Raitasuo V, Lehtovaara R, Huttunen MO. Effect of switching carbamazepine to oxcarbazepine on the plasma levels of neuroleptics. Psychopharmacology. 1994;117:115–6.
45. Loga S, Curry S, Lader M. Interactions of orphenadrine and phenobarbitone with chlorpromazine: plasma concentrations and effects in man. Br J Clin Pharmacol. 1975;2:197–208.
46. Raitasuo V, Lehtovaara R, Nuttunen MO. Carbamazepine and plasma levels of clozapine. Am J Psychiatry. 1993;150:169.
47. Junghan U, Albers M, Woggon B. Increased risk of haematological side-effects in psychiatric patients treated with clozapine and carbamazepine? Pharmacopsychiatry. 1993;26:262.
48. Tiihonen J, Hallikainen T, Ryynanen OP, Repo-Tiihonen E, Kotilainen I, Eronen M, Toivonen P, Wahlbeck K, Putkonen A. Lamotrigine in treatment-resistant schizophrenia: a randomized placebo-controlled crossover trial. Biol Psychiatry. 2003;54:1241–8.
49. Spina E, D'Arrigo C, Migliardi G, Santor V, Muscatello MR, Mico U, D'Amico G, Perucca E. Effect of adjunctive lamotrigine treatment on the plasma concentrations of clozapine, risperidone and olanzapine in patients with schizophrenia or bipolar disorder. Ther Drug Monit. 2006;28:599–602.
50. Yousra H, Pierrick L, Laurent L, Daniele D. Interaction between clozapine and oxcarbazepine: A case report. Ther Adv Psychopharmacol. 2017;7:95–9.
51. Miller DD. Effect of phenytoin on plasma clozapine concentrations in two patients. J Clin Psychiatry. 1991;52:23–5.
52. Facciola F, Avenoso A, Spina E, Perucca E. Inducing effect of phenobarbital on clozapine metabolism in patients with chronic schizophrenia. Ther Drug Monit. 1998;20:628–30.
53. Schjerning O, Lykkegaard S, Damkier P, Nielsen J. Possible drug-drug interaction between pregabalin and clozapine in patients with schizophrenia: clinical prospectives. Pharmacopsychiatry. 2015;48:15–8.
54. Migliardi G, D'Arrigo C, Santoto V, Bruno A, Cortese L, Campolo D, Cacciola M, Spina E. Effect of topiramate on plasma concentrations of clozapine, olanzapine, risperidone, and quetiapine in patients with psychotic disorders. Clin Neuropharmacol. 2007;30:107–13.
55. Centorrino F, Baldessarini RJ, Kando J, Frankenburg FR, Volpiccelli SA, Puopolo PR, Flood JG. Serum concentrations of clozapine and its major metabolites: effects of cotreatment with fluoxetine or valproate. Am J Psychiatry. 1994;151:123–5.
56. Facciola F, Avenoso A, Scordo MG, Madia AG, Ventimiglia A, Perucca E, Spina E. Small effects of valproic acid on the plasma concentration of clozapine and its major metabolites in patients with schizophrenia or affective disorders. Ther Drug Monit. 1999;21:341–5.
57. Jann MW, Fidone GS, Hernandez JM, Amrung S, Davis CM. Clinical implications of increased antipsychotic plasma concentrations upon anticonvulsant cessation. Psychiatry Res. 1989;28:153–9.
58. Jann MW, Ereshefsky L, Saklad SR, Seidel DR, Davis CM, Neil R, Bowden CL. Effects of carbamazepine on plasma haloperidol levels. J Clin Psychopharmacol. 1985;5:106–13.
59. Linnoila M, Viukari M, Vaisanen K, Auvinen J. Effect of anticonvulsants on plasma haloperidol and thioridazine levels. Am J Psychiatry. 1980;137:819–21.
60. Doose DR, Kohl D, Desai-Krieger D, Natarajan J, van Kammen DP. No clinically significant effect of topiramate on haloperidol plasma concentration. Eur Neuropsychopharmacol. 1999;9(Suppl 4):S357.
61. Hesslinger B, Normann C, Langosch JM, Klose P, Berger M, Walden J. Effects of carbamazepine and valproate on haloperidol plasma levels and on psychopathologic outcome in schizophrenic patients. J Clin Psychopharmacol. 1999;19:310–5.
62. Skogh E, Reis M, Dahl ML, Lundmark J, Bengtsson F. Therapeutic drug monitoring data on olanzapine and its N-desmethyl metabolite in the naturalistic clinical setting. Ther Drug Monit. 2002;24:518–26.

63. Haslemo T, Olsen K, Lunde H, Molden E. Valproic acid significantly lowers serum concentrations of olanzapine-an interaction effects comparable with smoking. Ther Drug Monit. 2012;34:512–7.
64. Sidhu J, Job S, Bullman J, Francis E, Abbott R, Asher J, Theis JGW. Pharmacokinetics and tolerability of lamotrigine and olanzapine coadministration to healthy subjects. Br J Clin Pharmacol. 2006;61:420–6.
65. Muscatello MR, Pacetti M, Cacciola M, La Torre D, Zoccali R, D'Arrigo C, Migliardi G, Spina E. Plasma concentrations of risperidone and olanzapine during coadministration with oxcarbazepine. Epilepsia. 2005;46:771–4.
66. Arroyo S. Rufinamide Neurotherapeutics. 2007;4:155–62.
67. Yasui-Furukori N, Kubo K, Ishioka M, Tsuchimine S, Inoue Y. Interaction between paliperidone and carbamazepine. Ther Drug Monit. 2013;35:649–52.
68. Grim SW, Richard NM, Winter HR, Stams KR, Reele SB. Effects of cytochrome P450 3A modulators ketoconazole and carbamazepine on quetiapine pharmacokinetics. Br J Clin Pharmacol. 2005;61:58–69.
69. Nickl-Jockschat T, Paulzen M, Schneider F, Grozinger M. Drug interaction can lead to undetectable serum concentrations of quetiapine in the presence of carbamazepine. Clin Neuropharmacol. 2009;32:55.
70. Andersson ML, Bjorkhem-Bergman L, Lindh JD. Possible drug-drug interaction between quetiapine and lamotrigine – evidence from a Swedish TDM database. Br J Clin Pharmacol. 2011;72:153–6.
71. McGrane IR, Loveland JG, Zaluski HJ, Foster KD. Serum quetiapine concentration changes with concomitant oxcarbazepine therapy in a boy with autism spectrum disorder. J Child Adolesc Psychopharmacol. 2015;25:729–30.
72. Wong YWJ, Yeh C, Thyrum PT. The effects of concomitant phenytoin administration on the steady-state pharmacokinetics of quetiapine. J Clin Psychopharmacol. 2001;21:89–93.
73. Aichhorn W, Marksteiner J, Walch T, Zernig G, Saria A, Kemmler G. Influence of age, gender, body weight and valproate comedication on quetiapine plasma concentrations. Int Clin Psychopharmacol. 2006;21:81–5.
74. Spina E, Avenoso A, Facciola G, Salemi M, Scordo MG, Giacobello T, Madia AG, Perucca E. Plasma concentrations of risperidone and 9-hydroxyrisperidone: effect of comedication with carbamazepine and valproate. Ther Drug Monit. 2000;22:481–5.
75. Sanderson DR. Drug interaction between risperidone and phenytoin resulting in extrapyramidal symptoms. J Clin Psychiatry. 1996;57:177.
76. Yoshimura R, Shinkai K, Ueda N, Nakamura J. Valproic acid improves psychotic agitation without influencing plasma risperidone levels in schizophrenic patients. Pharmacopsychiatry. 2007;40:9–13.
77. Otani K, Ishida M, Kanneko S, Mihara K, Ohkubo T, Osanai T, Sugawara K. Effects of carbamazepine coadministration on plasma concentrations of trazodone and its active metabolite, m-chlorophenylpiperazine. Ther Drug Monit. 1996;18:164–7.
78. Miceli JJ, Anziano RJ, Robarge L, Hansen RA, Laurent A. The effect of carbamazepine on the steady-state pharmacokinetics of ziprasidone in healthy volunteers. Br J Clin Pharmacol. 2000;49(Suppl 1):65S–70.
79. Arena GW, Epstein S, Molloy M, Greenblatt DJ. Carbamazepine-induced reduction in alprazolam concentrations: a clinical case report. J Clin Psychiatry. 1988;49:448–9.
80. Furukori H, Otani K, Yasui N, Kondo T, Kaneko S, Shimoyama R, Ohkubo T, Nagasaki T, Sugawara K. Effect of carbamazepine on the single oral dose pharmacokinetics of alprazolam. Neuropsychopharmacology. 1988;18:364–9.
81. Sennoune S, Mesdjian E, Bonneton J, Genton P, Dravet C, Roger J. Interactions between clobazam and standard antiepileptic drugs in patients with epilepsy. Ther Drug Monit. 1992;14:269–74.
82. Falcao A, Fuseau E, Nunes T, Almeida L, Soares-da-Silva P. Pharmacokinetics, drug interactions and exposure-response relationships of eslicarbazepine acetate in adult patients with

partial-onset seizures: population pharmacokinetic and pharmacokinetic/pharmacodynamic analysis. CNS Drugs. 2012;26:79–91.
83. Contin M, Riva R, Albani F, Baruzzi A. Effect of felbamate on clobazam and its metabolite kinetics in patients with epilepsy. Ther Drug Monit. 1999;21:604–8.
84. Perucca E, Baltes E, Ledent E. Levetiracetam: absence of pharmacokinetic interactions with other antiepileptic drugs (AEDs). Epilepsia. 2000;41(Suppl):150.
85. Perucca E, Cloyd J, Critchley D, Fuseau E. Rufinamide: clinical pharmacokinetics and concentration-response relationships in patients with epilepsy. Epilepsia. 2008;49:1123–41.
86. Giraud C, Treluyer JM, Rey E, Chiron C, Vincent J, Pons G, Tran A. In vitro and in vivo inhibitory effect of stiripentol on clobazam metabolism. Drug Metab Dispos. 2006;34:608–11.
87. Lai AA, Levy RH, Cutler RE. Time-course of interaction between carbamazepine and clonazepam in normal man. Clin Pharmacol Ther. 1978;24:316–23.
88. Colucci R, Glue P, Banfield C, Reidenberg P, Meehan J, Radwanski E, Korduba C, Lin C, Dogterom P, Ebels T, Hendriks G, Jonkman JHG, Affrime M. Effect of felbamate on the pharmacokinetics of clonazepam. Am J Ther. 1996;3:294–7.
89. Halasz P, Kalviainen R, Mazurkiewicz-Beldzinska M, Rosenow F, Doty P, Hebert D, Sullivan T. Adjunctive lacosamide for partial-onset seizures: efficacy and safety results from a randomized controlled trial. Epilepsia. 2009;50:443–53.
90. Eriksson AS, Hoppu K, Nergardh A, Boreu L. Pharmacokinetic interactions between lamotrigine and other antiepileptic drugs in children with intractable epilepsy. Epilepsia. 1996;37:769–73.
91. Khoo KC, Mendels J, Rothbart M, Garland WA, Colburn WA, Min BH, Lucek R, Carbone JJ, Boxenbaum HG, Kaplan SA. Influence of phenytoin and phenobarbital on the disposition of a single oral dose of clonazepam. Clin Pharmacol Ther. 1980;28:368–75.
92. Nanda RN, Jihnson RH, Keogh HJ, Lambie DG, Melville ID. Treatment of epilepsy with clonazepam and its effect on other anticonvulsants. J Neurol Neurosurg Psychiatry. 1977;40:538–43.
93. Dhillon S, Richens A. Pharmacokinetics of diazepam in epileptic patients and normal volunteers following intravenous administration. Br J Clin Pharmacol. 1981;12:841–4.
94. Dhillon S, Richens A. Valproic acid and diazepam interaction in vivo. Br J Clin Pharmacol. 1982;13:553–60.
95. Samara EE, Granneman RG, Witt GF, Cavanaugh JH. Effect of valproate on the pharmacokinetics and pharmacodynamics of lorazepam. J Clin Pharmacol. 1997;37:442–50.
96. Stockis A, Watanabe S, Scheen AJ. Effect of brivaracetam on CYP3A activity, measured by oral midazolam. J Clin Pharmacol. 2015;55:543–8.
97. Patsalos PN, Szaflarski JP, Gidal B, VanLandingham K, Critchley D, Morrison G. Clinical implications of trials investigating drug-drug interactions between cannabidiol and enzyme inducers or inhibitors or common antiseizure drugs. Epilepsia. 2020;61:1854–68.
98. Beckman JT, Olkkola KT, Ojala M, Laaksovirta H, Neuvonen PJ. Concentrations and effects of oral midazolam are greatly reduced in patients treated with carbamazepine or phenytoin. Epilepsia. 1996;37:253–7.
99. Summary of Product Characteristics: Everolimus. Accord Healthcare Ltd. Last update 9th November 2020.
100. Patsalos PN. The clinical pharmacology profile of the new antiepileptic drug perampanel: a novel noncompetitive AMPA receptor antagonist. Epilepsia. 2015;56:12–27.
101. Gay C, Plas J, Granger B, Olie JP, Loo H. Intoxication au lithium-Deux interactions: l'acetazolamide et l'acide. L'Encéphale. 1985;11:261–2.
102. Mayan H, Golubev N, Dinour D, Farfel Z. Lithium intoxication due to carbamazepine-induced renal failure. Ann Pharmacother. 2001;35:560–2.
103. Shukla S, Godwin CD, Long LEB, Miller MG. Lithium-carbamazepine neurotoxicity and risk factors. Am J Psychiatry. 1984;141:1604–5.
104. McGinness J, Kishimoto A, Hollister EA. Avoiding neurotoxicity with lithium-carbamazepine combinations. Psychopharmacol Bull. 1990;26:181–4.

105. Koczerginski D, Kennedy SH, Swinson RP. Clonazepam and lithium – a toxic combination in the treatment of mania? Int Clin Psychopharmacol. 1989;4:195–9.
106. Frye MA, Kimbrell TA, Dunn RT, Piscitelli S, Grothe D, Vanderham E, Cora-Locatelli G, Post RM, Ketter TA. Gabapentin does not alter single-dose lithium pharmacokinetics. J Clin Psychopharmacol. 1998;18:461–4.
107. Chen C, Verones L, Yin Y. The effects of lamotrigine on the pharmacokinetics of lithium. Br J Clin Pharmacol. 2000;50:193–5.
108. Abraham G, Owen J. Topiramate can cause lithium toxicity. J Clin Psychopharmacol. 2004;24:565–7.
109. Granneman GR, Schneck DW, Cavanagh JH, Witt GF. Pharmacokinetic interactions and side effects resulting from concomitant administration of lithium and divalproex sodium. J Clin Psychiatry. 1996;57:204–6.

Steroids

Corticosteroids

Cortisol/Hydrocortisone

Phenobarbital	Phenobarbital enhances the metabolism of cortisol and can decrease plasma cortisol levels [1]
Phenytoin	Phenytoin enhances the metabolism of cortisol and can decrease mean plasma cortisol half-life values by 37% [2]

Dexamethasone

Carbamazepine	Carbamazepine enhances the metabolism of dexamethasone and can increase plasma dexamethasone clearance [3]
Phenobarbital	Phenobarbital enhances the metabolism of dexamethasone and can increase plasma dexamethasone clearance [4]
Phenytoin	Phenytoin decreases mean dexamethasone half-life values by 46% and increases mean plasma dexamethasone clearance values by 190% [5]
Primidone	Primidone enhances the metabolism of dexamethasone and can decrease plasma dexamethasone levels [6]

Methylprednisolone

Carbamazepine	Carbamazepine enhances the metabolism of methylprednisolone and can increase mean plasma methylprednisolone clearance by 342% [7]
Phenobarbital	Phenobarbital enhances the metabolism of methylprednisolone and can increase mean plasma methylprednisolone clearance by 209% [7]
Phenytoin	Phenytoin enhances the metabolism of methylprednisolone and can increase mean plasma methylprednisolone clearance by 479% [7]

P. N. Patsalos, *Antiseizure Medication Interactions*,
https://doi.org/10.1007/978-3-030-82790-8_74

Prednisolone

Carbamazepine	Carbamazepine enhances the metabolism of prednisolone and can decrease mean plasma prednisolone half-life values by 28% and can increase mean plasma prednisolone clearance by 42% [8]
Phenobarbital	Phenobarbital enhances the metabolism of prednisolone and can increase mean plasma prednisolone clearance by 41% [7]
Phenytoin	Phenytoin enhances the metabolism of prednisolone and can decrease mean plasma prednisolone half-life values by 45% and can increase mean plasma prednisolone clearance by 77% [9]

Oral Contraceptives

Acetazolamide	The interaction has not been investigated. Theoretically, a pharmacokinetic interaction would not be anticipated
Brivaracetam	Brivaracetam does not affect the metabolism of oral contraceptives [10]
Cannabidiol	The interaction has not been investigated. Theoretically, a pharmacokinetic interaction would not be anticipated
Carbamazepine	Carbamazepine enhances the metabolism of oral contraceptives, thereby reducing the efficacy of the contraceptive pill and causing contraceptive failure. This loss of effectiveness relates to enhancement of the metabolism of the ethinylestradiol and levonorgestrel components of oral contraceptives. Typically, mean plasma ethinylestradiol AUC values can decrease by ~45%, and mean plasma levonorgestrel AUC values can decrease by ~44% [11]
Cenobamate	Cenobamate enhances the metabolism of oral contraceptives, thereby reducing the efficacy of the contraceptive pill and causing contraceptive failure. This loss of effectiveness relates to the enhancement of the metabolism of the ethinylestradiol component of oral contraceptives [12]
Clobazam	The interaction has not been investigated. Theoretically, a pharmacokinetic interaction would not be anticipated
Clonazepam	Clonazepam does not affect the metabolism of oral contraceptives [13]
Eslicarbazepine Acetate	Eslicarbazepine acetate enhances the metabolism of oral contraceptives, thereby reducing the efficacy of the contraceptive pill and causing contraceptive failure. This loss of effectiveness relates to the enhancement of the metabolism of the ethinylestradiol and levonorgestrel components of oral contraceptives. Typically, plasma ethinylestradiol AUC values can decrease by up to 32%, and plasma levonorgestrel AUC values can decrease by up to 25% [14]
Ethosuximide	Ethosuximide does not affect the metabolism of oral contraceptives [15]
Everolimus	The interaction has not been investigated. Theoretically, a pharmacokinetic interaction would not be anticipated
Felbamate	Felbamate enhances the metabolism of oral contraceptives, thereby reducing the efficacy of the contraceptive pill and causing contraceptive failure. Typically, plasma gestodene (progestin) AUC values can decrease by 42%, and plasma ethinylestradiol AUC values can decrease by 13% [16]
Fenfluramine	The interaction has not been investigated. Theoretically, a pharmacokinetic interaction would not be anticipated
Gabapentin	Gabapentin does not affect the metabolism of oral contraceptives [17]

Lacosamide	Lacosamide does not affect the metabolism of oral contraceptives [18]
Lamotrigine	Lamotrigine does not affect the metabolism of oral contraceptives
	The interaction between lamotrigine and oral contraceptives has been extensively studied, and while lamotrigine does not affect the estrogen component of the oral contraceptives pill, it produces a modest 12% reduction in the progesterone level, which, although probably of no clinical significance in most patients, this may result in contraceptive failure in some patients – particularly if they are prescribed the progesterone-only pill [19]
Levetiracetam	Levetiracetam does not affect the metabolism of oral contraceptives [20]
Oxcarbazepine	Oxcarbazepine enhances the metabolism of oral contraceptives, thereby reducing the efficacy of the contraceptive pill and causing contraceptive failure. This loss of effectiveness relates to the induction of the metabolism of the ethinylestradiol and levonorgestrel components of oral contraceptives. Typically, mean plasma ethinylestradiol AUC values can decrease by 47% and mean plasma levonorgestrel AUC values can decrease by 47%, possibly due to induction of UGT1A4 by estrogen [21]
Perampanel	Perampanel (>8 mg/day) enhances the metabolism of oral contraceptives, thereby reducing the efficacy of the contraceptive pill and causing contraceptive failure. This loss of effectiveness relates to the induction of the metabolism of the ethinylestradiol and levonorgestrel components of oral contraceptives. Typically, mean plasma ethinylestradiol and levonorgestrel Cmax values are decreased by 18% and 40%, respectively [22]
Phenobarbital	Phenobarbital enhances the metabolism of oral contraceptives, thereby reducing the efficacy of the contraceptive pill and causing contraceptive failure. This loss of effectiveness relates to the induction of the CYP3A4-mediated metabolism of ethinylestradiol and levonorgestrel. Typically, plasma ethinylestradiol and levonorgestrel AUC values can decrease by 40% [23]
Phenytoin	Phenytoin enhances the metabolism of oral contraceptives, thereby reducing the efficacy of the contraceptive pill and causing contraceptive failure. This loss of effectiveness relates to the induction of the CYP3A4-mediated metabolism of ethinylestradiol and levonorgestrel. Typically, plasma ethinylestradiol and levonorgestrel AUC values can decrease by 50% [24]
Piracetam	The interaction has not been investigated. Theoretically, a pharmacokinetic interaction would not be anticipated
Pregabalin	Pregabalin does not affect the metabolism of oral contraceptives [25]
Primidone	Primidone enhances the metabolism of oral contraceptives, thereby reducing the efficacy of the contraceptive pill and causing contraceptive failure. This loss of effectiveness relates to the induction of the CYP3A4-mediated metabolism of ethinylestradiol and levonorgestrel. Typically, plasma ethinylestradiol and levonorgestrel AUC values can decrease by 40% [23]
Rufinamide	Rufinamide enhances the metabolism of oral contraceptives, thereby reducing the efficacy of the contraceptive pill and causing contraceptive failure. This loss of effectiveness relates to induction of the CYP3A4 and/or UGT-mediated metabolism of ethinylestradiol and levonorgestrel. Typically, plasma ethinylestradiol and norethindrone levels are decreased by 22% and 14%, respectively [26]
Stiripentol	It is not known whether stiripentol affects hormonal contraception, but theoretically, it can increase plasma levels of hormonal contraceptives and thus necessitate lower doses to be prescribed

Sulthiame	It is not known whether sulthiame affects hormonal contraception, but theoretically, it can increase plasma levels of hormonal contraceptives and thus necessitate lower doses to be prescribed
Tiagabine	Tiagabine does not affect the metabolism of oral contraceptives [27]
Topiramate	Topiramate caused a dose-dependent decrease in mean plasma ethinylestradiol AUC values (200 mg—18%; 400 mg—21%; 800 mg—30%) but no change in plasma norethindrone levels. The interaction is minimal (mean plasma ethinylestradiol AUC values decrease by 12%) or absent at topiramate daily dosages of 100 mg or less. Nevertheless, because contraceptive effectiveness may be affected, caution is advised in patients receiving topiramate and oral contraceptives [28, 29]
Valproic acid	Valproic acid does not affect the metabolism of oral contraceptives [30]
Vigabatrin	Vigabatrin does not affect the metabolism of oral contraceptives [31]
Zonisamide	Zonisamide does not affect the metabolism of oral contraceptives [32]

References

1. Brooks SM, Werk EE, Ackerman SJ, Sullivan I, Thrasher K. Adverse effects of phenobarbital on corticosteroid metabolism in patients with bronchial asthma. N Engl J Med. 1972;286:1125–8.
2. Evans PJ, Walker RF, Peters JR, Dyas J, Diad-Fahmy D, Thomas JP, Rimmer E, Tsanaclis L, Scanlon MF. Anticonvulsant therapy and cortisol elimination. Br J Clin Pharmacol. 1985;20:129–32.
3. Ma RCW, Chan WB, So WY, Tong PCY, Chan JCN, Chow CC. Carbamazepine and false positive dexamethasone suppression tests for Cushing's syndrome. Br Med J. 2005;330:299–300.
4. Keitner GI, Fruzzetti AE, Miller IW, Norman WH, Brown WA. The effect of anticonvulsants on the dexamethasone suppression test. Can J Psychiatr. 1989;34:441–3.
5. Chalk JB, Ridgeway K, Brophy T, Yelland JDN, Eadie MJ. Phenytoin impairs the bioavailability of dexamethasone in neurological and neurosurgical patients. J Neurol Neurosurg Psychiatry. 1984;47:1087–90.
6. Young MC, Hughes IA. Loss of therapeutic control in congenital adrenal hyperplasia due to interaction between dexamethasone and primidone. Acta Paediatr Scand. 1991;80:120–4.
7. Bartoszek M, Brenner AM, Szefler SJ. Prednisolone and methylprednisolone kinetics in children receiving anticonvulsant therapy. Clin Pharmacol Ther. 1987;42:424–32.
8. Olivesi A. Modified elimination of prednisolone in epileptic patients on carbamazepine monotherapy, and in women using low-dose oral contraceptives. Biomed Pharmacother. 1986;40:301–8.
9. Petereit LB, Meikle AW. Effectiveness of prednisolone during phenytoin therapy. Clin Pharmacol Ther. 1977;22:912–6.
10. Stockis A, Watanabe S, Fauchoux N. Interaction between brivaracetam (100 mg/kg) and a combination oral contraceptive: a randomized, double-blind, placebo-controlled study. Epilepsia. 2014;55:e27–31.
11. Davies AR, Westhoff CL, Stanczyk FZ. Carbamazepine coadministration with an oral contraceptive: effects on steroid pharmacokinetics, ovulation, and bleeding. Epilepsia. 2011;52:243–7.
12. Bialer M, Johannessen SI, Koepp MJ, Levy RH, Perucca E, Perucca P, Tomson T, White HS. Progress report on new antiepileptic drugs: A summary of the fifteenth Eilat conference on new antiepileptic drugs and devices (EILAT XV). II Drugs in more advanced clinical development Epiepsia. 2020;61:2365–85.

13. Reddy DS. Clinical pharmacokinetic interactions between antiepileptic drugs and hormonal contraceptives. Expert Rev Clin Pharmacol. 2010;3:183–92.
14. Falcao A, Vaz-da-Silva M, Gama H, Nunes T, Almeida L, Soares-da-Silva P. Effect of eslicarbazepine acetate on the pharmacokinetics of a combined ethinylestradiol/levonorgestrel oral contraceptive in healthy women. Epilepsy Res. 2013;105:368–76.
15. Goren MZ, Onat F. Ethosuximide; from bench to bedside. CNS Drug Rev. 2007;13:224–39.
16. Saano V, Glue P, Banfield CR, Reidenberg P, Colucci RD, Meehan JW, Haring P, Radwanski E, Nomeir A, Lin CC, Jensen PK, Affrime MB. Effects of felbamate on the pharmacokinetics of a low-dose combination oral contraceptive. Clin Pharmacol Ther. 1995;58:523–31.
17. Eldon MA, Underwood BA, Randinitis EJ, Sedman AJ. Gabapentin does not interact with a contraceptive regimen of norethindrone acetate and ethinyl estradiol. Neurology. 1998;50:1146–8.
18. Cawello W, Rosenkranz B, Schmid B, Wierich W. Pharmacodynamic and pharmacokinetic evaluation of lacosamide and an oral contraceptive (levonorgestrel plus ethinylestradiol) in healthy female volunteers. Epilepsia. 2013;54:530–6.
19. Sidhu J, Job S, Singh S, Philipson R. The pharmacokinetic and pharmacodynamic consequences of the co-administration of lamotrigine and a combined oral contraceptive in healthy female subjects. Br J Clin Pharmacol. 2006;61:191–9.
20. Ragueneau-Majlessi I, Levy RH, Janik F. Levetiracetam does not alter the pharmacokinetics of an oral contraceptive in healthy women. Epilepsia. 2002;43:697–702.
21. Fattore C, Cipolla G, Gatti G, Limido GL, Sturm Y, Bernasconi C, Perucca E. Induction of ethinylestradiol and levonorgestrel metabolism by oxcarbazepine in healthy women. Epilepsia. 1999;40:783–7.
22. Patsalos PN. The clinical pharmacology profile of the new antiepileptic drug perampanel: a novel noncompetitive AMPS receptor antagonist. Epilepsia. 2015;56:12–27.
23. Back DJ, Orme ML. Pharmacokinetic drug interactions with oral contraceptives. Clin Pharmacokinet. 1990;18:472–84.
24. Crawford P, Chadwick DJ, Martin C, Tjia J, Back DJ, Orme M. The interaction of phenytoin and carbamazepine with combined oral contraceptive steroids. Br J Clin Pharmacol. 1990;30:692–6.
25. Bockbrader HN, Posvar EL, Hunt T, Randinitis EJ. Pregabalin does not alter the effectiveness of an oral contraceptive. Neurology. 2004;62(Suppl 5):A314. Abstract P04.097
26. Perucca E, Cloyd J, Critchley D, Fuseau E. Rufinamide: clinical pharmacokinetics and concentration-response relationships in patients with epilepsy. Epilepsia. 2008;49:1123–41.
27. Mengel HB, Houston A, Back DJ. An evaluation of the interaction between tiagabine and oral contraceptives in female volunteers. J Pharm Med. 1994;4:141–50.
28. Rosenfeld WE, Doose DR, Walker SA, Nayak RK. Effect of topiramate on the pharmacokinetics of an oral contraceptive containing norethindrone and ethinyl estradiol in patients with epilepsy. Epilepsia. 1997;38:317–23.
29. Doose DR, Wang SS, Padmanabhan M, Schwabe S, Jacobs D, Bialer M. Effect of topiramate or carbamazepine on the pharmacokinetics of an oral contraceptive containing norethindrone and ethinyl estradiol in healthy obese and nonobese female subjects. Epilepsia. 2003;44:540–9.
30. Crawford P, Chadwick DJ, Cleland P, Tjia J, Cowie A, Back DJ, Orme M. The lack of effect of sodium valproate on the pharmacokinetics of oral contraceptive steroids. Contraception. 1986;33:23–9.
31. Bartoli A, Gatti G, Cipolla G, Barzaghi N, Veliz G, Fattore C, Mumford J, Perucca E. A double-blind, placebo-controlled study on the effect of vigabatrin on in vivo parameters of hepatic microsomal enzyme induction and on the kinetics of steroid oral contraceptives in healthy female volunteers. Epilepsia. 1997;38:702–7.
32. Griffith SG, Dai Y. Effect of zonisamide on the pharmacokinetics and pharmacodynamics of a combination ethinyl estradiol-norethindrone oral contraceptive in healthy women. Clin Ther. 2004;26:2056–65.

Miscellanea

Alcohol

Brivaracetam	Brivaracetam does not affect the pharmacokinetics of alcohol [1]
	Brivaracetam approximately doubled the effect of alcohol on psychomotor function, attention, and memory consequent to a pharmacodynamic interaction [1]
Cenobamate	Cenobamate does not affect the pharmacokinetics of alcohol [2] The effect of perampanel on the pharmacokinetics of alcohol is not known
Perampanel	Perampanel in combination with alcohol results in impairment of psychomotor performance, working memory, and executive function. These effects are considered to be the consequence of a pharmacodynamic interaction [3]
Piracetam	Piracetam does not affect the pharmacokinetics of alcohol [4]
Pregabalin	Pregabalin does not affect the pharmacokinetics of alcohol [5]

Armodafinil

Carbamazepine	Carbamazepine enhances the metabolism of armodafinil, via an action on CYP3A4, and can decrease mean plasma armodafinil AUC values by 39% [6]

Dexmedetomidine

Carbamazepine	Carbamazepine enhances the metabolism of dexmedetomidine and can increase mean plasma dexmedetomidine clearance by 43% [7]
Phenytoin	Phenytoin enhances the metabolism of dexmedetomidine and can increase mean plasma dexmedetomidine clearance by 43% [7]

P. N. Patsalos, *Antiseizure Medication Interactions*,
https://doi.org/10.1007/978-3-030-82790-8_75

Dextromethorphan

Clobazam	Clobazam inhibits the metabolism of dextromethorphan and can increase mean plasma dextromethorphan AUC values by 60% [8]

Dihydroergotamine

Topiramate	Topiramate does not affect the pharmacokinetics of dihydroergotamine [9]

Fexofenadine

Carbamazepine	Carbamazepine decreases mean plasma fexofenadine C_{max} values by 42% and mean plasma fexofenadine AUC values by 43%. The mechanism of this interaction is considered to be induction of P-glycoprotein in the small intestine [10]

Gamma-Hydroxybutyrate

Topiramate	Topiramate can increase plasma gamma-hydroxybutyrate levels by up to 185% [11]

Glibenclamide (Glyburide)

Topiramate	Topiramate decreases mean plasma glibenclamide AUC values by 25% and decreases mean plasma AUC values of its two pharmacologically active metabolites (4-trans-hydroxy-glibenclamide and 3-cis-hydroxy-glibenclamide) by 13% and 15%, respectively [12]

Isoxicam

Phenytoin	Phenytoin increases the rate and extent of absorption of isoxicam and increases mean plasma isoxicam values by 19% [13]

Levodopa

Perampanel	Perampanel does not affect the pharmacokinetics of levodopa [3]

Lidocaine (Lignocaine)

Carbamazepine	Carbamazepine enhances the metabolism of lidocaine, probably via an action on CYP3A4, and can increase mean plasma lidocaine clearance by 196% and can decrease mean plasma lidocaine AUC values by 60% [14]
Phenobarbital	Phenobarbital enhances the metabolism of lidocaine, probably via an action on CYP3A4, and can increase mean plasma lidocaine clearance values by 196% and can decrease mean plasma lidocaine AUC values by 60% [14]
Phenytoin	Phenytoin enhances the metabolism of lidocaine, probably via an action on CYP3A4, and can increase mean plasma lidocaine clearance values by 196% and can decrease mean plasma lidocaine AUC values by 60% [14]
Primidone	Primidone enhances the metabolism of lidocaine, probably via an action on CYP3A4, and can increase mean plasma lidocaine clearance values by 196% and can decrease mean plasma lidocaine AUC values by 60% [14]

Metformin

Eslicarbazepine Acetate	Eslicarbazepine acetate decreases mean plasma metformin C_{max} values by 13% and mean plasma metformin AUC values by 6% [15]
Lacosamide	Lacosamide does not affect the pharmacokinetics of metformin [16]
Topiramate	Topiramate decreases mean plasma metformin clearance values by 20% and increases mean plasma metformin AUC values by 25% [17]

Metyrapone

Phenytoin	Phenytoin enhances the metabolism of metyrapone and decreases metyrapone plasma levels [18]

Oxiracetam

Carbamazepine	Carbamazepine decreases the plasma half-life of oxiracetam [19]
Valproic acid	Valproic acid decreases the plasma half-life of oxiracetam [19]

Pioglitazone

Topiramate	Topiramate can increase mean plasma pioglitazone clearance values by 18% and decrease mean plasma pioglitazone AUC values by 15% and can decrease mean plasma AUC values of its two pharmacologically active metabolites (a hydroxy-metabolite and a keto-metabolite) by 15% and 60%, respectively [17]

Pizotifen

Topiramate	Topiramate does not affect the pharmacokinetics of pizotifen [10]

Propofol

Pregabalin	Pregabalin does not affect the pharmacokinetics of propofol [20]
Valproic acid	Valproic acid reduces the dose of propofol required for sedation [21]

St John's Wort (Hypericum perforatum)

Carbamazepine	Carbamazepine enhances the metabolism of pseudohypericin but not hypericin (the two main constituents of St John's wort), via an action on glucuronidation, and can decrease mean plasma pseudohypericin levels by 29% [22]

Sumatriptan

Topiramate	Topiramate can enhance mean plasma sumatriptan clearance by 11% and decrease mean plasma sumatriptan levels by 10% [9]

Theophylline

Carbamazepine	Carbamazepine enhances the metabolism of theophylline and can decrease plasma theophylline half-life values by 48% [23]
Phenobarbital	Phenobarbital enhances the metabolism of theophylline and can increase mean plasma theophylline clearance values by 35% and decrease mean plasma theophylline levels by 30% [24]
Phenytoin	Phenytoin enhances the metabolism of theophylline and can increase plasma theophylline clearance by up to 75% [25, 26]
Tiagabine	Tiagabine does not affect the pharmacokinetics of theophylline [27]

Tirilazad

Phenobarbital	Phenobarbital enhances the metabolism of tirilazad, via an action on CYP3A4, and can decrease mean plasma tirilazad clearance by 25–29% and can decrease mean plasma U-89678, a pharmacologically active metabolite, AUC values by 51–69% [28]
Phenytoin	Phenytoin enhances the metabolism of tirilazad, via an action on CYP3A4, and can increase mean plasma tirilazad clearance by 92% and can decrease mean plasma U-89678, a pharmacologically active metabolite, AUC values by 93% [29]

Tolbutamide

Clobazam	Clobazam enhances the metabolism of tolbutamide and can decrease mean plasma tolbutamide AUC values by 11% [8]

Triazolam

Rufinamide	Rufinamide enhances the metabolism of triazolam and can decrease mean plasma triazolam C_{max} values by 24% and mean plasma triazolam AUC values by 36% [30]

Valnoctamide

Carbamazepine	Carbamazepine enhances the metabolism of valnoctamide and decreases valnoctamide plasma levels [31]

Zolpidem

Carbamazepine	Carbamazepine enhances the metabolism of zolpidem and can decrease mean plasma zolpidem C_{max} values by 39% and mean plasma zolpidem AUC values by 57% [32]
Valproic acid	Valproic acid does not affect the pharmacokinetics of zolpidem [33]
	A pharmacodynamic interaction has been suggested between zolpidem and valproic acid whereby somnambulism occurs [33]

References

1. Kruithof AC, Watanabe S, Peeters PA, de Kam ML, Zuiker RG, Stevens J, van Gerven JM, Stockis A. Pharmacological interactions between brivaracetam and healthy males. J Psychopharmacol. 2017;31:915–26.
2. Summary of Product Characteristics: Cenobamate (XCopri). SK Life Science Inc. Last update August 2020.
3. Patsalos PN. The clinical pharmacology profile of the new antiepileptic drug perampanel: a novel noncompetitive AMPA receptor antagonist. Epilepsia. 2015;56:12–27.
4. Summary of Product Characteristics: Piracetam (Nootropil). UCB Pharma Ltd. Last update 9th February 2017.
5. Summary of Product Characteristics: Pregabalin (Lyrica). Upjohn UK Ltd. Last update November 2020.
6. Darwish M, Bond M, Yang R, Hellriegel ET, Robertson P. Evaluation of the potential for pharmacokinetic drug-drug interaction between armodafinil and carbamazepine in healthy adults. Clin Ther. 2015;37:325–37.
7. Flexman AM, Wong H, Wayne Riggs K, Shih T, Garcia PA, Vacas S, Talke PO. Enzyme-inducing anticonvulsants increase plasma clearance of dexmedetomidine: a pharmacokinetic and pharmacodynamic study. Anaesthesiology. 2014;120:1118–25.

8. Walzer M, Bekersky I, Blum RA, Tolbert D. Pharmacokinetic drug interactions between clobazam and drugs metabolized by cytochrome P450 isoenzymes. Pharmacotherapy. 2012;32:340–53.
9. Bialer M, Doose DR, Murthy B, Curtin C, Wang SS, Twyman RE, Schwabe S. Pharmacokinetic interactions of topiramate. Clin Pharmacokinet. 2004;43:763–80.
10. Yamada S, Yasui-Furukori N, Akamine Y, Kaneko S, Uno T. Effects of the P-glycoprotein inducer carbamazepine on fexofenadine pharmacokinetics. Ther Drug Monit. 2009;31:764–8.
11. Weiss T, Muller D, Marti I, Happold C, Russmann S. Gamma-hydroxybutyrate (GHB) and topiramate-clinically relevant drug interaction suggested by a case of coma and increased plasma GHB concentration. Eur J Clin Pharmacol. 2013;69:1193–4.
12. Manitpisitkul P, Curtin CR, Shalayda K, Wang SS, Ford L, Heald SL. An open-label drug-drug interaction study of the steady-state pharmacokinetics of topiramate and glyburide in patients with type-2 diabetes mellitus. Clin Drug Investig. 2013;33:929–38.
13. Caille G, Du Souich P, Lariviere L, Vezina M, Lacasse Y. The effect of administration of phenytoin on the pharmacokinetics of isoxicam. Biopharm Drug Dispos. 1987;8:57–61.
14. Perucca E, Richens A. Reduction of oral bioavailability of lignocaine by induction of first pass metabolism in epileptic patients. Br J Clin Pharmacol. 1979;8:21–31.
15. Rocha JF, Vaz-da-Silva M, Almeida L, Falcao A, Tunes T, Santos AT, Martins F, Fontes-Ribeiro C, Macedo T, Soares-da-Silva P. Effect of eslicarbazepine acetate on the pharmacokinetics of metformin in healthy volunteers. Int J Clin Pharmacol Ther. 2009;47:255–61.
16. Thomas D, Scharfenecker U, Schiltmeyer B, Koch B, Rudd D, Cawello W, Horstmann R. Lacosamide has a low potential for drug-drug interactions. Epilepsia. 2007;48(Suppl 5):562.
17. Manitpisitkul P, Curtin CR, Shalayda K, Wang SS, Ford L, Heald D. Pharmacokinetic interactions between topiramate and pioglitazone and metformin. Epilepsy Res. 2015;108:1519–32.
18. Meikle AW, Jubiz W, Matsukura S, West CD, Tyler FH. Effect of diphenylhydantoin on the metabolism of metyrapone and release of ACTH in man. J Clin Endocrinol Metab. 1969;29:1553–8.
19. van Wieringen A, Meijer JWA, van Emde BW, Vermeij TAC. Pilot study to determine the interaction of oxiracetam with antiepileptics. Clin Pharmacokinet. 1990;18:332–8.
20. Moreau-Bussiere F, Gaulin J, Gagnon V, Sansoucy J, de Medicis E. Preoperative pregabalin does not reduce propofol ED_{50}: a randomized controlled trial. Can J Anesthesiol. 2013;60:364–9.
21. Ishii M, Higuchi H, Maeda S, Tomoyasu Y, Egusa M, Miyawaki T. The influence of oral VPA on the required dose of propofol for sedation during dental treatment in patients with mental retardation: a prospective observer-blinded cohort study. Epilepsia. 2012;53:e13–6.
22. John A, Perloff ES, Bauer S, Schmider J, Mai I, Brockmoller J, Roots I. Impact of cytochrome P-450 inhibition by cimetidine and induction by carbamazepine on the kinetics of hypericin and pseudohypericin in healthy volunteers. Eur J Clin Pharmacol. 2004;60:617–22.
23. Rosenberry KR, Defusco CJ, Mansmann HC, McGeady SJ. Reduced theophylline half-life induced by carbamazepine therapy. J Pediatr. 1983;102:472–4.
24. Saccar CL, Danish M, Ragni MC, Rocci ML, Greene J, Yaffe SJ, Mansmann HC. The effect of phenobarbital on theophylline disposition in children with asthma. J Allergy Clin Immunol. 1985;75:716–9.
25. Marquis JF, Carruthers SG, Spence JD, Brownstone YS, Toogood JH. Phenytoin-theophylline interaction. N Engl J Med. 1982;307:1189–90.
26. Sklar SJ, Wagner JC. Enhanced theophylline clearance secondary to phenytoin therapy. Drug Intell Clin Pharm. 1985;19:34–6.
27. Mengel H, Jansen JA, Sommerville K, Jonkman JHG, Wesnes K, Cohen A, Carlson GF, Marshal LR, Snel S, Dirach J, Kastberg H. Tiagabine: evaluation of the risk of interaction with theophylline, warfarin, digoxin, cimetidine, oral contraceptives, triazolam, or ethanol. Epilepsia. 1995;36(Suppl 3):S160.
28. Fleishaker JC, Pearson LK, Peters GR. Gender does not affect the degree of induction of tirilazad clearance by phenobarbital. Eur J Clin Pharmacol. 1996;50:139–45.

29. Fleishaker JC, Pearson LK, Peters GR. Induction of tirilazad clearance by phenytoin. Biopharm Drug Dispos. 1998;19:91–6.
30. Perucca E, Cloyd J, Critchley D, Fuseau E. Rufinamide: clinical pharmacokinetics and concentration-response relationships in patients with epilepsy. Epilepsia. 2008;49:1123–41.
31. Pisani F, Haj-Yehia A, Fazio A, Artesi C, Oteri G, Perucca E, Kroetz DL, Levy RH, Bialer M. Carbamazepine-valnoctamide interaction in epileptic patients: in vitro/in vivo correlation. Epilepsia. 1993;34:954–9.
32. Vlace L, Popa A, Neag M, Muntean D, Baldea I, Leucuta SE. Pharmacokinetic interaction between zolpidem and carbamazepine in healthy volunteers. J Clin Pharmacol. 2011;51:1233–6.
33. Sattar SP, Ramaswamy S, Bhatia SC, Petty F. Somnambulism due to probable interaction of valproic acid and zolpidem. Ann Pharmacother. 2003;37:1429–33.

29. [illegible] K, [illegible], Peters CR. Induction of [illegible] and clearance of phenytoin. Biopharm Drug Dispos. 1998;19:37–42.
30. [illegible] L, Cloyd J, [illegible] D, Pascal E, [illegible] clinical pharmacokinetic and concentration-response relationships in patients with epilepsy. Epilepsia. 2008;49:1123–1[illegible]
31. [illegible] E, [illegible] A, [illegible] A, Arter C, Chen G, [illegible] F, [illegible] OF, [illegible] RH, Bialer M. [illegible] administered in epileptic patients [illegible]
32. [illegible] L, [illegible] A, Wong M, [illegible] D, [illegible] [illegible]. Pharmacokinetic interaction between [illegible] and carbamazepine in healthy volunteers. J Clin Pharmacol. 2013;[illegible]
33. Sattar SP, Ramaswamy S, Bhatia SC, Petty F. Somnambulism due to probable interaction of valproic acid and zolpidem. Ann Pharmacother. 2003;37:1429–33.

Index

P. N. Patsalos, *Antiseizure Medication Interactions*,
https://doi.org/10.1007/978-3-030-82790-8

MIX
Papier aus verantwortungsvollen Quellen
Paper from responsible sources
FSC® C105338
FSC
www.fsc.org

If you have any concerns about our products,
you can contact us on
ProductSafety@springernature.com

In case Publisher is established outside the EU,
the EU authorized representative is:
Springer Nature Customer Service Center GmbH
Europaplatz 3, 69115 Heidelberg, Germany

Printed by Libri Plureos GmbH
in Hamburg, Germany